AF745492

# POSITRON EMISSION TOMOGRAPHY - RECENT DEVELOPMENTS IN INSTRUMENTATION, RESEARCH AND CLINICAL ONCOLOGICAL PRACTICE

Edited by **Sandro Misciagna, Kelly P Cosgrove, Karmen K Yoder** and **Bradley T Christian**

**Positron Emission Tomography - Recent Developments in Instrumentation, Research and Clinical Oncological Practice**
http://dx.doi.org/10.5772/57537
Edited by Sandro Misciagna, Kelly P Cosgrove, Karmen K Yoder and Bradley T Christian

## Contributors

Massimiliano Mistrangelo, Todd Faasse, Sandro Misciagna, Evan Morris, Kelly P. Cosgrove, Shigeto Ueda, Toshiaki Saeki, Amélie Lothe, Sandrine Bouvard, Philippe Ryvlin, Stefano Pallanti, Daniela Santoro, Suzana Alexandra Corciova, Inga Grills, Victor Mangona, Raimundo Garcia, Karmen Yoder

**Published by InTech**
Janeza Trdine 9, 51000 Rijeka, Croatia

**Copyright © 2013 InTech**
All chapters are distributed under the Creative Commons Attribution 3.0 license, which allows users to download, copy and build upon published articles even for commercial purposes, as long as the author and publisher are properly credited, which ensures maximum dissemination and a wider impact of our publications. However, users who aim to disseminate and distribute copies of this book as a whole must not seek monetary compensation for such service (excluded InTech representatives and agreed collaborations). After this work has been published by InTech, authors have the right to republish it, in whole or part, in any publication of which they are the author, and to make other personal use of the work. Any republication, referencing or personal use of the work must explicitly identify the original source.

**Notice**
Statements and opinions expressed in the chapters are these of the individual contributors and not necessarily those of the editors or publisher. No responsibility is accepted for the accuracy of information contained in the published chapters. The publisher assumes no responsibility for any damage or injury to persons or property arising out of the use of any materials, instructions, methods or ideas contained in the book.

**Publishing Process Manager** Sandra Bakic
**Technical Editor** InTech DTP team
**Cover** InTech Design team

Additional hard copies can be obtained from orders@intechopen.com

Positron Emission Tomography - Recent Developments in Instrumentation, Research and Clinical Oncological Practice, Edited by Sandro Misciagna, Kelly P Cosgrove, Karmen K Yoder and Bradley T Christian
p. cm.
ISBN 978-953-51-1213-6

# We are IntechOpen, the world's leading publisher of Open Access books

## Built by scientists, for scientists

**4,200+**
Open access books available

**116,000+**
International authors and editors

**125M+**
Downloads

**151**
Countries delivered to

Our authors are among the
**Top 1%**
most cited scientists

**12.2%**
Contributors from top 500 universities

WEB OF SCIENCE™

Selection of our books indexed in the Book Citation Index in Web of Science™ Core Collection (BKCI)

Interested in publishing with us?
Contact book.department@intechopen.com

Numbers displayed above are based on latest data collected.
For more information visit www.intechopen.com

For EU product safety concerns:
IN TECH d.o.o., Prolaz Marije Krucifikse Kozulić 3, 51000 Rijeka, Croatia,
info@intechopen.com or visit our website at intechopen.com.

# Meet the editors

Doctor Sandro Misciagna was born on March 15, 1969 in Italy. He received degree in medicine in 1995 and in Neurology in 1999 at Catholic University in Rome. From 1993 to 1995 he attended research laboratory involving in cerebellar functions in mice. From 1994 to 2003 he attended Neuropsychological department of Catholic University involving in human cognitive and behavioural disorders, writing various publications and book chapters. In 2003 he took PhD in Neuroscience. He has been teacher of clinical neuropsychology, neurology, neurological and cognitive rehabilitation mainly at Catholic University. As clinician he has worked as neurologist in Alzheimer's clinics, Neuropsychiatric clinics and Neuropsychological departments. Currently he works as clinical neurologist and neuropsychologist at rehabilitation department of Don Gnocchi Foundation in Rome.

Dr. Cosgrove is an Associate Professor of Psychiatry and Diagnostic Radiology at Yale University. She uses PET brain imaging to examine the chemical changes that occur during the recovery from tobacco smoking and alcohol dependence in human subjects and in preclinical models.

Dr. Yoder utilizes PET to study neurochemistry in both humans and small animal models of psychiatric and neurological disorders.  Dr. Yoder's background is in neuropharmacology and neurochemistry, with additional training in PET tracer kinetic modeling. The main focus of her laboratory is understanding the role of dopamine in cognitive processes that subserve addiction and pain disorders.  Dr. Yoder's scope of research also includes traumatic brain injury, Alzheimer's Disease, and other dementias. Molecular targets of interest include dopaminergic receptors (primarily to study relative changes in dopamine levels), markers for neuroinflammation, amyloid and tau, and tracers for blood flow and glucose utilization.

Dr. Brad Christian serves as faculty with the departments of Medical Physics and Psychiatry at the University of Wisconsin-Madison where he serves as Director of PET Physics and Co-director of the Waisman Brain Imaging Core Laboratory. His research focuses on developing and translating novel PET methods for the study of neurodevelopment and neuropsychiatric illness. This involves using PET methodologies to investigate neurochemical changes in the brain and studying novel radioligands to characterize neurotransmitter-protein interactions and how they are influenced by development, genes, environment and drugs.

# Contents

# Preface

Positron emission tomography (PET) is a minimally invasive method and relatively safe diagnostic procedure of nuclear medicine imaging that uses short-lived radiopharmaceutical to detect and assess perfusion and metabolic activity in various organs and systems.

The majority of radioactive isotopes used in medical imaging decay by releasing energy as single gamma rays (photons). PET is based on use of radioisotopes which decay by emitting a positively charged electron (positron) from the nucleus. The positron collides with a negatively charged electron, resulting in two high-energy photons (511 kiloelectron-volts, KeV) that travel in opposite directions. The high-energy photon is subjected to less absorption or scatter by tissue than in comparatively lower-energy photons released during conventional imaging, meaning potential image degradation with PET is less likely, so there is superior image quality.

Charged particle accelerators (e.g. generators and cyclotrons) produce the radiopharmaceutical used for PET scanning that includes primarily $^{18}$FDG, but also $^{1}$C-$CO_2$, $^{11}$C-methionine, $^{13}$N-$NH_3$ and $^{15}$O-$H_2O$. PET radiotracers are generally used in microgram quantities, so the incidence of adverse reactions to very small amounts of labelled molecules is likely to continue to be low.

The first successful PET scan using the radionuclide 2-[$^{18}$F]fluoro-2-deoxy-D-glucose ($^{18}$FDG), a radio-labelled analogue of glucose, was applied in 1976 by Reivich et al. After that time several PET centres concentrated on studying brain metabolism and brain function.

The methodology for PET whole body imaging was only developed in early 1990s and since that time there have been improvements in both scanner performance and processing techniques. The number of detector elements has increased from about 20 to about 20,000, the axial field of view from about 2 to about 20 cm, the spatial resolution has improved from about 25 to about 5mm and the sensitivity has increased about 1000 fold.

Modern PET instrumentation are also multi-modality scanners, combining high-performance state-of-the-art PET and Computed Tomography (CT) scanners in a single device. These instruments provide near-perfect registration of both images of anatomy (with CT) and in vivo functions (with PET). Spiral CT scanners incorporated into PET-CT devices are extremely fast, potentially allowing the completion of a whole-body scan in a matter of seconds or even a single breath hold.

Most clinical PET imaging uses the FDG and are a potentially valuable means of diagnosis for a range of clinical conditions including oncology, cardiology and neuropsychiatric disorders. During the 1990s international experience recognized that oncology is the area where FDG PET shows greatest potential as a clinical tool.

On current clinical practice the disease areas covered by PET are: (1) differentiation of benign from malignant lesions in the case of isolated lung nodules, (2) preoperative staging of non-small cell lung cancer, (3) guiding biopsy to the highest area in primary brain tumours, (4) diagnosis of radiation necrosis, residual or recurrent mass in patients treated with radiotherapy for malignant glioma, (5) diagnosis of suspected recurrence of colorectal cancer, (6) preoperative evaluation of patients being considered for surgical resection of hepatic or lung metastases from colorectal cancer, (7) detection of metastatic disease potentially respectable in patients with melanoma, (8) evaluation of medically refractory epilepsy who are being considered for surgery, (9) assessment of viable myocardium that may respond to reperfusion in patients with ischemic hearth disease being considered for coronary revascularization. However the availability of PET is still quite limited, as evidenced by low numbers of scanners in each country.

In this book, divided into three sections, authors review some of the recent developments in PET, concentrating on factors influencing instrumentation development and the acceptance of PET as a research and clinical tool.

In the first section of the book authors review the technical basic design and performance characteristics of PET scanning emphasing on data acquisition, processing and image reconstruction. In particular authors present an historical review of Time-Of-Flight (TOF) systems, discuss their main advantages and describe requirements on the scintillation crystals and detectors suitable for TOF-PET design. Authors review recent development in acquisition, processing and archiving of PET-CT raw data and image data in clinical PET-CT environment primarily centred on oncology and neurology and illustrate key points of basic PET imaging processing and data analyses, using data and images from several neurolegands.

In the second section authors expose examples of use of PET imaging for human research purposes such as (1) study of cognitive function in normal subject, (2) study of cerebral metabolism in patients with cognitive decline related to cerebrovascular or degenerative diseases, (3) study of nicotine acetylcholine receptors in tobacco smoking, (3) imaging of dopamine release in response to alcohol consumption, (4) imaging of serotoninergic system in neuropsychiatric disorders such as temporal lobe epilepsy, depression, schizophrenia, (5) imaging of dopaminergic system in emotional, motivational, stress responses as in pathological gambling.

The third section of the book is centred around PET imaging techniques and assessment of response to oncologic treatment. In particular authors discuss assessment of response with early and late post-radiotherapy PET imaging for head and neck cancer, non-small cell lung cancer, lymphoma and gastrointestinal malignancies such as oesophageal cancer and anal cancer. The authors also expose how PET could be useful to predict tumour response, individualizing treatments, to avoid ineffective chemotherapies in particular in the management of chemotherapy in breast cancer.

**Dr. Sandro Misciagna**
Don Gnocchi Foundation
Rome, Italy

Section 1

# PET Instrumentation and Imaging Processing

Chapter 1

# Implementation of TOF-PET Systems on Advanced Reconfigurable Logic Devices

J. Torres, R. García, A. Aguilar, J. Soret, J. Martos, A.J. González, F. Sánchez, J.M. Benlloch and M.J. Rodríguez

Additional information is available at the end of the chapter

http://dx.doi.org/10.5772/57123

## 1. Introduction

The ability to resolve the Time-Of-Flight (TOF) of the gamma particles resulting after the positron annihilation until their absorption by the detector material has a strong impact on the performance of the Positron Emission Tomography (PET) systems. This occurs because, by reducing the noise level, it becomes possible to also reduce the total amount of data required to reconstruct the medical image to a given quality degree. This furthermore translates into a reduction of the time required for the image acquisition or into a reduction of the radioactive dose employed. Additionally, the capability to resolve the TOF is critical for image reconstruction in situations where the detectors cannot be completely deployed around the point of interest [1].

In Figure 1 it is shown the improvement on the image quality as a function of the TOF resolution and the solid angle covered by the detectors. As it can be seen from the figure, the importance of the TOF-PET measurement is greater as the solid angle covered by the detectors becomes smaller. According to this, the TOF capability is essential to any PET system that cannot completely surround the patient, like it could be the case of specific-application PET systems developed for particular applications, as for instance the approach for nuclear cardiology depicted on Figure 2.

Current PET scanners are built around analog subsystems implemented with discrete circuits. The electronic advances have allowed replacing the analog circuits by digital equivalents. Some of the reasons are that digital circuits present higher throughput; digital circuits also increase self-test and diagnostic capability; they present higher reliability and they also present

INTECH
open science | open minds

© 2013 Torres et al.; licensee InTech. This is a paper distributed under the terms of the Creative Commons Attribution License (http://creativecommons.org/licenses/by/3.0), which permits unrestricted use, distribution, and reproduction in any medium, provided the original work is properly cited.

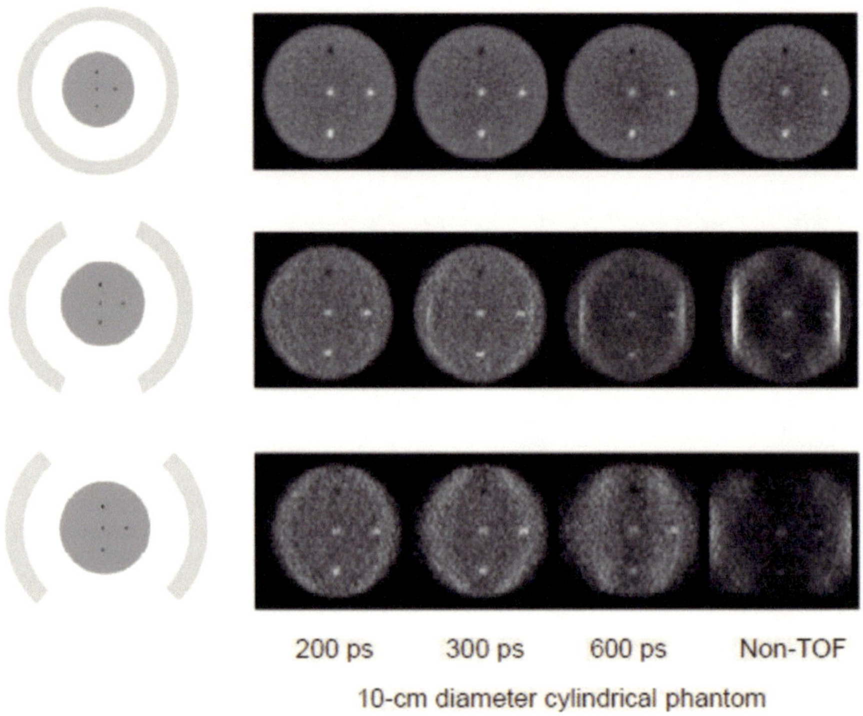


**Figure 1.** Improvement on image quality provided for TOF-PET scanners as a function of time resolution and covered solid angle [1]

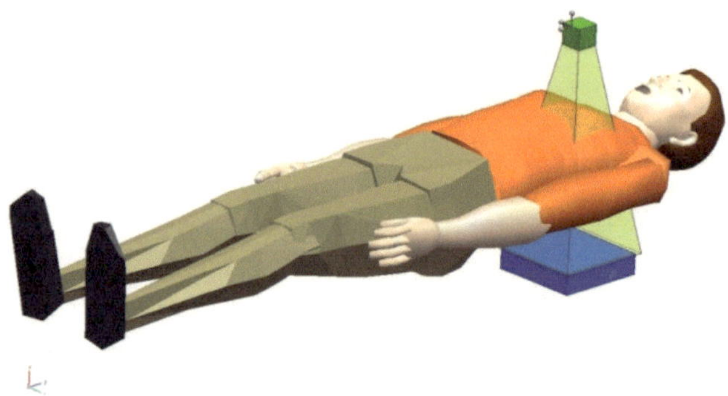

**Figure 2.** Example of a TOF-PET system setup for cardiology applications.

higher security of intellectual proprieties. In contrast to these advantages, uncertainties on the time determination appear due to the discretization and the rounding effect of the digital systems. Moreover, the complexity of the design tools is considerably higher [2].

http://dx.doi.org/10.5772/57123

PET systems contain trigger units responsible to identify true coincidences. These units are typically based on Complex Programmable Logic Device (CPLD) or Application Specific Integrated Circuit (ASIC) devices combined with Digital Signal Processors (DSPs).

On one hand, DSPs are designed to support high-performance, repetitive and numerically complex sequential tasks. They are specialized on execution of repetitive algorithms, which involve multiplication and accumulation operations. The execution of several operations with one instruction are the features that accelerate the performance in state of the art DSPs [3]. Such a performance strongly relies on pipelining, which increases the number of instructions that can be executed in a time unit. However, parallelism in DSP is not very extensive; DSP is limited in performance by the clock rate and the number of useful operations that can be performed at each clock cycle. For instance, the TMS320C6202 processor, a well-known DSP, has two multipliers and a 200 MHz clock, so it can achieve at most 400 $10^6$ multiplications per second, which is much less than a programmable logic device counterpart.

On the other hand, CPLDs are very simple reconfigurable logic devices, with a few tens of input channels and quite small logic units for data processing. They have gradually been replaced for more complex devices with higher amount of resources. For instance, ASICs present a better optimization of logic size and power management. For many high-volume designs the cost-per-gate for a given performance level is lower than that of high speed CPLDs or DSPs. However, the inherently fixed nature of ASICs limits their flexibility, and the long design cycle may not justify the cost for low-volume or prototype implementation, unless the design would be sufficiently general to adapt to many different applications. Moreover, the development of very high performance reconfigurable logic devices, as Field Programmable Gate Arrays (FPGAs), has allowed its successful application in a wide number of areas.

First FPGAs lacked the gate capacity to implement demanding DSP algorithms and did not have specific tools well enough for implementing DSP tasks. They were also perceived as being expensive and with a relatively poor power management. But these limitations are being overcome with the introduction of new DSP-oriented products from Altera and Xilinx, the two leading companies for FPGAs. High throughput and design flexibility have positioned FPGAs as a solid silicon solution over traditional DSP devices in high-performance signal processing applications. FPGAs can provide more raw data processing power than traditional DSP processors by using massive parallelism.

Since FPGAs can be hardware reconfigured, they offer a complete customization while implementing various DSP applications. All these features are, nowadays, easy to implement by means of a new generation of specific tools. FPGAs also have features that are critical to DSP applications, such as embedded memory, DSP blocks and embedded processors. Current FPGAs provide more than 96 embedded DSP blocks, delivering at least 384 multipliers operating at 420 MHz. This results on over 160 billion multiplications per second, a performance improvement of over 30 times what is provided by the fastest DSPs. This configuration leaves the programmable logic elements on the FPGAs available to implement additional signal processing functions and a system logic, including interfaces to high-speed chips and external memory interfaces such as DDR2 controllers. Using high bandwidth embedded memory, FPGAs can in certain cases suppress the need for external memory.

Summarizing, FPGAs present a high speed data transfer; fast data processing capabilities; the ability to handle simultaneously a huge number of electronic signals; and the possibility to reconfigure itself to adapt to the very wide range of applications without the need of modifying the hardware design. They additionally include hardware (Xilinx PowerPC) or software (Xilinx MicroBlaze) processor cores, depending on the model; they offer a huge storage capacity with dedicated RAM blocks and look-up table memories; and large logic capacity with tens of millions of system gates. All these features make FPGAs to be great candidates to replace CPLD or ASIC devices on PET trigger units.

Besides the advantages of PET systems based on FPGAs, recent advances in digital electronic design allows to use FPGAs for TOF determination with very high accuracy, less than 100 ps [4, 5]. This timing resolution opens the door to the development of trigger units for PETs systems with TOF capabilities built on them at a very competitive cost. Moreover, the reconfiguration characteristics of these devices allow to easily modify the PET setup (number of channels, detector coincidence map, etc) and to adapt it to different environments or physical requirements. In this chapter the main considerations for the design of TOF-PET systems based on advanced reconfigurable logic devices will be presented.

In the first section, the main advantages of TOF-PET systems will be highlighted and a historical review of these systems will be presented. In the second section, the requirements on the scintillation crystals and detectors suitable for TOF-PET designs will be described. Details of the electronic TOF implementation on FPGAs will be provided in the third section. In the fourth section, the impact of the TOF information on the reconstruction algorithms will be discussed and, finally, the conclussions will be pointed out in the fifth section.

## 2. Historical perspective

In this section, a brief description of the evolution of TOF-PET scanners from its origin to nowadays is presented.

The idea of TOF information for PET was already suggested by Anger [6] and Brownell [7] in the 1960s. However, it was rejected since the available scintillators crystals, photo-sensors and electronics were not fast enough. It was considered again when the type of crystals like CsF or $BaF_2$ appeared in early 1980s. Several TOF-PET scanners were built at that time by leading groups as by CEA-LETI in Grenoble [8, 9], by Ter-Pogossian's group at Washington University [10,11] and by Wong's group at University of Texas [12, 13]. This first generation of TOF-PET devices achieved time resolutions ranging from 470 to 750 ps [14-16]. The decay time of these scintillator materials (CsF and $BaF_2$) was very short (see Table 1 below), but their low density, low photoelectric fraction and low light output resulted on a poor spatial resolution and sensitivity.

At the same time, Bismuth Germanate ($Bi_4Ge_3O_{12}$ or BGO) began to also be used for PET designs. This scintillator has much better characteristics for PET systems, as high detector efficiency due to its increase effective atomic number (*Z*). However, its long decay time made it hardly suitable for TOF-PET systems. It is also remarkable in 1980s that is the time span in which two major companies (i.e., General Electric and Computer Technology Imagery) entered into the PET industry and gave credence to the clinical application of PET, because prior to this time (the late 1980s) most PET applications had been research applications [17,18].

The development improvement of TOF-PET systems was stopped until the discovery in 1990s of new scintillators based on Cerium-doped Lutetium Orthosilicate ($Lu_2SiO_5$ or LSO). LSO quickly revolutionized PET imaging systems because it excelled in three fundamental detector material parameters: high density, high effective $Z$ and a relatively high light yield with a short decay time of around 40 ns, allowing very narrow coincidence windows. The short decay time (LSO decays 7.5 times faster than BGO) permitted to decreased patient scan times and, thus, supposed an improvement that made patients more comfortable during the procedure and from a clinical standpoint increased patient throughput. The increase in patient throughput made the procedure accessible to more patients and subsequently increased the testing revenue for hospitals and PET imaging centers. The short decay time also lowered the level of random noise in these scans [5]. In terms of resolution, systems based on LSO scintillators permitted a new generation of TOF-PET scanners with timing resolutions as small as 300 ps [19]. The decade of the 1990s, thus, is known as the decade in which the extended use of PET progressed and made strong in the clinical sector. As more and more members of the medical community became acquainted with the utility of PET and its present and future benefits, PET imaging became increasingly popular and was available in more hospitals, diagnostic clinics, mobile systems, and physician practices.

Recently, the discovery of new materials as Cerium-doped Lanthanum Bromide ($LaBr_3$) with shorter decay time (16 ns) and excellent energy resolution has led to the development of TOF-PET systems also reaching time resolutions of 420 ps, and it is expected to reduce this resolution to 315-330 ps [20]. $LaBr_3$ present the drawback of being hygroscopic and, thus, requiring a tedious manipulation and montage.

Finally, from a commercial point of view, only two TOF-PET scanners have been introduced in the market by Philips and Siemens. The Gemini TF PET-CT is commercialized by Philips since 2006, it uses LYSO scintillator crystals (similar to LSO but with slightly lower density) and achieves a time resolution of 585 ps [21]. Recently, there has been presented results for the Siemens TOF-PET scanner, called mMR, showing a time resolution of 550 ps [22].

Currently, in parallel with advances in scintillator materials, new fast and cost-effective photosensors are being developed. Silicon Photomultipliers (SiPMs) are at the forefront of this development. They are almost unaffected by magnetic fields [23], are very fast and have high gain. SiPMs aim to improve TOF resolution due to their fast timing [24]. Single-photo-electro timing resolutions close to 50 ps root-mean-square have been reported [25]. It is expected that a new generation of TOF-PET scanners based on fast scintillators and SiPMs would be able to achieve unprecedented time resolutions.

For additional information about the historical development of TOF-PET systems, excellent reviews can be found in the literature, for instance in [26-28].

## 3. Crystals and detectors for TOF-PET scanners

The capability of PET systems to return highly accurate TOF performances strongly depends on the read-out electronics but also on the detector block itself. In this section, the main considerations about this block namely the type of crystal and the photosensor, will be presented paying special attention to its timing properties.

### 3.1. Crystals for TOF-PET systems

PET devices containing scintillators crystals must be as denser as possible since they have to stop the photons of 511 keV energy produced in the positron-electron annihilation. Such crystals need to generate high amounts of scintillation light to be detected with the photosensors. The crystal light yield is very important since it directly relates with the energy resolution of the system but also with the spatial resolution and later with the timing performance. To increase the photon emission probability in the visible range during the relaxation process, most of the crystals are doped with small quantities of impurities which generate intermediate states of energy.

In order to obtain fast output signals from the scintillation light, it is also important to account for a decay time of such light as short as possible. Moreover, the emission light wavelength should match the sensitivity of the photo-sensor utilized for electronic conversion.

NaI(Tl) has been one of the first types of crystals used for PET design. It generates significant amounts of scintillation light providing a high energy resolution and, thus, allowing to distinguish for instance photons of similar energies. One of the drawbacks when using this material has been its hygroscopic property, which requires using it in dry environments. In contrast to NaI, as stayed before, BGO crystal have been the most used scintillation crystal for PET applications, especially due to its high density, but with the lack of a good light yield and, therefore, time response.

GSO (Gadolinium-orthosilicate) has also been considered for PET designs although the light yield is also low compared to others. In this ranking, LSO (Lutetium oxyorthosilicate) appears to be good positioned offering a similar stopping power than BGO but also generating a high light yield compared to NaI. Nowadays, a LSO variant, commercially named LYSO is being widely used since its performances are very similar to LSO but at lower prices.

We will focus now in the decay time of the scintillation light since it is the dominant property in order to accurately achieve a TOF determination. As shortly introduced above, the scintillation light is described by a fast increase of the intensity followed by an exponential decrease of this emission. Here, it is called scintillation decay time to the one reached after the light pulse intensity reduces to 1/e of its maximum.

The time resolution is conditioned by the rise time, decay time and absolute light output. The rise time is negligible compared to the decay time, only the decay time and light output determine the intrinsic limits of the time resolution. In particular, faster decay times and higher light outputs reduce, i.e. improve, the time resolution. The shortest the decay time the lower the sensor dead time to process more events. The high initial rate suggests that LSO should return excellent timing properties.

| | NaI | BGO | GSO | LSO | LYSO |
|---|---|---|---|---|---|
| **Density (gr/cm$^3$)** | 3.67 | 7.1 | 6.7 | 7.4 | 7.1 |
| $1/\mu$ **a** 511 **keV (mm)** | 29.1 | 10.4 | 14.1 | 11.4 | 12.0 |
| $Z_{eff}$ | 51 | 75 | 59 | 66 | 64,5 |
| **Light yield (γ /MeV)** | 41000 | 9000 | 8000 | 31000 | 32000 |
| **Initial rate (γ/ns/MeV)** | | 37 | 232 | 676 | |
| **Time constant (ns)** | 230 | 300 | 30 – 60 | 40 – 47 | 40 – 48 |
| **Refraction index** | 1.85 | 2.15 | 1.85 | 1.82 | 1.81 |
| **Emission peak (nm)** | 410 | 480 | 430 | 420 | 420 |
| **Naturally radioactive** | No | No | No | Yes | Yes |
| **Hygroscopic** | Yes | No | No | No | No |

**Table 1.** Scintillation crystals for TOF-PET systems.

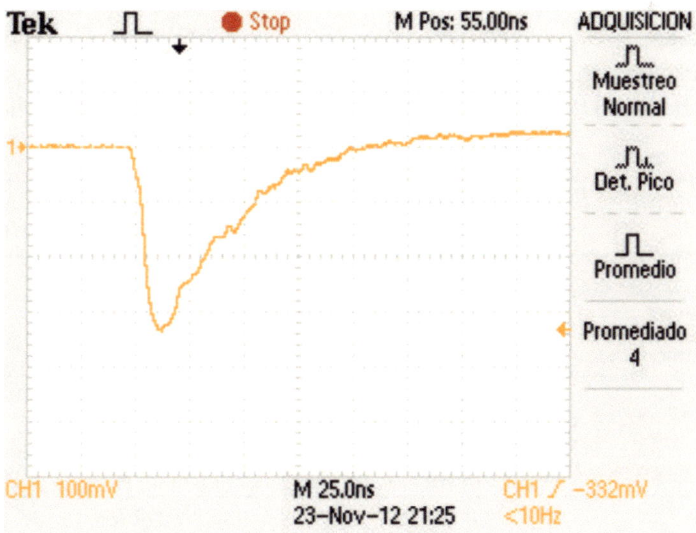


**Figure 3.** Scintillation signal and decay time (τ).

However, the timing properties of a scintillator depend on both the energy deposited in the crystal and the geometry of the scintillation crystal.

### 3.2. Photosensor, detectors capable of TOF and signal types

The photosensors are the next part of the puzzle in order to reach high time resolutions. Two main groups of photosensors are currently under use in PET technology namely Photomultiplier Tubes (PMT) and solid state photo-diodes.

PMTs use the external photo-electric effect. The scintillation photon enters the PMT through the crystal window, deposits its energy in the photocathode, and excites the electrons in the photocathode coating. The photoelectrons are accelerated and focused to the first anode with the help of an electric field. The photoelectrons are multiplied after impacting the first dynode, and this structure is sequentially repeated. A typical PMT gain is of about $10^6$ from anode to last dynode. It is possible to increase the gain with the high voltage difference and the number of stages or dynode sequence.

Most scintillators emit in the 400 nm range, allowing the use of Borosilicate glass-windowed PMTs. Many of the PMTs that are used in commercial PET cameras have transit times that vary significantly across the face of the PMT. Such a time corresponds to the interval between the light pulse striking the photocathode and the pulse signal at the anode. The transit time inversely depends with the square root of the supplied voltage. However, concerning the time resolution of the PMTs, this is better defined as the mean transit time. TOF measurements with PET scanners based on PMTs require a transit time variation very small among the different PMTs used in the design but also across the different PADs (anodes) of each individual device.

The coupling of PMTs and scintillation crystals permit to recover the photon impact position. In the case of multi-anode PMTs it is somehow easier to derive such an incidence position. The location of the interaction is achieved by measuring the light detected on each anode. This is referred as Anger-logic. In the following table, the characteristics of typical signals of a PMT are shown, together with the specifications of those for Silicon Photomultipliers.

| | **PMT**<br>**H8500 Hamamatsu** | **SiPM**<br>**S10362-11-050 Hamamatsu** |
|---|---|---|
| **Spectral response** | 300 to 650 nm | 320 to 900 nm |
| **Typical peak wavelength** | 420 nm | 420 nm |
| **Window (material, thickness)** | Borosilicate glass, 1.5 mm | Epoxy, 300 μm |
| **Anode pixels** | 64 (8 x 8) | 20 x 20 (50 x 50 um each) |
| **Active area** | 49 x 49 mm | 1 x 1 mm |
| **Supply voltage** | -1100 V | 70 V |
| **Quantum efficiency** | 24% | 50 % |
| **Gain** | $1.5x10^6$ | $7.5x10^5$ |
| **Time (rise, transit, transit spread)** | 0.8 ns, 6 ns, 0.4 ns | NA, NA, < 0.3 ns |
| **Anode dark current** | 0.1 nA | 400 kcps |

**Table 2.** PMT and SiPM comparison.

Semiconductor detectors and, in particular, Avalanche Photodiodes (APDs) have proven to be suitable photosensors for PET detectors since the mid-1990s. These compact and reliable silicon-based devices have successfully been used to replace bulky photomultiplier tubes in high-resolution PET systems. Since arrays of small dimensions crystals are most commonly used as the scintillation block, these crystal pixels may be used individually coupled to single small area APDs. These sensors are very thin and, because of the high internal electric field and the short transit distances of the charge carriers, they are quite immune to magnetic fields. This characteristic allows them to be placed inside a magnet and to operate quite normally. APDs have been tested in high magnetic fields of up to 7 or 9.4 T without showing any performance degradation [29].

Although APDs are compact and insensitive to magnetic fields, they present limitations for optimal PET performance. In particular, they can be hardly used for TOF measurements due to their slow response time. They also show low gains in the order of a few hundreds, and therefore, require sophisticated preamplifiers. These drawbacks seem to be overcome by the so-called Silicon Photomultipliers (SiPMs). Note that they are differently named depending on the manufacturer.

A SiPM consists of multiple tiny (currently up to about 20 microns side length) avalanche photo-diodes (so-called microcells) connected to a common electrode structure. When a reverse bias is applied to the SiPM at a voltage higher than the breakdown, each microcell operates in Geiger mode providing single photon counting capability. However, one photo-electron saturates the microcell limiting the linear response of the device as a function of the quantity of photoelectrons to about half the number of microcells. Similarly to APDs, they are compact, exhibit good photon detection efficiency (PDE) and do not need high voltage power supply. In advantage to APDs, they require simpler electronics and provide a high gain ($10^5$-$10^6$).

Due to their excellent timing resolution (hundreds of picoseconds), SiPMs are currently considered as the best choice for future TOF-PET applications. Their insensitivity to magnetic fields makes them ideal for the development of hybrid PET-MRI scanners. Moreover, their costs are expected to diminish rapidly in the near future due to increasing competition (there is no patent for the main invention) and automated massive production.

## 4. Design and implementation of a TOF-PET system based on a FPGA

In this section, several electronic techniques for TOF measurement will be described, also introducing the concept of FPGAs. The main features of this technology will be identified and their impact on the total system performance will be discussed. Once the use of FPGAs has been justified, the multiple implementation techniques, advantages and benefits for TOF measurements will be exposed.

### 4.1. Electronic techniques enabling TOF calculation

There exist several techniques for electronically measuring the photons TOF. In a first approach, TOF systems were based on analog circuits, using extremely uniform current sources and converting the electrical charge accumulated by a capacitor into voltage values, proportional to the charging time, that later were digitalized [30], as illustrated in Figure 4.

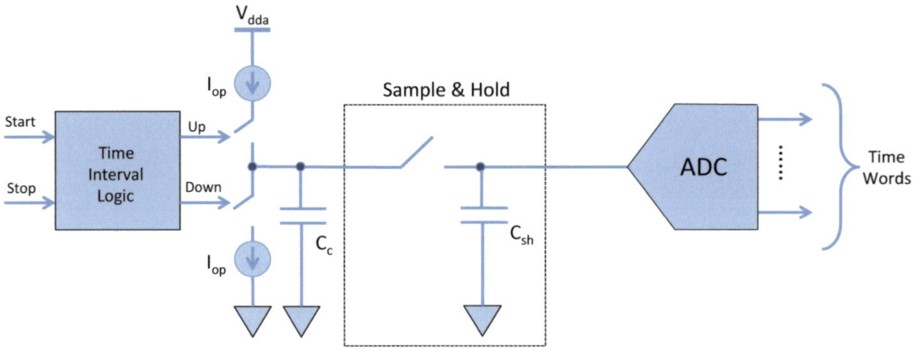


**Figure 4.** Analog TDC based on current integration and analog-to-digital conversion.

This technique presents several drawbacks, mainly related with scalability, design complexity and static power dissipation. Nowadays, most of TOF measurement devices are based on digital circuits using delay lines in different configurations. These devices use the propagation delay across the individual digital blocks to measure TOF [31-33], so they are able to measure it with a resolution lower than the system clock period. Figure 5 represents a digital delay line used to measure TOF.

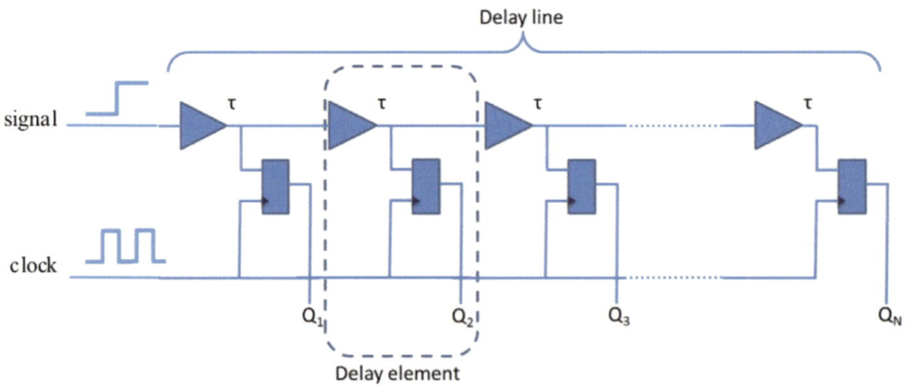


**Figure 5.** Digital delay line for TOF calculation.

The digital TDCs (Time to Digital Converters) overcome the inconvenient of the analog approach and, if properly designed, they can even compensate the effect of temperature and/or power supply fluctuations. However, most of them are built on ASICs, so they are expensive, have a reduced number of available channels, and their functionality is limited. Here, the development in recent years of very sophisticated reconfigurable logic devices opens the possibility to integrate digital TDCs on high performance FPGA.

### 4.2. FPGAs overview

FPGAs are pre-fabricated silicon devices that can be electrically programmed to carry out multiple digital functions. Unlike Microprocessors or Computers in which programming means change the incoming instructions to the device, programming an FPGA consist of change the internal logic of the device.

Historically, their strongest competitors in the market were the ASICs. They are designed for specific application using CAD (Computer-Aided Design) tools. Developing an ASIC takes much time but they have a great advantage in terms of recurring costs as very little material is wasted due to the fixed number of basic elements in the design. With an FPGA, a certain number of basic elements are always wasted, as these packages are standard. This means that the cost of an FPGA is often higher than that of a comparable ASIC. Although the recurring cost of an ASIC is quite low, its non-recurring cost is relatively high and often reaching into the millions. Since it is non-recurring though, its value per IC (Integrated Circuit) decreases with increased volume. If the cost of production in relation to the volume is analyzed, it will be find that going lower in production numbers, using FPGA actually becomes cheaper than using ASICs [34]. Furthermore, it is hardly possible to correct errors after fabrication.

In contrast to ASICs, FPGAs are configured after fabrication allowing the user for further reconfigurations. This is done with a hardware description language (HDL), which is compiled to a bit stream and downloaded to the FPGA. The disadvantages of FPGAs are that the same application needs more space on chip and the application runs faster on the ASIC counterpart. Due to the size reduction of the basic components, FPGAs were getting more powerful over the years. Herein, the development of ASICs was decreasing and becoming more expensive. Figure 5 shows the design flow of the two mentioned devices.

From Figure 6 it is easy to observe the highest complexity involved in an ASIC design as for instance:

- Design for Testability (DFT) Insertion. This technique is used to check whether the manufacturing process has added defects to the chip. DFT insertion means incorporating an additional logic to improve the testability of the internal nodes of the design.
- Hand-off to foundry. The process takes several months due to the "personalized" design.
- Equivalency checking. A system design flow requires comparison between a Transaction Level Model (TLM) and its corresponding Resistor-Transistor Logic (RTL) specification.
- Verification of 2$^{nd}$ and 3$^{rd}$ order effects. This stage is not included in the FPGA design flow because is carried out by the manufacturer.

An FPGA design flow eliminates the complex and time-consuming floorplanning (design and interconnection of the internal blocks), place and route, timing analysis, and other stages of the ASIC design project since the design logic is already synthesized to be placed onto an already verified, characterized FPGA device. However, when needed, manufacturers provide the advanced floorplanning, hierarchical design, and timing tools to allow users to maximize the performance for the most demanding designs. Furthermore, FPGA technologies are

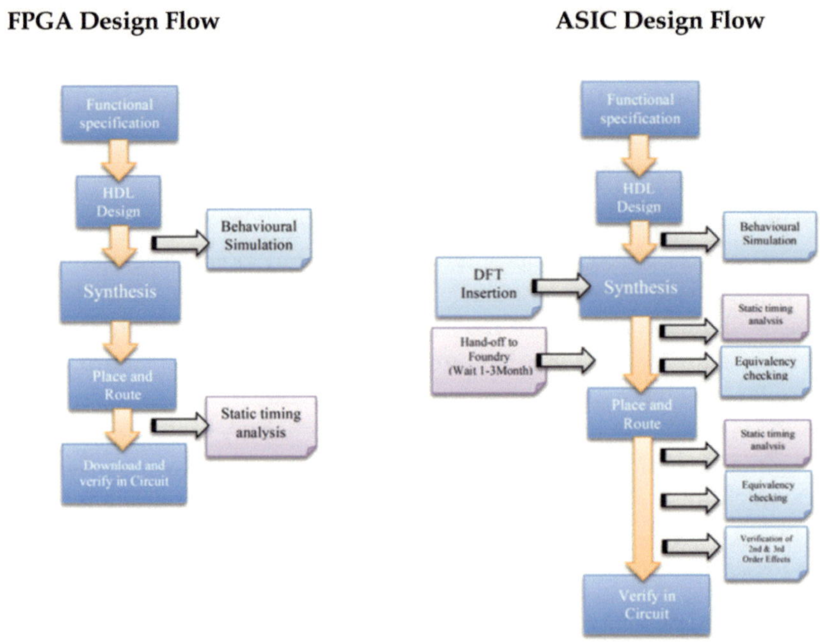


**Figure 6.** Design flow comparison: FPGA and ASIC.

considered very competitive due to the wide specification ranges. Each manufacturer provides FPGAs with different capabilities that adapt to the desired application. There are families for high performance applications, for high volume of production and even radiation tolerant families.

CPLDs are, in some cases, a good alternative to FPGA. They have a similar internal architecture to the FPGAs, as shown in the Figure 6. CPLDs are composed of digital blocks, which implement digital functions, analogous to the FPGA, IOBs (Input Output Block) and Interconnection Matrices. In general terms, CPLDs have less internal resources than FPGAs but they are able to achieve better speeds. However, when a considerable number of resources such as memory blocks and multipliers are required, FPGAs are still the best choice. In fact most of the current FPGAs incorporate Digital System Processing blocks, which have internal Multipliers. FPGAs have become more popular and, thus, CLPDs have experienced a noticeable decrease in its production, which gives FPGAs more guarantee of continuity. Therefore, FPGAs are increasingly applied to high performance embedded systems.

### 4.3. FPGA internal architecture

In the following, a basic description of the internal blocks of an FPGA is presented. Its basic structure is composed of three main blocks:

- CLBs (Configurable Logic Blocks). Generic blocks, which contain digital logic for implementing specific functions.

- IOBs. They are used to connect the FPGA to other systems of the whole application.
- Programmable Interconnect. Enables the communication between CLBs and IOBs.

Additionally to these basic blocks, FPGAs incorporate:

- Distributed memory blocks that store the user-programmed configuration.
- Clock blocks that are intended to additional clock signal generation for using either in internal blocks or external purposes.
- Other blocks that manage the proper coexistence of all the resources.

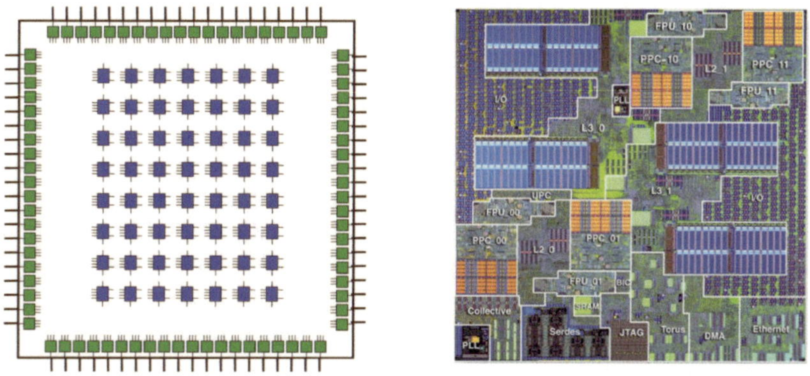


**Figure 7.** FPGA internal blocks (left) and typical example of an ASIC internal structure (right).

Figure 7 (left) shows the internal block distribution of a conventional FPGA. It is easy to appreciate how the blocks are uniformly placed in order to make possible multiple applications. Green blocks represent the IOBs, located on the boundary of the device to facilitate the interaction off-chip. Blue blocks represent the CLBs, centered with respect to the device and close to each other. They are connected through an Interconnection Matrix (not showed) which path would go over the white spaces between CLBs. Figure 6 (right) represents the internal part of an ASIC. Unlike Figure 7 (left), in this case there are not blocks uniformly distributed but different specific blocks placed optimizing the speed and space. These two figures highlight the mentioned features. The following table summarizes the commented characteristics of the three technologies.

| | Speed | Integration density | Reconfiguration capability | Time until cost-effective |
|---|---|---|---|---|
| **ASIC** | High | High | Hardly | High |
| **CPLD** | Medium | Low | Yes | Low |
| **FPGA** | Medium | Medium | Yes | Low |

**Table 3.** Programmable logic devices comparison.

### 4.4. FPGA design for TOF measurement

As commented above, there are several alternatives for implementing the TOF determination, many of them based on ASICs, that are expensive, hardly reconfigurable, and they need to be produced in high volumes to be cost-effective. However, reconfiguration capabilities of FPGAs and their low cost compared to other solutions have made them the ideal candidates for the development of complex electronic equipment, as PET systems [35]. Additionally, it is technically possible to use FPGAs to measure TOF with a very high time resolution [36], much better than the resolution of current commercial PET systems whose resolution is around 600 ps. Thus, the electronic device responsible for the TOF measurement must be able to distinguish events between time periods in the order of few-tens hundreds of picoseconds to be competitive enough in the market. In this subsection, the main considerations for TOF calculation using an FPGA will be presented.

#### *4.4.1. Time to digital converter*

TDC is a well-known technique traditionally used for TOF determination [37]. The TDC goal is to recognize events and to provide a digital representation of the time they occurred. There are many TDC implementation possibilities. Focusing in digital TDCs and leaving aside the analog TDC, the simplest is a high-frequency counter, which value is incremented at each clock cycle. When an event occurs, the accumulated amount of clock periods are stored and presented. The drawback of this approach is that the stored counter is a number of integer clock cycles and, therefore, the resolution is restricted to the clock system. Thus, in order to get accurate resolution, the use of a faster clock is required. Thus, the larger the frequency the more the signal integrity problems, translating into a complex system design. Moreover, the stability of the clock system becomes critical.

Interpolation circuits emerged as a necessity to measure events below the clock period. These circuits measure the time between a clock event and the event being measured. One of the problems is the TDC time required to perform a measurement, blocking new measurements for a certain period of time. One of the most implemented structures based on interpolating circuits is the Vernier Delay line.

Until recently, TDCs were ASIC implemented either by companies which launched the product to the market or by owners who wanted a specific design. Nowadays, the use of FPGAs aimed at this purpose is getting more popular [36-38]. Low cost, fast development cycle and commercial availability are some of the motivations of this fact. Other trade-offs of using FPGAs compared to ASICs have been amply discussed in previous sections. Sometimes a TDC is completely included within an FPGA but, depending on the application, some parts may be outside FPGA. Beyond the delay line, current TDCs contain many other elements. An example of a TDC block diagram is depicted in Figure 8.

Figure 8 represents a basic scheme of a modern TDC. The most complex block corresponds to the delay line, which will be deeply discussed below. A simplified description of a TDC follows:

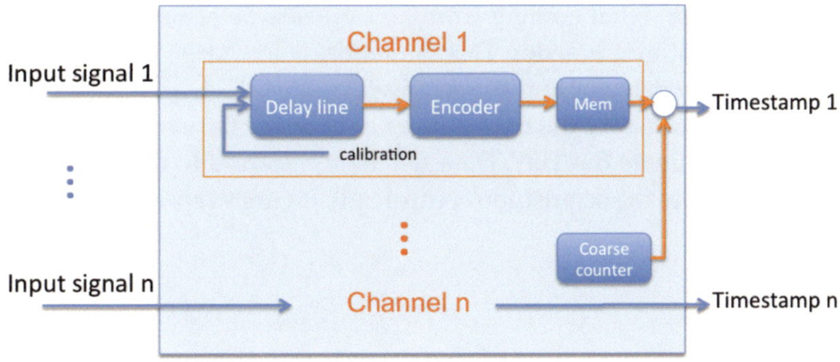


**Figure 8.** Digital TDC basic scheme.

- A calibration signal is initially selected for the system calibration. This is a necessary task to determine the individual delay of the elements from which the delay line is composed by. The raw counter (not yet in terms of time) is stored into the histogram memory.
- Each raw time element previously booked into the histogram memory is converted into a real time value and booked again into a look up table (LUT).
- The system is ready to receive an event through the "signal" connection, which is selected by the "select" signal.
- When the time event is greater than the clock period, a number of entire clock cycles must be stored, performed by the coarse counter block.
- Then, when an event occurs the "signal" is bypassed into the delay line. The encoder counts the number of elements reached by the signal and provides this number to the LUT, which convert this number to time and, after this value is combined with the coarse counter value, a final timestamp is generated.

*4.4.2. System architecture*

TDCs may incorporate more than one channel. In the block diagram previously described, a multiple channel TDC is referred. In this case, the proposed TDC channels will share the histogram memory block and coarse counter block. At the time to get the final timestamp, the coarse counter block will store each coarse time associated to each channel number. Analogously, the histogram memory block will store, after the initial calibration, the time delay of each tap for each channel.

The importance of channels lays in the possibility of group in one single device the TOF measurement of a complete PET system [35]. The outputs of the detectors placed on the PET ring system have to be fed into a trigger unit, which will be the responsible of data processing. When a signal coming from one detector is received, the system waits certain time with the purpose of receiving another signal coming from an opposite detector (or a defined set of them). The block CFD (Constraint Fraction Discriminator) is in charge to adapt the voltage values of the signals from the detector to those required by the FPGA, without disturbing the timing information. A TDC measures the time difference between the events coming from the two detectors in order to estimate the TOF. Data will be transferred to the co-processor unit (see below) to be further sent to the acquisition control unit. Figure 9 represents the mentioned architecture.

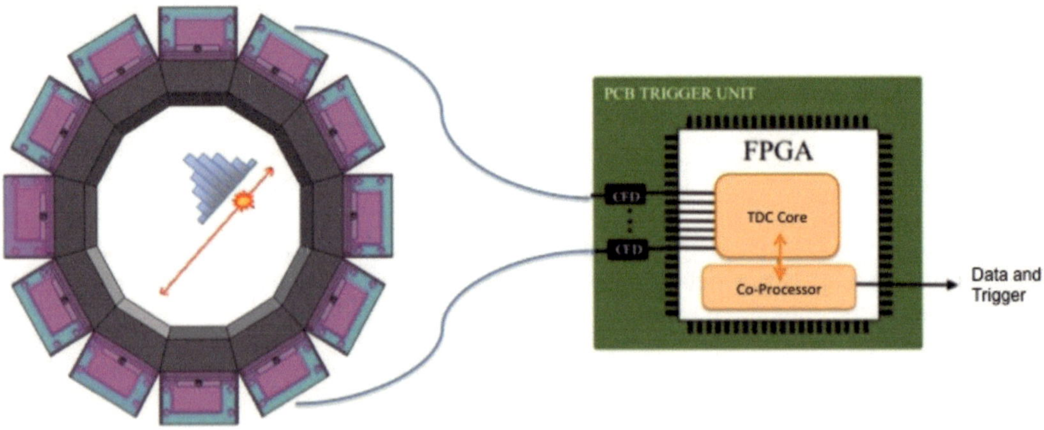


**Figure 9.** TOF-PET architecture.

The selected FPGA must account for enough resources to accommodate the required channels. Key resources that have to be considered are those that are going to be part of the delay line. Depending on the total amount of channels needed by the application, it will be mandatory focusing on the resources, which delay elements will be placed, and a proper FPGA selection.

Concerning the channel implementation in FPGA compared to other devices, FPGAs offer flexibility at the time of providing high number of channel inputs. These channels can be dynamically defined by software and enable/disable some of them if required. This means that those resources that are now free can be used for other purposes.

*4.4.3. Delay line*

Basically, a delay line is a set of interconnected elements whereby a signal is passed through. It is normally used to count the time between two or more events. Each delay element (also referred as tap or bins) has a propagation delay ($\tau$) and a storage block (see Figure 5). At certain time instant, the incoming signal is stopped and the total amount of reached taps is counted. Since the propagation delay of each element was previously measured, the time interval from the input signal arriving to the delay line until the signal is halted, can be determined.

It is very important to be taken into account that the total delay of the delay chain must be equal or greater than the clock period. Additionally, when high accuracy in TOF measurements is required (below 100 ps), any change on the propagation feature of the delay elements or the delay line path (path which join the bins) becomes critical. There are three major issues that threaten them [37, 38]:

**a. PVT**

The propagation features of the delay elements are temperature and voltage dependent. This means that the variation of the temperature inside the device and the variations of the supplied voltage have to be controlled. In ASIC-based TDCs is possible compensating the delay variation through analog method, more exactly, generating a control voltage internal circuit ad-hoc. In FPGAs, analog calibration is not suitable and a digital compensation is adopted [39]. The two more popular approaches already proposed are:

- *Double registration*. In this approach the total delay time of the delay line is designed to be longer than the system clock period. After a random time, the incoming signal is stored twice in order to take the average time value. This solution presents a fast time response but the drawback of this configuration is that does not provide a calibration of every bin independently since the average is taken when the bins have different width.

- *Statistical*. In this other approach the calibration process provides a compensated delay to each bin. The calibration process is, in many cases, automatically designed through a specific feedback. For instance, a certain component, which is also affected by PVT (Process Voltage and Temperature induced variations), is implemented and placed close to the delay line in order to resemble the temperature and voltage variations. This component might be, for example, a ring oscillator whose oscillator frequency is temperature and voltage dependent. Initially, the ring oscillator frequency is measured and stored as well as the initial time delay of each tap. Then, once the system has been calibrated, it remains continuously checking if the ring oscillator frequency has changed. If it has, the time values of each tap are interpolated according to the ring oscillator frequency differences.

**b. Delay line placement.**

A design tool often places delay elements of TDC automatically, what sometimes triggers imbalanced delays [37]. FPGAs dispose of repetitive structures commonly known as chain structures. FPGA designers place these sorted structures for general-purpose applications. The benefit is the short path connection between them what makes their use appropriate for TDC delay line implementation. Some of the different kinds of chain structures that the vendors include in many FPGAs are carry chain structures, sum-of-products chain, cascade chains, etc. Figure 10 depicts a deployed carry chain structure.

Figure 10 shows an internal view of a commercial FPGA. Red blocks corresponds to the delay line, which in this case if composed of carry logic structures. This is one possible placement of many. Depending on the length of the delay line, it is possible to locate the carry chain in multiples areas as long as the region contains carry elements (they are not present in all FPGA blocks). In this case, the carry chain occupancy is almost 400 slices. Often it occurs that there is not space enough to accommodate all the carry chains in a single column and additional columns are required. This fact will make the delay line less uniform. Therefore, in some designs a possible placement restriction must be taken into account.

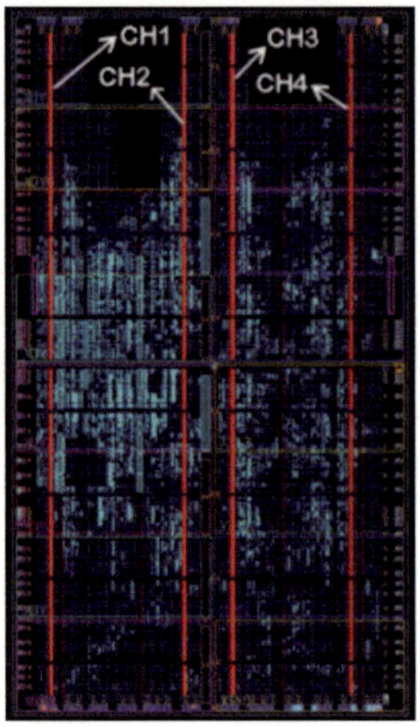


**Figure 10.** Carry chain structure.

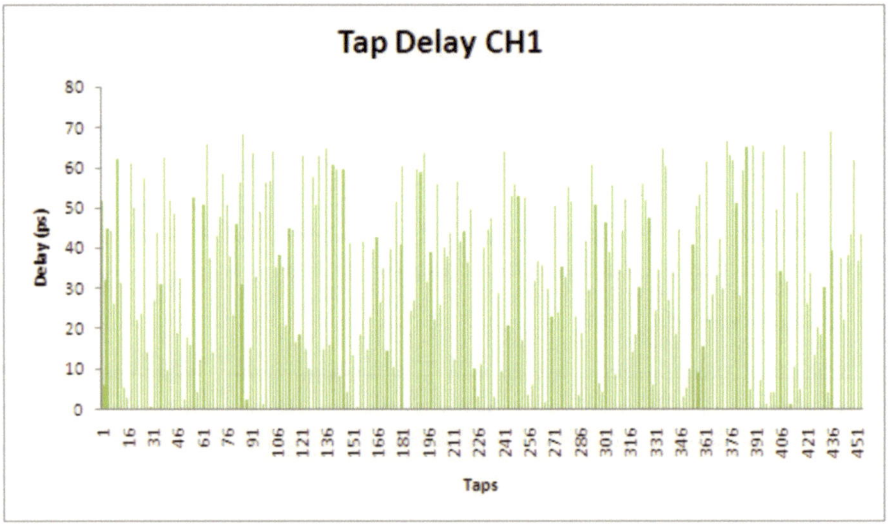


**Figure 11.** Time delay of each delay element.

## c. Differential non linearity (DNL).

The problem of the non-uniformity of tap delays is the greatest disadvantage of the FPGA delay line implementation. Its origins come from the internal way whereby the delay taps are connected, which in some cases is made by a CAD tool. Moreover, the discordances relate to the special features of some FPGAs. More specifically when the input signal passes across Logic Array Block boundaries and extra delays added cause ultra-wide bins [38]. An example of this effect is depicted in Figure 11.

Figure 11 plots an FPGA delay line time distribution. The delay line is composed of 456 taps. A calibration process determines the delay of each tap. The maximum delay is about 70 ps and the minimum delay is about 2 ps, what exhibits a big discordance between the tap uniformity. It is easy to appreciate the DNL (Differential Non Linearity of the delay bins) effect. This effect deteriorates the time resolution of the TOF measurement system but, fortunately, there exist some techniques to reduce this negative effect if required [38].

#### *4.4.4. Co-processor*

An important part of the system intended to measure the TOF is the co-processor. The goal of this component is to manage the information coming from the TDC and to provide with a timestamp to the next part of the system. Traditionally, it is not included in the trigger system but it as an extra module.

Trigger systems have currently become more complex, integrating more sub-systems in it. With the advent of modern devices, co-processors have been integrated into the main part of this trigger system, namely, FPGAs or ASICs. Either in ASIC or last decade in FPGAs, the co-processor was hardware integrated, what meant that certain resources were already used and there were no chance to make user-defined architecture. However, new generation FPGAs provide software-defined co-processors, which are liable to be dimensioned according to the application requirements. This relatively new feature has given FPGAs even more advantages and, thus, more relevance when it deals with TOF calculation systems.

## 5. Impact of TOF information on reconstruction algorithms

To finalize this chapter, we will it will be described how the algorithms currently used for image reconstruction are affected by the TOF information.

Conventional PET (or non TOF-PET) reconstruction uses TOF only to determine if two detected photons are in the same time coincidence $\Delta t$ and therefore belong to the same positron annihilation event. Here, a positron annihilation event would be registered along the line at which the event occurred, but it is unable to identify which voxel is the source of the event, thus all the voxels along the path are suggested to have the same probability of emission.

However, in TOF-PETs, the faster detectors are able to measure the difference in the arrival time of the two gamma rays, providing better localization of the annihilation event along the line formed by each detector pair. In fact, the position is blurred by a time measurement uncertainty named "time resolution", the time resolution of a detector is defined as the minimum time interval between two subsequent photon events in order for these to be recorded as separate events and depends on several instrumental factors. The smaller time resolution $\Delta t$, the smaller error on the localization of the source $\Delta x$. In fact the FWHM of the probability function is the localization uncertainty $\Delta x$ (FWHM) = $c\Delta t/2$. This results in an overall improvement in signal to noise ratio (SNR) of the reconstructed image. In particular, the SNR in an image including TOF information improves with decreasing time resolution $\Delta t$ (or the corresponding spatial uncertainty $\Delta x$). Therefore, such an uncertainty is larger for bigger patients (being related to the effective diameter D). The TOF SNR is proportional to the non-TOF SNR, through the following relationship:

$$SNR_{TOF} = \sqrt{\frac{D}{\Delta x}} SNR_{non-TOF}$$

Nowadays, the image reconstruction problem for fully 3D TOF-PET is challenging because of the large data sizes involved. Thus, it produces a high degree of redundancy in 3D TOF-PET data which can be exploited in multiple ways as reducing data storage and thereby accelerating image reconstruction, or to reject missing or inconsistent data. These unmeasured data samples can be caused either by defective detectors, or incomplete angular coverage of the patient due to special PET scanner architectures like it could be the case of a dedicated ring PET with an aperture aiming to allow for biopsy procedures.

Mathematically, redundancy is expressed by consistency conditions which can be visualized in terms of the 3D Fourier Transform and employed for compensation of missing data, using Fourier rebinning of PET data from TOF to non TOF. Thus, TOF-PET systems require less data to provide higher quality images, so the doses to the patient could be reduced. Moreover, redundancy of information can be used to overcome missing data either from defective detectors or to special scanner architectures.

Current TOF-PETs timing resolutions of about 550-600 ps do not directly lead to an improvement in the spatial resolution of the reconstructed image. It actually reduces noise propagation by localizing events along segments of each Line of Response (LOR) rather than spreading statistical noise across the full length of each LOR. At the ultimate limit, TOF-PET could potentially localize annihilation events to within a single image voxel, effectively measuring the activity distribution directly and eliminating the need for tomographic reconstruction. However, this would require a timing-resolution of approximately 10 ps to isolate events to within a 3-mm voxel. With the current TOF-PET devices, inclusion of TOF information provides a degree of improvement similar to that obtained with the Point Spread Function (PSF) model. Moreover, TOF information can lead to an artifact-free image reconstruction when the number of angular samplings is reduced. This fact is important if PET devices with limited angle coverage are considered. Partial ring PET devices can have advantages over full ring geometries in future dedicated PET systems designed for imaging specific organs. However, partial ring design leads to an incomplete sampling of the polar angles, producing artifacts in image reconstruction. Nevertheless, the number of angular views necessary for an artifact-free image reconstruction is reduced as TOF-PET timing resolution improves (*i.e.* the additional TOF information can recover some of the missing information and reduce or eliminate the artifacts). In this sense, with TOF information, the angular sampling requirements are reduced. [40]

TOF-PET approaches put challenges in the field of image reconstruction algorithms. The first challenge is to make the reconstruction time clinically viable, as TOF-PET implies a non-negligible increase on the image reconstruction computational cost. A variety of reconstruction methods already exist for TOF-PET data. These image reconstruction procedures can be divided in two groups: analytical and iterative algorithms. This division is normally made whatever the tomography technique is considered (computed tomography, Single Photon Emission Computed Tomography (SPECT), and PET).

**Analytical methods**

Analytical (*i.e.* Filtered Back Projection, FBP) reconstruction methods were the only reconstruction methods available at the beginning of TOF-PET development and were originally described in the 1980s for 2D data [41, 42]. In an analytical TOF-PET approach, the image is reconstructed by using a one dimensional time-of-flight weight along the time-of-flight line [43]. In this reconstruction, the TOF response kernel *k(l)* is usually taken to be a Gaussian where *l* is a scalar variable [44]:

$$k(l)=\frac{1}{\sqrt{2\pi}\sigma}\exp(-\frac{l^2}{2\sigma^2}),$$

whose spatial FWHM, Δx=(2σ2(4ln2))1/2, is related to the FWHM time resolution Δt as described above. The convolution of the function describing the "unknown" emitter distribution e(r) with the kernel function *k(l)* is directly related to the TOF projection data d(θ,r) as:

$$d(\theta, r)=\int_{-\infty}^{+\infty} e(r+l\hat{u})k(l)\,dl,$$

where $\hat{u}$ is the unit vector in the projection direction at angle $\theta$. It can be demonstrated [44] that the function describing the emitter in the frequency domain, E(ν), can be obtained from:

$$E(\nu)=\int H(\hat{u}, \nu)D(\theta, \nu)\,d\theta,$$

where $D(\theta,\nu)$ is the Fourier Transform (FT) of the projection data at angle $\theta$, and

$$H(\hat{u}, \nu)=\frac{W(\hat{u}, \nu)}{\int W(\hat{u}, \nu)K(\nu\cdot\hat{u})\,d\theta}$$

with $K(\nu\ \hat{u})$ the FT of the TOF kernel *k(l)*. The function $W(\hat{u}, \nu)$ is the filtering function, which is normally used if we consider FBP-like approaches. Distinct reconstruction filters normally differ only in the way they propagate noise or artifacts. Different TOF reconstruction filters can be considered (*i.e.* Most Likely Position, Confidence Weighting, Transverse Ramp, Convolved Ramp and Gaussian, Convolved Ramp and Gaussian With Confidence Weighting) being the Confidence Weighting (CW) the most widely used. In this case the filtering function is chosen as $W(\hat{u}, \nu)=K(\nu, \hat{u})$. The CW reconstruction TOF filter has been shown to be optimal in terms of minimizing image noise variance when working with Poisson data from an infinite uniform source distribution [43], but could not be optimal in other situations. In the above discussion we have considered the 2D tomography problem and the continuous domain. These expressions can be discretized for practical implementation on real TOF-PET data. The 2D approach has been also extended to 3D data. Axial single-slice and Fourier rebinning approaches followed by 2D reconstruction have been described [45-47]. Moreover, techniques based on rebinning the TOF data into non-TOF arrays have been also developed [48].

### Iterative Methods

Although analytical reconstruction methods are generally faster than the iterative ones, these last generate higher quality images, in terms of spatial resolution and image noise [49]. Iterative reconstruction methods such as the Ordered Subsets Expectation Maximization (OSEM) algorithm have to be modified in order to take into account TOF information. This is done by including a PSF along the LOR in the projector, with a width directly related to the time resolution of the scanner. Despite of the high computational cost of the iterative algorithms with respect to the analytical ones, current iterative reconstruction methods are the standard in clinical PET, and also appear to be the natural choice for TOF-PET in both present and future clinical TOF scanners [50]. Moreover, TOF-PET adds complexity to data organization and computation time to the reconstruction algorithm. If the reconstruction is sinogram based, TOF information adds a "4th" dimension to the 3D sinogram representation, changing data storage and dynamic memory requirements. In contrast to these drawbacks, if the reconstruction is list-mode based, the data are stored as a list of detected events [51]. However, 3D list-mode iterative TOF reconstruction allows for the modeling of all physical effects of the scanner system, thus retaining the resolutions of the data in the spatial and temporal domains without any binning approximation. In this sense, this approach is much more flexible and powerful than the sinogram approach at the cost of a computationally effort, being slower, since back- and forward- projections are independently executed for each event of the list. In this case, the reconstruction time depends not only on the length of the list, *i.e.* the number of detected events, but also on the sizes of the spatial and TOF kernels. Fully 3D implementations of the TOF-OSEM algorithm from list-mode data have been described in [52, 53].

In order to get image reconstruction times compatible with the daily clinic routine, 3D list-mode TOF-OSEM algorithms use multiple (10–20) processors and non-optimized reconstruction parameter choices (*e.g.*, stopping criteria determined by the reconstruction time rather than convergence and use of a truncated TOF kernel to speed up the forward- and back-projection steps) [54]. However, great effort has been put in optimizing timing requirements for TOF-PET iterative reconstruction algorithms. In reference [55] a new formulation for computing line projection operations on graphics processing units (GPUs) using the compute unified device architecture (CUDA) framework, is described. When applied to 3D list-mode TOF-OSEM image reconstruction this procedure is >300 times faster than the single-threaded reference CPU implementation[51].

Recently [56], a new TOF-PET list-mode based algorithm has been developed (DIRECT, direct image reconstruction for TOF) to speed up TOF-PET reconstruction that takes advantage of the reduced angular sampling requirement of TOF data by grouping list-mode data into a small number of azimuthal views and co-polar tilts. In terms of computing time, the total processing and reconstruction time for the DIRECT approach seems to be about 25%–30% that of list-mode 3D TOF-OSEM for comparable image quality. In addition, the total processing and reconstruction time is roughly constant with DIRECT, regardless of the sizes of the TOF and LOR resolution kernels, while the times for list-mode TOF-OSEM strongly depend on these kernel sizes. The reconstruction time per iteration for DIRECT is also independent of the number of events, while the per-iteration time for list-mode TOF-OSEM is almost linear with the number of counts [57].

http://dx.doi.org/10.5772/57123

Data corrections concerning randoms, attenuation and possibly also normalization for TOF-PET devices seem not to have a TOF structure. Thus, the current approach is to apply conventional non-TOF corrections to the new TOF data. However, scatter correction is clearly identified as the component that definitely has a TOF structure and requires an appropriate TOF computation [58].

Finally, it should be pointed out that TOF reconstruction is much less sensitive to errors and improper approximations. The redundant information present in TOF data naturally corrects the data inconsistencies during the reconstruction. It has been observed that TOF reconstruction reduces artifacts due to incorrect normalization, approximated scatter correction, truncated attenuation map, to name but a few [59].

## 6. Conclusion

In this chapter a complete review of the main design characteristics of TOF-PET systems based on reconfigurable logic devices has been performed. These systems have been presented from a historical perspective, and the main advantages of recovery timing information have been discussed. The goodness of the application of reconfigurable logic devices for TOF-PET systems have been described as well as digital electronics designs that would allow to accurate measure the timing information. Finally, the impact of timing information on image reconstruction algorithms has also been discussed.

As a conclusion, the implementation of the electronic hardware of PET systems on reconfigurable devices, including the TOF measurement capability, seems to offer several advantages over conventional approaches based on ASICs or CPLDs, mainly in terms of cost-effectiveness, time-to-market and re-configurability. Modern programmable logic devices present the necessary features to compete with the traditional used devices in terms of TOF calculation as technology of fabrication reaches high speeds and smaller sizes. For the time being, time resolutions in FPGAs are limited by the propagation time of the digital gates that conform the digital internal blocks of the device. But, due to the fast advances in fabrication processes, it is envisaged that these limitations will be overcome in the near future.

## Author details

J. Torres[1], R. García[1], A. Aguilar[1], J. Soret[1], J. Martos[1], A.J. González[2], F. Sánchez[2], J.M. Benlloch[2] and M.J. Rodríguez[2]

1 Communications and Digital Systems Design Group, Department of Electronic Engineering, University of Valencia, Valencia, Spain

2 Institute for Instrumentation in Molecular Imaging, UPV-CSIC, Valencia, Spain

## References

[1] Surti, S., Karp, J.S., "Design considerations for a limited angle, dedicated breast, TOF PET scanner", Phys. Med. Biol. 2008, 53(11), pp. 2911-2921

[2] Kuo, S.M., Gan W.S., "Digital Signal Processors Architectures, Implementations, and Applications", PEARSON Education,Inc (2005).

[3] Phelps, M.E., Cherry, S.R., "The changing design of positron imaging systems", Clin Positron Imaging. 1998, Vol. 1, pp. 31-45.

[4] Wu, J. et al., "The 10-ps Wave Union TDC: Improving FPGA TDC Resolution beyond Its Cell Delay" Nuclear Science Symposium Conference Record, 2008 IEEE.

[5] Torres J. et al., Nuclear Instruments & Methods In Physics Research A (2012), Vol. 702, 21 February 2013, Pages 73-76

[6] Anger H.O., "Survey of radioisotope cameras", J. Nucl. Med., Vol. 5, pp. 311-334, 1966.

[7] Brownell G.L. et al., "New developments in positron scintigraphy and the application of cyclotron-produced positron emitter", Medical Radioisotope Scintigraphy (IAEA Proceedings of a Symposium (Austria, 1968)), pp. 163-176.

[8] Gariod R., Allemand R., Carmoreche E., et al. "The LETI Positron tomograph architecture and time of flight improvements". Proceeding of the Workshop on Time-of-Flight tomography. IEEE Publication: Washington University; 1982. p. 25-29.

[9] Bendriem B., Soussaline F, Campagnolo R, Verrey B, Wajnberg P, Syrota A. A technique for the correction of scattered radiation in a PET system using Time-of-Flight information. J. Comput Assist Tomogr 1986;10(2):287e95.

[10] Ter-Pogossian M.M., Ficke D.C., Yamamoto M., et al. "Super PETT I: a positron emission tomograph utilizing photon time-of-flight information". Trans Med Imaging 1982, Vol 1, pp. 179-186.

[11] Yamamoto M., Ficke D.C., Ter-Pogossian M.M., "Experimental assessment of the gain achieved by the utilization of time-of-flight information in a positron emission tomograph (Super PETT I)", IEEE Trans Med Imaging, 1982, Vol. 1, pp.187-192.

[12] Wong W.H., Mullani N.A., Philippe E.A., Hartz R.K., Gould K.L., "Image improvement and design optimization of the Time-of-Flight PET", J Nucl Med, 1983, Vol. 24, pp. 52-60.

[13] Wong W.H., Mullani N.A., Philippe E.A., Hartz R.K., Bristow D., Yerian K., et al. "Performance characteristics of the University of Texas TOFPET-I PET camera", J Nucl Med, 1984, Vol. 25, pp. 46-47.

[14] Ishii K., Orihara H., Matsuzawa T., Binkley D.M., Nutt R., "High resolution time-of-flight positron emission tomograph", Rev Sci Instr., 1990, Vol. 61(12), pp. 3755-3762.

[15] Soussaline S., Comar D., Allemand R., Campagnolo R., Laval M., Vacher J., et al., "New developments in positron emission tomography instrumentation using the time-of-flight information", In: Gretz T, editor. The metabolism of the human brain studied with positron emission tomography. New York: Raven Press, 1985. p. 1-11.

[16] Lewellen T.K., "Time-of-flight PET". Semin Nucl Med, 1998, Vol 28(3), pp 268-275

[17] Phelps M.E., Cherry S.R., "The changing design of positron imaging systems", Clin Positron Imaging, 1998, Vol 1, pp. 31-45.

[18] Coleman R.E., rev. "What is PET?" About Nuclear Medicine Webpage. Society of Nuclear Medicine Website. Available at: http://interactive.snm.org/index.cfm?PageID=972&RPID=31 06. Accessed August 17, 2011.

[19] Moses W.W., Derenzo S.E., "Prospects for time-of-flight PET using LSO scintillator", IEEE Trans Nucl Sci, 1999, Vol. 46(3), pp. 783-788.

[20] Kyba C.C.M., Wiener R.I., Newcomer F.M., Van Berg R., Dressnandt N., Karp J.S., "Timing measurements from a TOF-PET scanner using local PMT triggering", IEEE 2007 Nuclear Science Symposium Conference Record, Honolulu, Hawaii, October 27 - November 3, 2007.

[21] Zaidi, H. et al., "Design and performance evaluation of a whole-body Ingenuity TF PET-MRI system", Phys. Med. Biol., Vol. 56, 2011. Pp. 3091-3106.

[22] Delso, G. et al., J Nucl Med December 1, 2011 vol. 52 no. 12 1914-1922.

[23] Espana, S., et al., "Performance evaluation of SiPM detectors for PET imaging in presence of magnetic fields", 2008 IEEE Nuclear Science Symposium Conference Record, 2008, pp. 3591-3595.

[24] Kim, Ch.L., Wang, G-Ch., Dolinsky, S., "Multi-pixel photon counters for TOF PET detector and its challenges", IEEE Tran. Nucl. Sci., Vol. 56(5), 2009, pp 2580-2585.

[25] Collazuol G., et al., Nucl. Instr. and Meth. A 581 (2007) 461.

[26] Conti, M., "State of the art and challenges of time-of-flight PET", Physica Medica, Vol. 25, pp. 1-11, 2009.

[27] Moses W.W., "Time of flight in PET revisited", IEEE Trans Nucl Sci, 2003, Vol. 50(5), pp. 1325-1330.

[28] Muehllehner G., Karp J.S., "Positron emission tomography", Phys Med Biol, 2006, Vol. 51, pp. 117-137.

[29] Pichler, B.J. et al., "Performance test of an LSO-APD Detector in a 7-T MRI scanner for simultaneous PET/MRI", J. Nucl. Med., Vol. 47, 2006. pp. 639-647.

[30] Napolitano, P. et al., "A novel sample-and-hold-based time-to-digital converter architecture", IEEE Transactions on Nuclear Science, pp. 1019-1026

[31] M. Bogdan et al., NIM A, 554(1-3), pp. 444 – 457 (2005).

[32] C. Chen et al., IEEE Transactions on Nuclear Science 52(4), pp. 954–958 (2005).

[33] M. Straayer et al., IEEE Jounal of Solid-State Circuits 44(4), pp. 1089–1098 (2009).

[34] W. Jerry. The field programmable gate array (FPGA): expanding its boundaries. In-Stat Market Research; 2006. p. 1-42. http://www.instat.com/abstract.asp?id=68&SKU=IN0603187-SI

[35] M.D. Haselman, et al., CiteSeerX—Scientific Literature Digital Library, (2010) http://dx.doi.org/10.1.1.152.3344.

[36] S. S. Junnarkar, P. O'Connor and R. Fontaine "FPGA based self calibrating 40 picosecond resolution, wide range Time to Digital Converter", 2008 IEEE Nuclear Science Symposium Conference Record.

[37] J. Wu, Z. Shi & I. Y. Wang, "Firmware-only implementation of time-to-digital converter (TOC) in field programmable gate array (FPGA)", in Nuclear Science Symposium Conference Record, 2003 IEEE, 19-25 Oct. 2003 Page(s):177 - 181 Vol. 1.

[38] J. Wu et al., "An FPGA Wave Union TDC for Time-of-Flight Applications", Nuclear Science Symposium Conference Record (NSS/MIC), 2009 IEEE

[39] J. Wu et al., "The l0-ps Wave Union TDC: Improving FPGA TDC Resolution beyond Its Cell Delay" Nuclear Science Symposium Conference Record, 2008 IEEE.

[40] S. Surti, J.S. Karp, " Design considerations for a limited angle, dedicated breast, TOF PET scanner," Phys. Med. Biol.,vol. 53, pp. 2911-2921, 2008.

[41] D. L. Snyder, L. J. Thomas, and M. M. Ter-Pogossian, "A mathematical model for positron-emission tomography systems having time-of-flight measurements," IEEE Trans. Nucl. Sci., vol. 28, no. 3, pp. 3575–3583, Jun. 1981.

[42] E. A. Philippe, N. A. Mullani, W.H. Wong, and R. Hartz, "Real-time image reconstruction for time-of-flight positron emission tomography (TOFPET)," IEEE Trans. Nucl. Sci., vol. 29, no., pp. 524–528, Feb. 1982.

[43] T. Tomitani, "Image reconstruction and noise evaluation in photon time-of-flight assisted positron emission tomography," IEEE Trans. Nucl. Sci., vol. NS-28, no. 6, pp. 4582–4588, Dec. 1981.

[44] C.C. Watson, "An Evaluation of Image Noise Variance for Time-of-Flight PET," IEEE Trans. Nucl. Sci., vol. 54, no. 5, pp. 1639-1647, October 2007.

[45] M. Defrise, M. E. Casey, C. Michel, and M. Conti, "Fourier rebinning of time-of-flight PET data," Phys. Med. Biol., vol. 50, pp. 2749–2763, 2005.

[46] M. Defrise, V. Panin, C. Michel, and M. E. Casey, "Discrete axial rebinning for time-of-flight PET," in Conf. Rec. IEEE Nucl. Sci. Symp. Med. Imag. Conf., 2006, pp. 2370–2374.

[47] S. Cho, S. Ahn, Q. Li, and R. M. Leahy, "Analytical properties of time-of-flight PET data," Phys. Med. Biol., vol. 53, pp. 2809–2821, 2008.

[48] S. Cho, S. Ahn, Q. Li, and R. M. Leahy, "Exact and approximate Fourier rebinning of PET data from time-of-flight to non time-of-flight," Phys. Med. Biol., vol. 54, pp. 467–484, 2009.

[49] D.G. Politte, "Image improvements in positron-emission tomography due to measuring differential time-of-flight and using maximum-likelihood estimation," IEEE Trans Nucl. Sci., vol. 37 pp. 737-742, 1990.

[50] M. Conti, "State of the art and challenges of time-of-flight PET," Physica Medica, vol. 25, pp. 1-11, 2009.

[51] L. Moliner, et al., Nuclear Instruments & Methods In Physics Research A (2012), http://dx.doi.org/10.1016/j.nima.2012.08.029

[52] L. M. Popescu, S. Matej, and R. M. Lewitt, "Iterative image reconstruction using geometrically ordered subsets with list-mode data," in Conf. Rec. IEEE Nucl. Sci. Symp. Med. Imag.Conf., Rome, Italy, 2004, pp. 3536–3540.

[53] C. J. Groiselle and S. J. Glick, "3-D PET list-mode iterative reconstruction using time-of-flight information," in Conf. Rec. 2004 IEEE Nucl. Sci. Symp, Med, Imag. Conf., Rome, Italy, 2004, pp. 2633–2638.

[54] W. Wang, et al., "Systematic and distributed time-of-flight list mode PET reconstruction," in Conf. Rec. IEEE Nucl. Sci. Symp. Med. Imag. Conf., San Diego, CA, 2006, pp. 1715–1722.

[55] J. Cui, G. Pratx, S. Prevrhal, andC. S. Levin, "Fully 3D list-mode time-of-flight PET image reconstruction on GPUs using CUDA," Med. Phys.,vol. 38, no. 12, pp. 6775-6786, December 2011.

[56] S. Matej, S. Surti, S. Jayanthi, M. E. Daube-Witherspoon, R. M. Lewitt, and J. S. Karp, "Efficient 3-D TOF PET reconstruction using view-grouped histo-images: DIRECT—Direct image reconstruction for TOF," IEEE Trans. Med. Imag., vol. 28, no. 5, pp. 739–751, May 2009.

[57] M. E. Daube-Witherspoon, S. Matej,M. E. Werner, S. Surti, and J. S. Karp, "Comparison of List Mode and DIRECT Approaches for Time-of-Flight PET Reconstruction," IEEE Trans. Med. Imag., vol. 31, no. 7, pp. 1461-1471, July 2012.

[58] C.C. Watson, " Extension of single scatter simulation to scatter correction of time-of-flight PET," IEEE Trans Nucl Sci,vol. 54, no. 5, pp. 1679-1686, 2007.

[59] M. E. Daube-Witherspoon, S. Surti, A. Perkins, C. C. M Kyba, R. Wiener, M. EWerner, R. Kulp, and J. S. Karp, "The imaging performance of a LaBr3-based PET scanner", Phys. Med. Biol., vol. 55, pp. 45-64, 2010.

# Chapter 2

# Positron Emission Tomography-Computed Tomography Data Acquisition and Image Management

Todd Faasse

Additional information is available at the end of the chapter

http://dx.doi.org/10.5772/57119

## 1. Introduction

Combined and optimized Positron Emission Tomography and Computed Tomography (PET-CT) exams are among the more complex of the radiographic modalities utilized in both body oncology and neurology settings. A distinct and targeted workflow is essential to successful data acquisition, processing, and related image management and reporting [1, 2]. This chapter will review the primary considerations involved in acquisition, processing, and archiving of PET-CT raw data and image data in a clinical PET-CT environment primarily centered on oncology and neurology.

## 2. Raw data acquisition

The method utilized for the creation of PET images is steeped in proprietary acquisition techniques available from a very limited number of PET-CT scanner manufacturers. Regardless of the manufacturer, successful PET-CT acquisition depends on a consistent quality assurance and quality control program as well as an attentive technologist staff and supportive physicist. Routine and careful quality control at daily intervals is at the center of any high performing PET-CT department. The pinnacle of PET quality control is the acquisition and evaluation of PET sinograms that comprise the raw data. PET-CT raw data consists of gigabyte sinogram data sets that are used to generate image sets consisting of transverse slices. Each transverse slice maps to a sine wave frequency. These frequencies on the sinogram can be practically visualized as displacements or rows on the x axis and an angle on the y-axis which represent a projection through the object being imaged. At the smallest level, each pixel in the sinogram corresponds to specific line-of-response (LOR) based on the byproducts of a positron

INTECH
open science | open minds

© 2013 Faasse; licensee InTech. This is a paper distributed under the terms of the Creative Commons Attribution License (http://creativecommons.org/licenses/by/3.0), which permits unrestricted use, distribution, and reproduction in any medium, provided the original work is properly cited.

annihilation event detected in the scanner PET crystals. The resulting pixel rendering is considered image data. Additional or revised reconstructions of different slice thickness or overlap can only be rendered from *raw* data. Image data slice thickness cannot be changed once rendered. Figure 1 illustrates a sinogram rendered from daily quality control procedures.

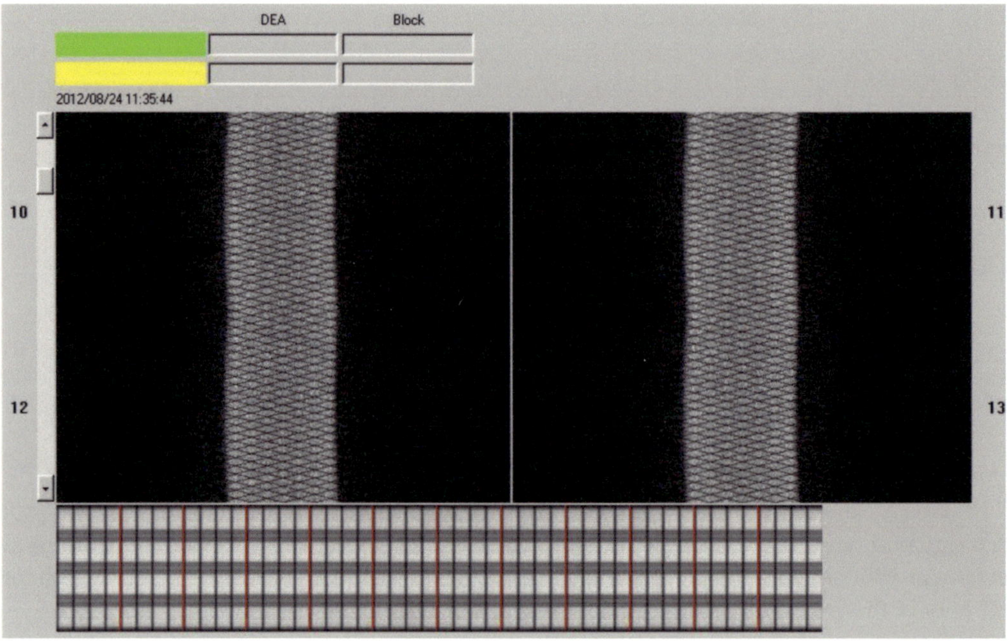


**Figure 1.** Normal PET sinogram

The PET sinogram will reveal excessive and non-uniform fluctuations occurring in the gantry crystal detector architecture. Any significant change in the detector crystals will be manifest as a "stripe" of non-uniformity. In most cases, this stripe indicates a detector block failure. The presence of a failed detector block will require a repeat of the quality control to attempt to verify scanner malfunction. Block failure is a serious malfunction that in most cases requires the intervention of a PET service engineer. The block will either need to have the corresponding electronics tuned or the block will require replacement in order to continue with scanning. Figure 2 depicts a PET sinogram with a failed block artifact.

PET scintillation crystals are especially susceptible to failure due to environmental conditions such as dramatic alterations in ambient temperature, humidity, or cooling infrastructure. As a result, the technologist should intermittently but frequently review a gantry interface that provides a continuous report of gantry status and conditions. In particular, the technologist should be mindful of alterations in gantry temperature or dew point as well as substantial changes in the voltage of the detector electronics. Maintaining vigilance in monitoring gantry conditions can be an important part of early troubleshooting to minimize delays and eventual

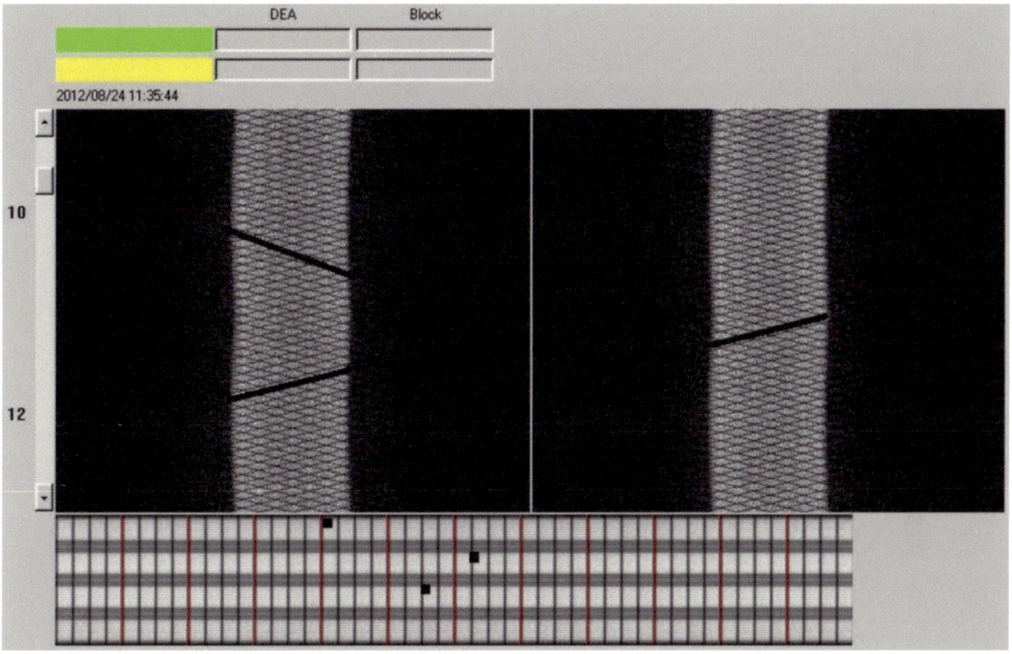


**Figure 2.** PET sinogram with failed block ("stripes" with no activity)

downtime. Figure 3 demonstrates a typical positron emission tomography acquisition interface.

## 3. Raw data reconstruction into processed image data

Once an appropriate sinogram data set has been acquired and confirmed as meeting the manufacturer and site-specific quality control requirements, reconstruction of slices from the data can be commenced. Common and clinically useful reconstructions include filtered back projection corrected and uncorrected images as well as iterative reconstructions. With iterative reconstructions, manufacturers are also bringing to bear time of flight capabilities made possible as a result of the very latest and most progressive reconstruction algorithms. Regardless of the vendor or reconstruction methodology employed, any actions necessary to correct for random events, scatter, decay, normalization, and dead time will be applied.

Two dimensional (2D) versus three dimensional (3D)acquisitions continue to play a role in image reconstruction management with 3D gaining primacy and near routine usage for all PET reconstructions [3]. In the earlier days of PET, 2D imaging was the most desirable and feasible means of imaging. This was true because, too many events would be detected within the PET crystal array with excessive dead time and image degradation in adjacent PET detector rings. This was overcome by placing septa comprised of tungsten or lead in between the detector rings. Along with these septa, the scanner electronics were configured to only detect

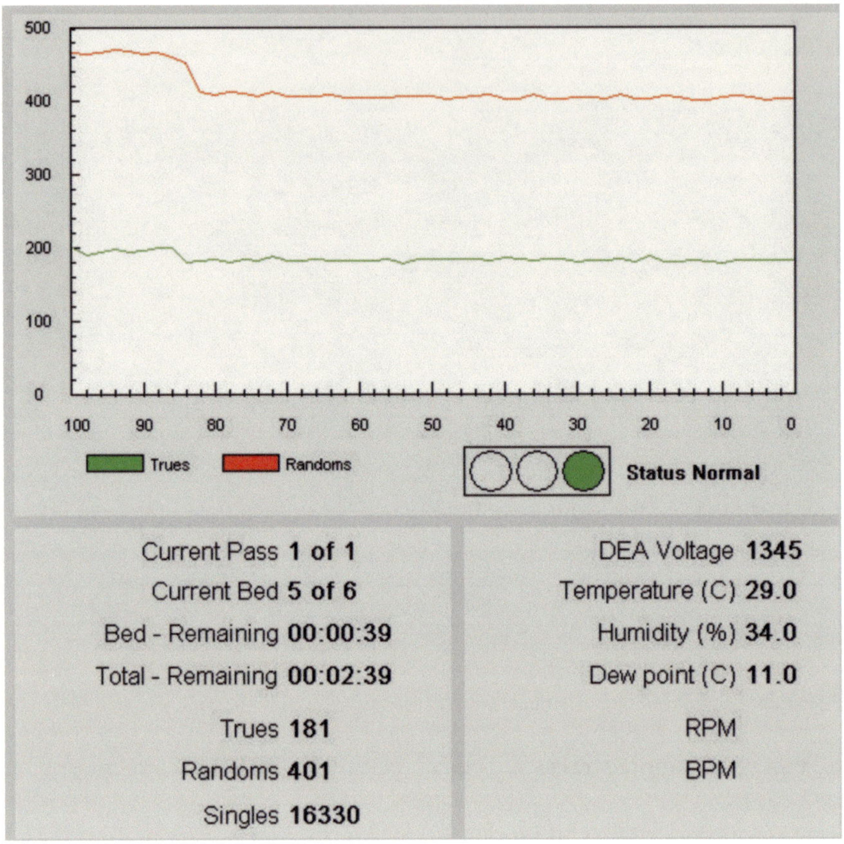


**Figure 3.** PET acquisition interface. In addition to critical benchmarks such as gantry temperature and dew point, the technologist may also view PET prompt information such as random, true, and single events.

coincidence events from within a limited plane to exclude non-collinear events. This also reduced the sensitivity of coincidence detection and corresponding image resolution. With improvements in crystal technology and detector electronics, it became possible to remove the septa that separated PET rings and detect collinear events in the adjacent PET rings. This could occur without concomitant dead time affects and allowed for a nearly quadruple increase in sensitivity. Figure 4 depicts 2D mode imaging (left) and 3D mode (right):

Attenuation corrections methods must also be implemented routinely or the PET axial images will have a muted or dim appearance for those structures that are more towards the center and deeper aspects of the patient's anatomy. The most simple attenuation correction method is that of filtered back projection whereby the body is assumed to be an ellipse of relatively uniform density. This "Chang technique" works well in uniformly dense anatomic structures but is woefully slow and inadequate in portions of the anatomy that contains variable density structures. Therefore, for both speed and accuracy, measured attenuation is preferable via the use a of a CT source. The historical arc of PET-CT attenuation projection has progressed from usage of an external transmission rod source to "modern" CT scanners that are now commer-

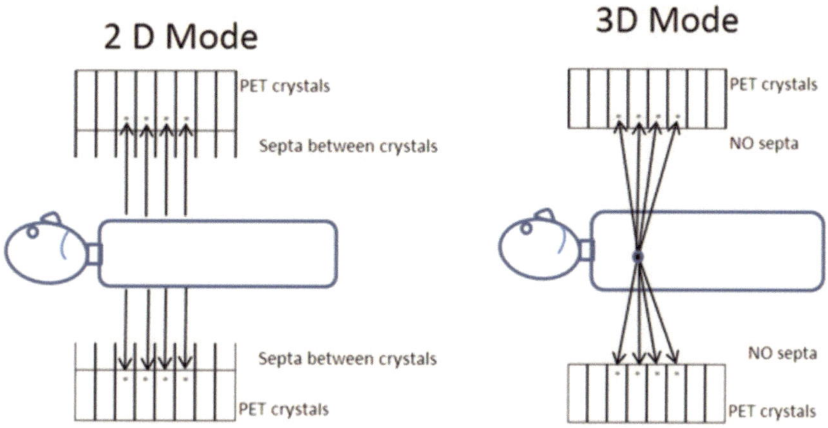


**Figure 4.** PET detection modes

cially available and integrated with PET-CT. CT detector architecture utilizing upwards of 128 rows can now be found on commercially available PET-CT scanners [4]. In the earlier days of PET, Ge-68 or Cs-137 rod sources were used to generate a transmission scan through each slice of the patient's body resulting in a measurement of attenuation correction for each pixel. Typically, the rod source was maintained within a shielded portion of the gantry. Upon the issuing of a transmission command from the scanner operating software, the shielded rod would be extended and rotated about the patient for a predefined time per bed position, usually 3-4 minutes per bed. This was a lengthy process that commonly took upwards of 30 minutes to complete. Modern PET scanners no longer utilize transmission rod sources and PET scanners containing CT infrastructure are the norm due to the dramatically increased speed of acquisition and resulting attenuation correction map [5]. Figure 5 depicts transmission scan created with a rotating radioactive rod source assembly.

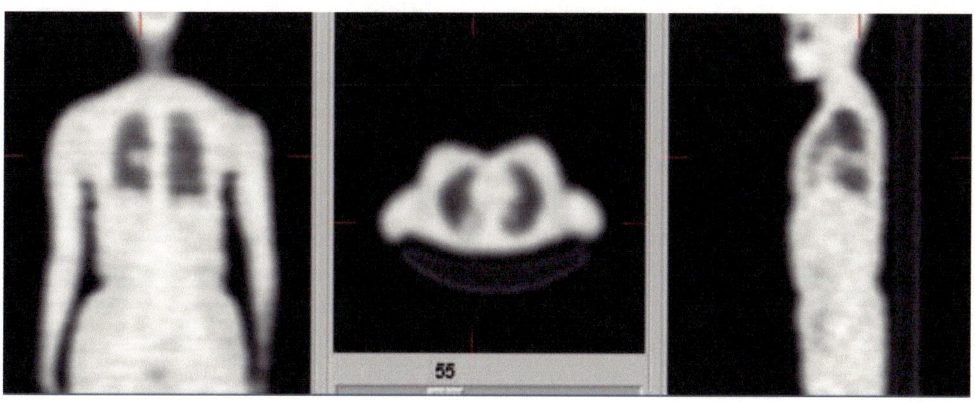


**Figure 5.** PET rod transmission source scan: Contemporary PET scanners no longer make use of rod-based transmission because CT has become the sole source of transmission-based attenuation correction.

The advantage of the traditional transmission rod source was that the patient received much less radiation dose with a transmission rod source compared to modern CT transmission methods [6]. Additionally, the transmission data were acquired in the native 511 keV energy obviating the need for segmentation that is required for CT. Segmentation involves smoothing the transaxial CT images to approximate the spatial resolution of the PET scanner. This segmentation is necessary because the energy settings of 80-140 keV inherent to CT are much lower than the 511 keV energies common to PET. The pixel values of these regions are altered and replaced with the known linear attenuation coefficient for the imaged tissue or other internal materials such as a prosthetic (joint replacement, pacemaker etc.). The process of replacing the pixel values eliminates a considerable amount of noise inherent in the "raw" image. The segmented CT attenuation map is scaled to the 511 keV and applied as attenuation correction to the PET images.

As mentioned previously, the PET-CT scanning acquisition results in the creation of raw projection data. This raw projection data is processed and rendered into reconstructed image sets. It is common practice at most clinical imaging institutions to retain the CT raw projection data for a limited number of days. This permits sufficient time to elapse such that the corresponding reconstructed images can be reviewed by the interpreting physician. It is particularly important to retain the raw data for those limited but important circumstances that the interpreting physician requests an additional reconstruction for better elucidation of a particular abnormality prior to generating the final scan interpretation. Reconstructed axial images may also be utilized to create additional projections including coronal and sagittal image sets. If the images are to be used outside of the oncology realm that PET-CT has principally been concerned with, the image data will be rendered into vertical and horizontal long axis images to accompany the usual transverse/transaxial image sets. However, certain institutions due to internal protocols or to adhere to specific research protocols must retain the raw data indefinitely. In this case, a reliable and timely means of archiving of all of the raw data generated by a scan will be necessary. There are myriad options available for archiving of said data. Reliable and timely archiving and retrievabililty will figure prominently in deciding which type of archiving solution is appropriate. Despite the increasing availability of robust and inexpensive computer memory, these data sets quickly deplete available hard drive space and create a pressing need for removal. This is because the CT raw data sets are much larger when compared to a corresponding PET acquisition of the same axial coverage. Archival and retrieval methods and strategies will be covered later in this chapter.

The amount of raw image data space required for each PET-CT examination depends on both the particular scanner configuration as well as the scan protocols in general usage by a facility. Each PET bed will require fewer than 10 megabytes (MB) of storage for lower matrix acquisitions. Lower matrices are usually those that are lower than 256. A lower matrix would be commonly used for axial coverage necessary for torso-based oncology such as breast, colorectal, and lymphoma staging and restaging. Higher matrices, such as those used for head & neck oncology or neurology imaging on the very latest and modern PET-CT scanners, are as high as 512. These high, fine matrices will require in excess of 70 MB for a single PET bed position. Figure 6 shows lower and higher matrix image examples.

http://dx.doi.org/10.5772/57119

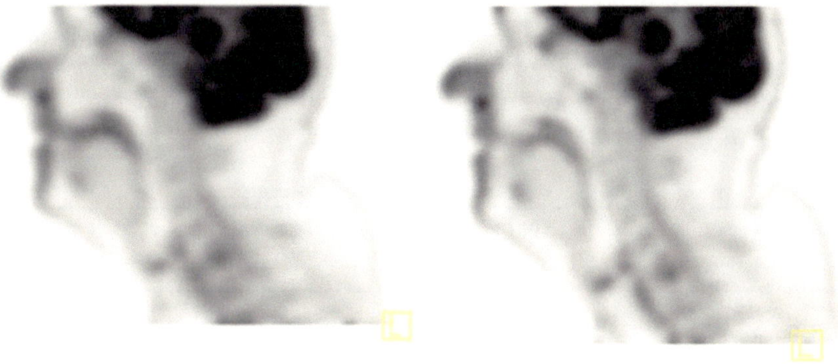

**Figure 6.** PET low (128 matrix) PET high (400 matrix)

CT raw data requires substantially more space, with modern 64-row scanner used in PET-CT generating upwards of 70 MB of projection data per second. As a result, the typical whole torso PET-CT examination can readily require in excess of 2 gigabytes (GB) of hard drive storage space for the raw data alone when there is a single CT acquisition created for the entire torso axial coverage (Table 1). With the addition of other CT acquisitions which may include lung breath hold, multiple contrast phases or longer axial coverage, the raw data space consumed increases accordingly to 4 GB and greater. The reconstructed images consume considerably less hard drive space; an entire image set, including different PET and CT image reconstructions occupy less than 500 MB. Common PET image reconstructions include attenuation corrected iterative and non-attenuation corrected filtered back projection. Figure 7 depicts the transaxial PET reconstructions commonly used in body oncology imaging.

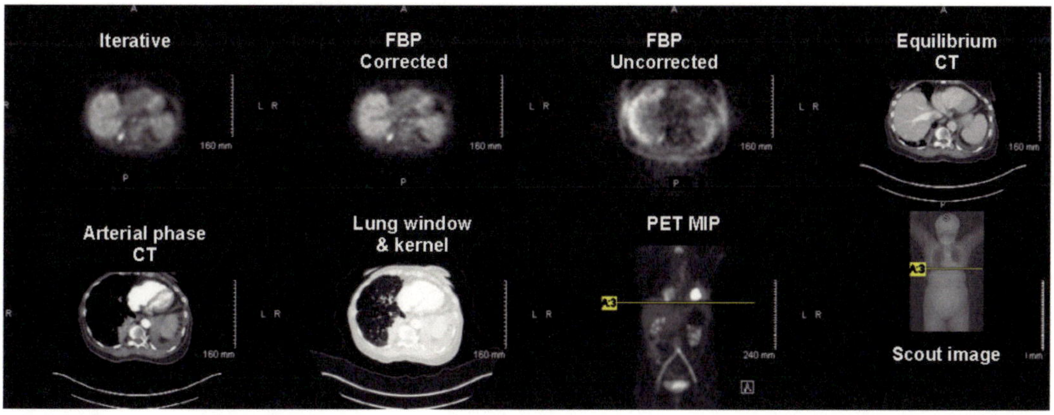


**Figure 7.** Typical transaxial PET-CT image reconstructions. Note CT was acquired with both arterial and equilibrium contrast phases and rendered in multiple kernels and windows

In a very active practice in which 10 or more patients are imaged per scanner, several GB of hard drive space can be easily filled in the course of a day [1]. If the PET-CT technologist does not routinely transfer raw data sets and reconstructed image sets to other storage sites or delete them from the hard drive space on a routine basis, system functionality can be severely hampered. In some cases, intensive hard drive utilization may cause database corruption resulting in significant interruptions and possibly downtime. Table 1 depicts a comparison of both PET and CT raw and reconstructed file sizes.

| # of PET beds | CT scanning time in seconds | PET raw data set size in MB | CT raw data set size in MB | Total PET-CT file size in MB |
|---|---|---|---|---|
| 1 | 3 | 70 | 210 | 280 |
| 2 | 6 | 140 | 420 | 560 |
| 3 | 9 | 210 | 630 | 840 |
| 4 | 12 | 280 | 840 | 1120 |
| 5 | 15 | 350 | 1050 | 1400 |
| ***6** | **18** | **420** | **1260** | **1680** |
| 7 | 21 | 490 | 1470 | 1960 |
| 8 | 24 | 560 | 1680 | 2240 |
| 9 | 27 | 630 | 1890 | 2520 |
| 10 | 30 | 700 | 2100 | 2800 |
| 11 | 33 | 770 | 2310 | 3080 |
| 12 | 36 | 840 | 2520 | 3360 |
| 13 | 39 | 910 | 2730 | 3640 |
| 14 | 42 | 980 | 2940 | 3920 |
| 15 | 45 | 1050 | 3150 | 4200 |

File size assumptions: A PET bed occupying approximately 10 cm of axial coverage requires 70 MB. A CT of the corresponding PET axial coverage is 3 times as large or ~ 210 MB. *The typical PET-CT would be of the torso ("skull base to thighs") and would be approximately 5-6 bed positions. Depending on the axial field of view, wholebody (skull vertex to toes) imaging may require as many as 15 or more bed positions to provide sufficient axial coverage.

**Table 1.** Comparison of both PET and CT raw and reconstructed file sizes

Common and scalable raw and image data archiving strategies and solutions will be discussed later in this chapter.

## 4. Time-of-flight PET

The PET scanner crystals remain the primary limiting factor in both image resolution and speed of acquisition capabilities [7]. The development and implementation of Time-of-Flight (ToF)

technology has been the primary strategy targeted at improving image resolution and acquisition speed [8, 9]. The concept of time of flight dates back many years and was utilized for limited applications employing very fast and expensive crystal arrays [8, 9]. The economics of crystal manufacture combined with more affordable and rapid computer processors and memory have made ToF feasible to deploy among virtually all of the mainstream PET-CT manufacturers. The crystal standard for many years in PET technology was the bismuth germinate crystal. It had the advantage of having good 511 keV stopping power, universal availability and was well-tested within PET gantry design. However, it lacked the fast scintillation capabilities that are essential to ToF PET. Lutetium oxyorthosilicate (LSO) or cerium-doped lutetium yttrium orthosilicate (LYSO) have emerged as the industry standard capable of the rapid scintillation times necessary to support ToF [10].

The principle advantage of ToF is the ability to dramatically improve the positioning of annihilation events that occur outside of the line of response (LOR). This is accomplished by locating the annihilation photon energy deposition on the opposing sides of the ring of crystals in the PET gantry and determining the difference in arrival times of those events.

It is important to understand that ToF allows for better lesion detectability not because of improvement in resolution but as a result of improved signal-to-noise definition inherent in improved timing resolution. For this to occur in contemporary PET scanners, the coincidence timing window must be configured to be very short (4-6 nanoseconds) to improve the fraction of randoms detected and resultant improvement in image contrast.

## 5. Quantitative PET imaging: Considerations for optimizing and rendering the standardized uptake value (SUV)

Provided accurate attenuation correction is performed, PET scanners provide the opportunity to generate semi-quantitative measurements of tumor metabolism. These measurements, known as standardized uptake values (SUVs) continue to be the primary and most universally accepted method for generating semi-quantitative measurements that depict tumor metabolism [11]. The default unit of measurement in all PET scanners is kilobecuerels per milliliter. This unit of measurement together with the quantity of injected radioactivity, patient weight, and decay time is used to compute the SUV. Considerable error inherent to all of the aforementioned criteria can result in badly flawed measurements and ultimately, false tumor metabolism quantification. In order to reduce the likelihood of introducing error in SUVs, at a minimum, the following must be evaluated and effectively implemented in the SUV calculation [11]:

- Scanner cross-calibration: procedure performed to ensure that dose calibrator dose assays match the radioactivity measured by the PET scanner.
- Measurement of residual syringe activity: This occurs immediately subsequent to administering the dose to the patient. The residual syringe activity is subtracted and the total

quantity administered is recorded in the radiopharmaceutical administration record. This same resulting quantity is used for all SUV calculations.

- Synchronization of all clocks utilized in reporting injection time
- Assurance of proper infusion of radiopharmaceutical (no dose extravasation)
- Accurate patient weight
- Accurate patient dose

The equation for SUV calculation is as follows:

**SUV= Region of interest of radiopharmaceutical concentration**

**(Tracer dose/patient weight)**

Because radiopharmaceutical dose and patient weight are in the denominator, these are among the 2 most important values to optimize to reduce the magnitude of error inherent to the calculation.

## 6. Computed Tomography acquisitions considerations for PET-CT

Prior to 1998 and the prototype development of the PET-CT at the University of Pittsburgh, PET-only systems had primacy given that those systems were the only offering available [3]. The genesis of PET combined with CT derived from the suggestion of a Swiss oncology surgeon. During the development of the PET-CT, the oncologist opined that a CT scanner in the voids between the banks of the PET detectors might provide useful anatomical information familiar to oncology surgeons. This suggestion was a catalyst to the advent of the modern-day PET-CT. Dr. David Townsend and Ron Nutt began creating a prototype PET-CT in 1991 but it would not be a viable device for use clinically until 1998 [3].

Since that time, the practice of PET-**CT** could be considered more largely to be PET-**ct** in which the CT portion of the scan is used primarily for attenuation correction and anatomic localization. However, the original intent of Townsend and colleagues was to generate *clinical* CT and *clinical* PET scans in the course of a single scanning session using a single machine. Moreover, the desired purpose of the CT was to provide clinical patient information rather than only attenuation correction and anatomic localization. Indeed, CT for attenuation correction was a secondary to the main purpose of developing a clinical PET-CT scanner [3]. High-quality, optimized CT was possible routinely even on 2 row CT units that were commonly available and interfaced with the PET gantry at that time [3].

There has been considerable divergence over the routine integration of optimized, contrast enhanced CT with PET. However, over the course of the past decade, the literature has repeatedly borne out the superior quality and efficacy of optimized CT used in conjunction with PET [12, 13]. The most strident objection to performing optimized, contrast-enhanced CT with PET is that the oral and/or intravenous contrasts utilized on the CT creates artifacts in the

PET images. More specifically, it was proposed that the intravenous contrast or oral barium sulfate attenuation correction artifacts diminished the readability of the PET [14, 15]. While there are limited examples of attenuation correction artifacts from oral or intravenous contrast, experienced PET-CT readers have learned to utilize filtered back projection uncorrected images to differentiate artifacts versus clinically relevant findings [16]. The emergence of routinely used dual syringe intravenous contrast injectors that permit the injection of a normal saline "chaser" after the initial intravenous contrast have virtually eliminated intravenous contrast artifacts on the attenuation corrected images [17].

There are substantial requirements and preparations necessary to incorporating optimized CT into PET-CT practice [2]. The most ideal approach has been to have truly-dually trained and boarded radiologists and technologists working together to produce the PET-CT images. Regrettably, this situation is rarely achievable given the time investment necessary to garner nuclear medicine physician and radiologist credentials or for similar circumstances to be available to nuclear medicine technologists. Nevertheless, it is possible to routinely incorporate optimized CT into the PET-CT practice provided there can be collaboration between nuclear medicine and CT departments.

Critical considerations for optimizing CT acquired along with PET include configuring scanner parameters for the best quality image while dosing the patient safely. Technologist staff should become knowledgeable regarding basic CT principles such as pitch and slice overlap, CT dose index (mGy and mAs or mA), slice thickness and noise inter-relationship, and x-ray penetration characteristics (keV setting). Intravenous contrast administration requires careful screening of each patient both at the time the patient's appointment is scheduled as well as during the actual appointment. Internal protocols should be developed to optimize the patient's ingestion of oral contrast, administration of intravenous contrast for optimized bolus timing, as well as persistent awareness of the potential for contrast reactions. Figure 8 illustrates a protocol for PET-CT incorporating optimized CT:

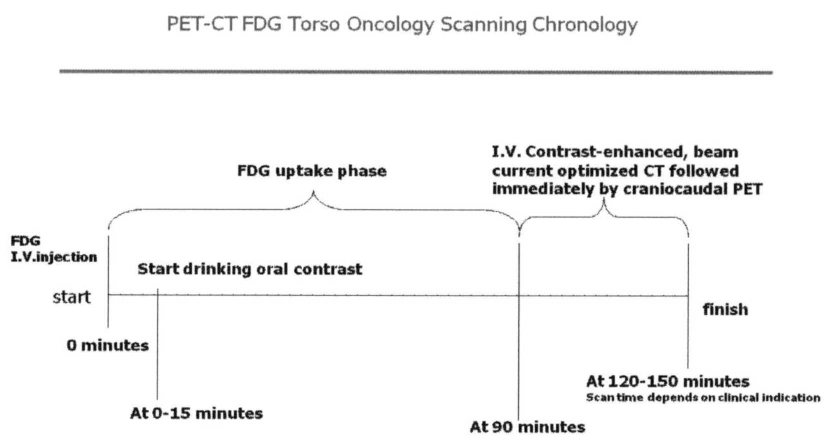


**Figure 8.** Optimized CT-PET protocol

A final consideration for performing optimized CT is patient safety given clinically significant findings. In the course of performing optimized CT, it is not uncommon to encounter a large pleural effusion (fluid in the lungs) or a pneumothorax (collapsed region of lung) or similar life-threatening circumstance. PET-CT technologists must be vigilant and trained to routinely evaluate the CT images for obvious significant findings and report these findings to a radiologist for appropriate follow up. Figure 9a illustrates a pleural effusion and Figure 9b shows a pneumothorax:

On rare occasions, pulmonary emboli are also encountered and must be reported but these findings are often extremely subtle even to the experienced imager.

Along with noticing clinically significant findings during and subsequent to the scan, it is vital that the technologist provide the utmost in safety while administering intravenous contrast. The threat of intravenous contrast extravasation, allergic reactions, or renal compromise are the foremost dangers for the patient. It has been well-documented that intravenous contrast extravasations of 100 milliliters or greater almost always require a plastic surgery consult as localized tissue necrosis may occur [18]. This is because the osmolality of commonly used non-ionic intravenous contrast (~650 mOsm/kg) is often vastly different from osmolality of blood (~285 mOsm/kg) creating conditions for unfavorable osmotic gradients to occur [19]. The majority of intravenous contrast extravasations can be avoided entirely by verifying venous patency prior to and during the administration of contrast [1]. Figure 10 demonstrates a graphical depiction of the venous patency both *before* (10a) and *during* (10b) contrast administration. Figure 10c reveals an example of a steeply sloped, worrisome curve that may indicate an extravasation event will occur.

Additionally, though uncommon, allergic reactions to intravenous contrast range from localized mild urticaria to anaphylactic shock [20]. Also, patients at risk for renal insufficiency such as those who have diabetes, hypertension, solitary kidney, or any combination of the aforementioned are at substantial risk for developing contrast induced nephropathy (CIN) [21]. Therefore, *all* patients must be carefully screened prior to receiving contrast. This will include a thorough review of the patient's medical history as well as assessment of creatinine and estimated glomerular filtration rate ideally within 30 days of administering intravenous contrast [22].

## 7. Image fusion

Prior to the introduction and routine utilization of modern PET-CT scanners, the technologist or similar staff used third party programs in post-processing attempts targeted at aligning PET and CT or PET and MR image sets that had been acquired on different scanners. In addition, the radiologist was also tasked with customary mental alignment of image metabolism structures, so called "mental fusion" [23]. The fully integrated and combined PET-CT has allowed for practical and real-time image fusion that is considered commonplace in contemporary imaging [24]. Unfortunately, this has not obviated the need for third party image fusion systems because fusion of IR, MR or other modality fusion is now considered standard-of-care.

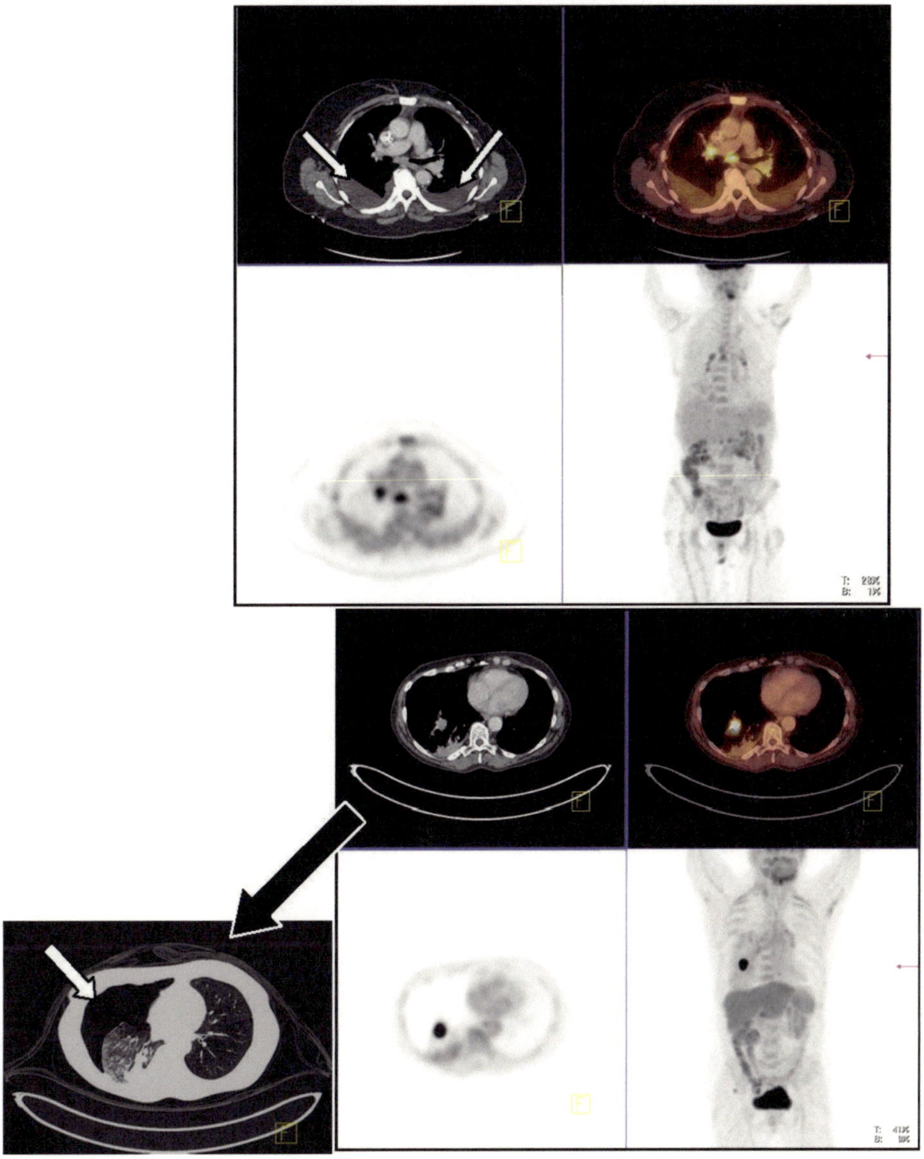

**Figure 9.** (a.) Bilateral pleural effusions encountered during viewing of CT images; (b.) Pneumothorax. Note that this clinically-significant finding is *only fully revealed* upon application of a CT kernel and appropriate windowing.

This is increasingly becoming the case in multidisciplinary oncology environments as well as neurology subspecialty environments that include an epileptologist as part of a multidisciplinary epilepsy team. Until recently, rigid fusion was the only possible fusion option. Rigid fusion involves image landmark matching to achieve the closest best fit among anatomic structures and metabolic activity. This is achievable by using software to co-register multiple image volumes against a reference volume. However, due to myriad alterations in patient

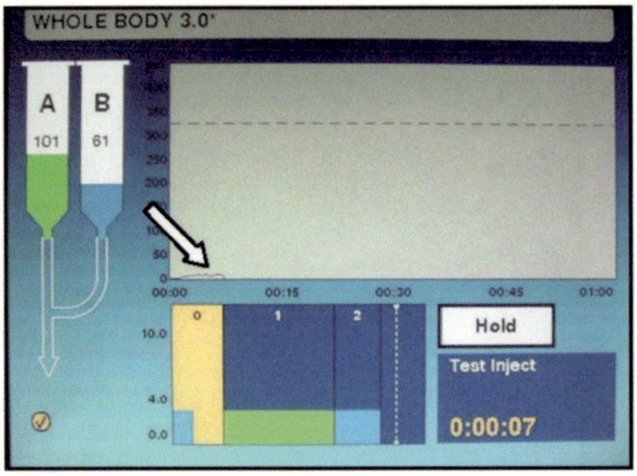


(a)

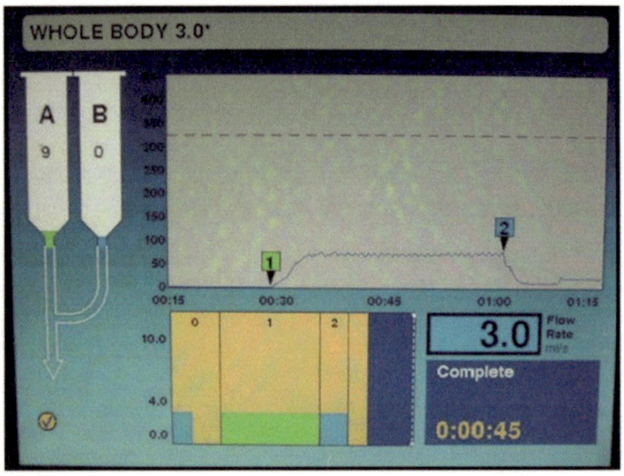


(b)

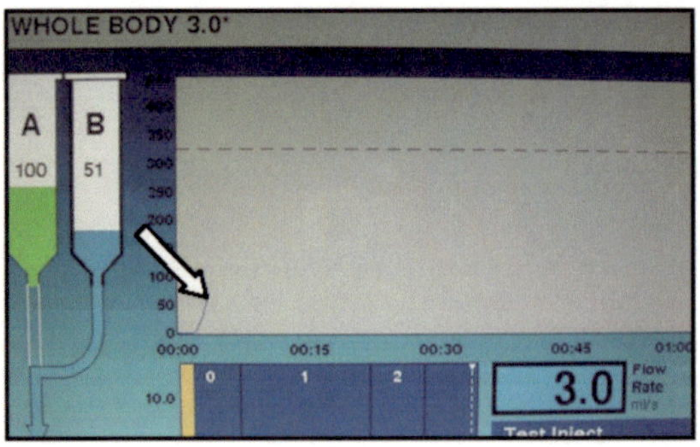


(c)

**Figure 10.** a. Saline test bolus phase, b. Intravenous contrast bolus phase, c. Non-patent I.V.: Administering intravenous contrast when the test bolus has a rapidly increasing slope that does not level off is an imminent indicator of extravasation Venous patency tracing viewed both during test bolus of saline (a), injection of intravenous contrast (b) and non-patent IV (c). For maximum safety, the technologist should actually palpate the injection site during an initial bolus of normal saline while also reviewing the time versus pressure tracing.

http://dx.doi.org/10.5772/57119

position between scanners, patient weight changes, and surgical variants rigid fusion frequently reveals undesirable matches between image sets. In contrast, deformable fusion has emerged and permits more favorable metabolic and structural alignment by incorporating virtual stretch algorithms. This involves mutual information algorithms that function at the pixel and/or voxel level to "warp" the image data [25].

Figure 11 demonstrates a post-processed PET-CT fusion image while Figure 12 illustrates a post-processed PET-MR deformably fused image.

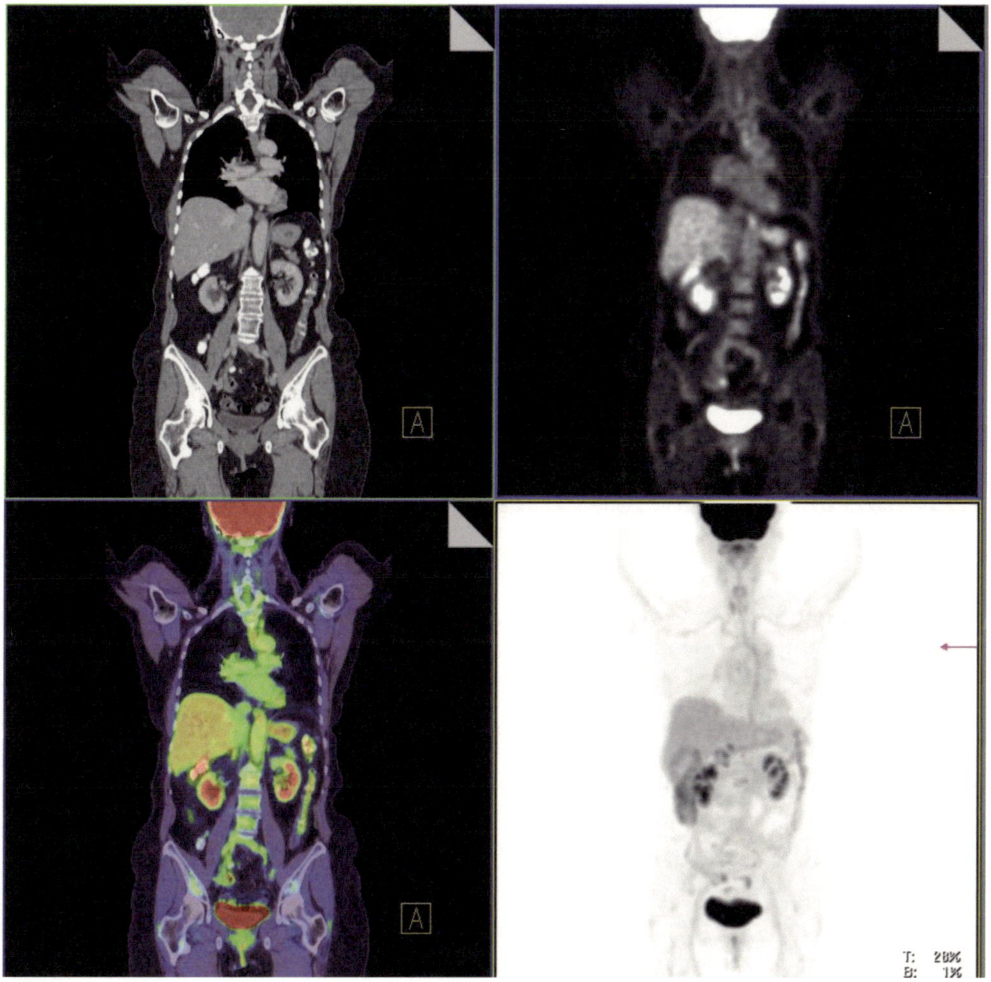


**Figure 11.** PET-CT fusion images: Images were acquired during co-registered acquisition and fused during post-processing

Provided the processed image matrices are similar, deformable fusion is routinely achievable and permits for favorable and clinically useful alignment of morphological and metabolic image sets across multiple cross-sectional modalities [26].

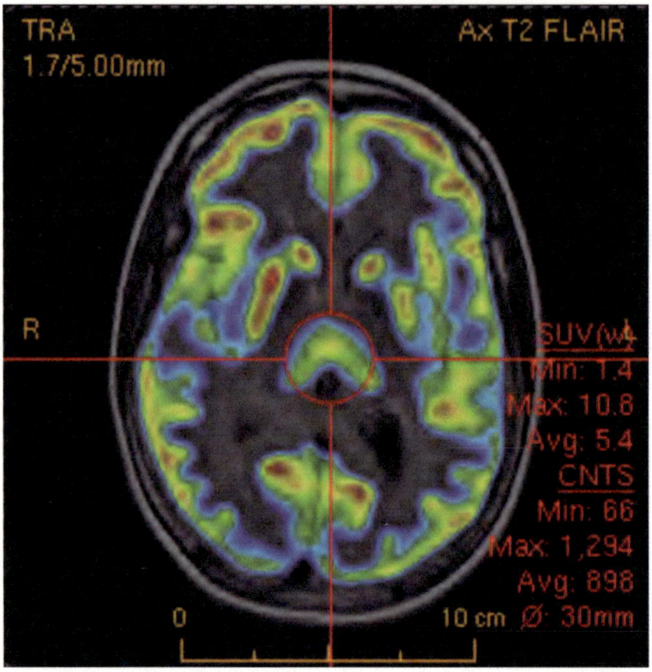


**Figure 12.** PET-MR fusion images-the PET and MR were acquired separately and fused utilizing deformable fusion post-process application software.

## 8. Workflow and the optimized PET-CT acquisition: The United States perspective

If PET-CT experienced a "golden age" it was immediately following more widespread adoption of PET-CT in the early 2000s. Numerous PET-CT facilities had business models based upon as few as 3 patients per day due to robust reimbursement that prevailed up until 2005. This was an ephemeral but important time of prosperity, growth, and development for PET-CT. At that time, the per scan fee provided by the Centers for Medicare and Medicaid Services (CMS) was at an all time high. This period was destined for an eventual phase out but was hastened by the implementation and enforcement of the Deficit Reduction Act (DRA) [26, 27, 28, 29].The DRA of 2005 (signed into law February of 2006) was implemented as part of a broader strategy targeted at limiting the unnecessary expenditure of funds thought to be redundant in patients' care [26]. The ultimate result of this policy was that reimbursement for PET-CT was reduced by nearly one half in the non-hospital, free-standing imaging environment [26]. Many independent imaging centers that once prospered by only performing 3 or 4 patients per day no longer could achieve a margin to sustain a solvent business model. In the ensuing aftermath of full phase in of DRA policy, many of these facilities were either assimilated by larger institutions or simply became insolvent and bankrupt.

In addition to the DRA of 2005, a second blow to PET-CT arrived in the form of the major economic downturn and crisis of 2008. This dramatically reduced the borrowing power of institutions as well as the number of patients with healthcare insurance who could afford to have PET-CTs. What emerged was a new paradigm of very efficient, higher volume imaging workflows in PET-CT in both public and private hospital industry. Institutions with targeted and efficient workflows have been able to weather the continued acrimonious economic conditions as funds for both full time equivalents (FTEs) and capital infrastructures such as scanners continues to diminish. PET-CT has continued to grow although the percentage increase has tended to decrease each year since 2005 [30]. This environment is indeed the new normal and will likely persist for several years to come.

## 9. Specialized acquisition circumstances: Pediatrics, radiation therapy planning, and inpatients

### 9.1. Pediatrics

Pediatric PET-CT acquisition requires all of the same precautions as those that accompany adult PET-CT *plus* specific considerations for PET emission times, matrix, and minimization of movement artifacts. Despite the fact that pediatric patients tend to be shorter and have much lower body mass than adult patients, acquisition paradoxically takes longer. This is because ideally, a higher and finer matrix will be used to image the smaller bodies of pediatric patients. As a general guideline, if the matrix size is doubled there should be concomitant quadrupling of acquisition time in order to achieve appropriate imaging statistics and image quality. Given these considerations, achieving high-quality, motion-free images may require coordination of sedation services, immobilization devices and/or considerable psychosocial support from the PET-CT staff as well as accompanying patient guardian(s) [31]. Within a conventional scheduling paradigm, high quality pediatric scanning invariably requires more planning and imaging time. These needs cannot be underestimated and should be an integral part of the pediatric PET-CT scheduling process.

In any pediatric PET-CT imaging environment, there should be age and weight-specific criteria for dosing the patient with radiopharmaceuticals. One method that can be used is to standardize the pediatric dose to the "standard man" of 70 kilograms while also setting absolute low and high dose limits. As an example, an institution might designate 74 MBq (2 mCi) as the minimum dose and 370 MBq (10 mCi) as the maximum dose. The dose would then be computed with the following equation:

**Pediatric radiopharmaceutical dose=370 MBq x child's weight in kg/150 kg**

It is helpful to use any number of commercially available spreadsheet programs to extrapolate all values of radiopharmaceutical dosing based on this equation for ease of reference.

Pediatric PET-CT will also require careful consideration of radiation dose delivered in the CT portion of the exam. This is of the utmost importance if the institution has incorporated optimized or diagnostic CT parameters because dose from CT will be nearly twice the radiation dose from the 511 keV emitting radiopharmaceutical such as fluorine-18 2-deoxy-2-fluoro-D-glucose ($^{18}$FDG) [32]. There are now well-established "Image Gently" protocols available from the American College of Radiology that can assist any facility in creating protocols that provide age-appropriate CT dosing. In recent years, these protocols have become increasingly common in many pediatric-based radiology departments although the adoption of optimized or diagnostic CT parameters in PET-CT has been slower to emerge [33]. Integrated applications to reduce CT dose should be routinely incorporated into the imaging of pediatric patients to maintain their dose as low as reasonably achievable (ALARA). Low dose pediatric CT is generally accepted to be 5 mSv or below for the typical torso axial coverage [34]. This is easily achievable in younger and smaller pediatric patients who possess a lower body mass index (BMI) but becomes considerably more difficult in imaging older and higher BMI pediatric patients. An ongoing and continuing dialogue with a health physicist and radiologist is essential to providing safe and lower dose CT in the pediatric PET-CT environment [35].

### 9.2. Radiation therapy planning

Similar to pediatric PET-CT, radiation therapy (RT) planning may be a very small portion of image volume but requires considerable additional time and attention to execute properly. PET-CT has been playing an increasingly important role in the radiation therapy process, especially in multidisciplinary oncology centers [36, 38]. One of the essential advantages that PET-CT offers over CT alone is the detection of smaller lymph nodes that would not likely be considered positive on CT by size criteria [36]. Additionally, there is now ample evidence that PET-CT consistently locates unsuspected distant metastatic disease that is not visible on CT alone [36]. There are several possible approaches to incorporating radiation therapy planning into the PET-CT environment but 2 primary methods have emerged in more routine PET-CT clinical practice. The simplest method is to complete the PET-CT on a flat RT therapy planning pallet with the patient positioned in a manner approximating the positioning established or anticipated in the patient's RT planning [36-39]. Figure 13 depicts a PET-CT scanner equipped with the RT pallet.

This approach requires no additional preparation other than the PET-CT staff receiving notification in advance to place the patient on the RT pallet. A more complex method is to position the patient in the same RT apparatus as created for the patient's original simulation. In this case, the patient is instructed to bring their simulation position device with them to their PET-CT appointment.

The primary limiting factor for this approach is usually the bore of the PET-CT gantry [36, 40]. Most manufacturers now offer RT-sized PET-CT gantries because of the emerging complementary nature of RT and PET-CT [36]. This approach permits the most accurate but also most complex and time-intensive approach with the simulation and PET-CT occurring all in one session. In this environment, the dosimetrist or radiation therapist will position the patient in their custom radiation therapy body cradle, thermoplastic mask, or similar radiation therapy simulation apparatus [36-38]. Figure 13 a and b depict a patient who has been fitted with the same thermoplastic mask as used in the patient's actual radiation therapy. Figure 14 shows the fiducials together with RT planning "B pillar" viewed on the reconstructed images. The PET-CT image sets are then migrated to the radiation therapy planning software

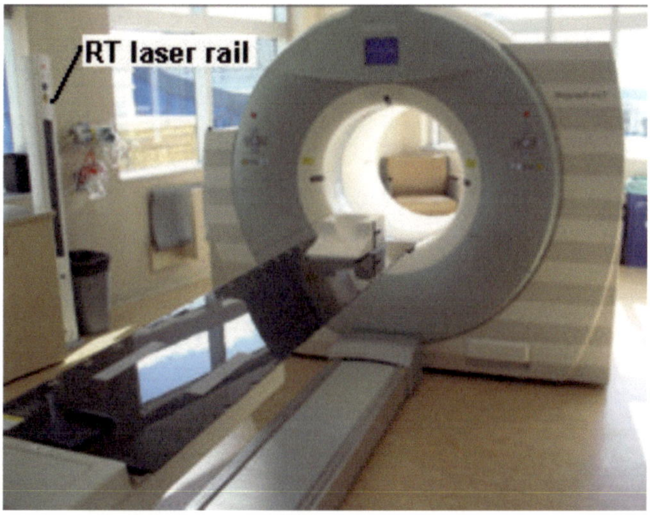


**Figure 13.** PET-CT equipped with RT pallet. Note radiation therapy planning laser adjacent to scanner (left) that will be used in aligning patient.

and used by the radiation oncologist and dosmetrist for the patient's radiation therapy sessions. The advantage of this approach is that the PET-CT images acquired are the *actual* simulation or planning images and PET with respect to a simulation CT will contain no error [36]. The disadvantage is that the additional time required to perform a full PET-CT simulation of this type can be upwards of 30 minutes. Moreover, the radiation exposure the dosimetrist and technologist receive while setting the patient up can be significant and unacceptable if performed routinely. Additionally, scanner time is expensive and in a busy institution, the additional time necessary for true PET-CT RT may create significant scheduling backlogs or patient scanning delays. For this approach to be practical, the PET-CT scanner may even be sited in the RT department.

### 9.3. Inpatients in the PET-CT environment

A final but important consideration for PET-CT acquisition is the additional maneuvers required for inpatient scanning. Inpatients will almost always require more time to ambulate, transition, and position in the PET-CT scanner. A corresponding increase in staff time must be planned for given the higher level of acuity inherent to inpatient scanning. A variety of imaging workflows and paradigms exist for incorporating inpatients into a busy imaging practice. One approach is to have an inpatient-only scanner dedicated exclusively to performing inpatient requests. This approach is more readily integrated in a large academic institution that has the resources for multiple scanners allocated for specific purposes. It is not well-suited to the typical, smaller imaging environment that relies on higher volume and more closely sequenced outpatients. Nevertheless, as the result of diminishing funds and resources, it has become increasingly common to perform inpatient studies in the outpatient setting. In any case, many institutions have found that a radiology RN is vital link in the preparation necessary to create

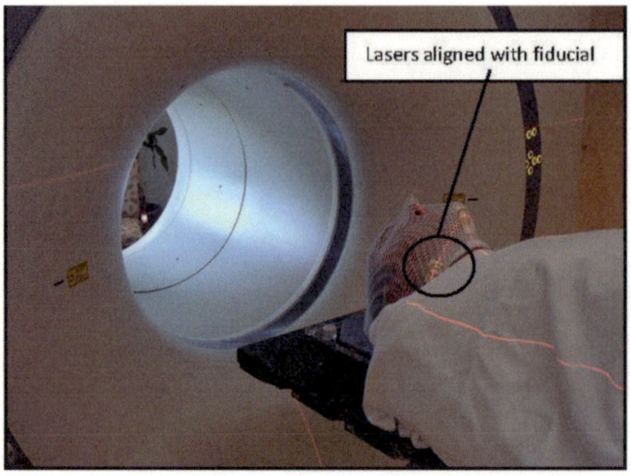


(a)

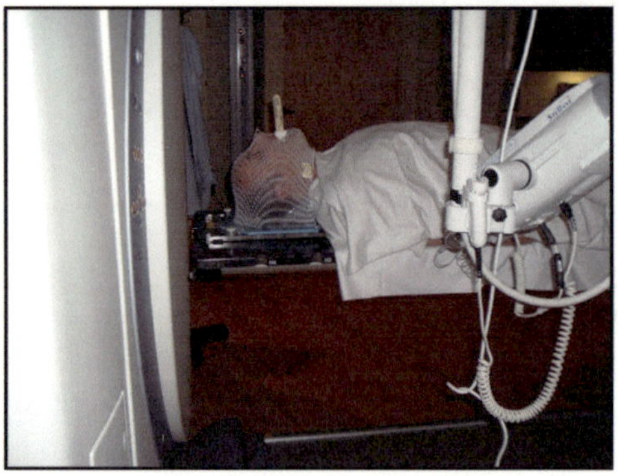

(b)

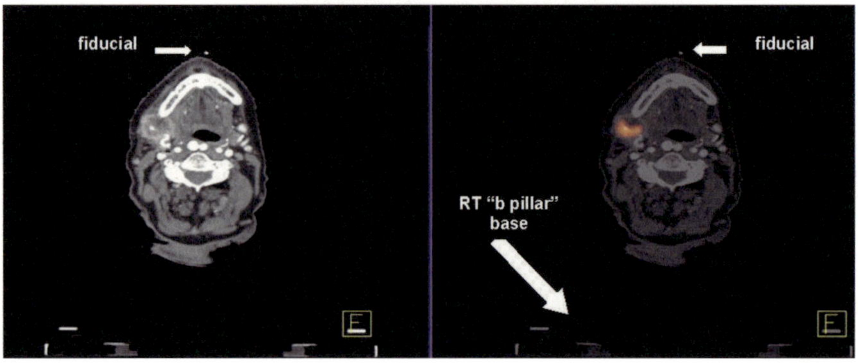


**Figure 14.** a: Patient positioned for RT planning on RT pallet with simulation position device. Note that external RT planning laser array has been aligned to patient's fiducials. b: Additional view of patient positioned for RT planning on RT pallet with simulation position device. Note patient has been fitted with thermoplastic mask that will be utilized for each RT treatment event. Intravenous contrast dual injector has also been positioned and is ready to use for optimized CT. Fiducials visualized on axial reconstructed images

a high-quality PET-CT scan. The RN should be available to perform a true peer-to-peer interaction with the patient's RN prior to the patient's actual arrival. This helps to insure the patient can be transported and maintained in the PET-CT department safely. Primary considerations include but are not limited to the following:

**Ambulation and falls:** Minimizing falls is at the center of patient safety in any clinical service and becomes especially important when caring for inpatients. The public health and hospital safety literature have repeatedly reported the poor outcomes and compromised care that falls cause in the hospital setting [41-43]. The prevention of falls has arisen to such a level that it has garnered the attention of the Joint Commission as a National Patient Safety Goal [44]. Preventing falls for inpatients undergoing PET-CT will require a peer-to-peer RN interaction whenever possible to reduce the likelihood of the patient falling upon transition to the PET-CT environment.

**Diabetes:** In an oncology setting, diabetes can be the single most challenging inpatient management regimen as the patient's medication schedule and diet must be carefully controlled to achieve a euglycemic state compatible with high quality $^{18}$FDG PET-CT imaging. If blood glucose levels exceed 200 mg/dL, the PET imaging cannot be undertaken [45]. This is true because image quality will be suboptimal as endogenous glucose competes with the same binding sites as exogenous $^{18}$FDG [45].

**Medications:** Many inpatients receive intravenous medications in an excipient such as dextrose that will make the PET-CT impossible to perform due to glucose receptor saturation. There are also numerous medications that create difficult circumstances for blood sugar control and achieving the desired serum glucose level prior to the PET-CT. These include but are not limited to corticosteroids, chemotherapy infusions, and insulin [45].

**Telemetry:** Contemporary higher acuity inpatient practice has incorporated routine usage of telemetry as a proactive means of discovering and treating cardiac events. In the peer-to-peer interaction, a plan must be formulated either for safely and temporarily discontinuing the telemetry or sending a specialized individual with the patient to monitor for cardiac events.

**Patient line status:** Inpatients will have a variety of ostomies, surgical drains, catheters and the like that will require maintenance and specialized positioning within the scanner. Because these devices will contain patient secretions that may be radioactive, additional caution to minimize the likelihood of contamination in the scanner will be required.

**Isolation:** In an era of increasingly resistant microorganisms, more and more inpatients will be discovered to be colonized with bacteria that cannot be treated with conventional antibiotics. The vast majority of hospital infection control protocols require that once a patient has been characterized as having a resistant microorganism, the patient must be isolated from other patients and staff. The more common resistant bacteria include methicillin resistant staph aureus (MRSA) and vancomycin resistant enterococcus (VRE) [46-48]. Clostridium difficile (C. diff.) isolation also has become problematic in these same hospital scenarios [49]. Since many hospital organizations cannot afford multiple PET-CT scanners, the prospect of needing to scan isolation patients in the midst of a busy outpatient workflow is not uncommon. Internal protocols that uphold cleaning the patient's uptake room, PET-CT scan room, and scanner itself must be consistently applied to reduce the likelihood that immuno-compromised outpatients do not contract a resistant bacterial strain from a scheduled inpatient.

**Attire:** Inpatients will typically be attired in standard hospital gowns which may contain metal snaps that can result in beam hardening and scatter on the CT phase of the imaging. This same metal can also introduce artifacts into the attenuation corrected PET-CT images. Therefore, it is beneficial to proactively remove said gowns or provide alternative attire such as scrubs prior to the scanning event.

**Pain management:** Given the higher acuity of inpatients as compared to outpatients, it is not surprising that a greater degree of patient pain management may be required. It is helpful to identify additional pain management needs in a peer-to-peer interaction prior to the inpatient's arrival. This will be paramount to maximizing patient comfort such that motion is minimized and a successful PET-CT scanning event will occur. Along with the pain evaluation, the RN can ascertain the patient's need for anxiolytics targeted at minimizing claustrophobia-related distress. To standardize the care of inpatients and enhance a safe time for the patient in PET-CT, it is highly desirable to collect, review, and access all of the aforementioned information prior to the patient's arrival. Figure 15 shows an example of an inpatient criteria sheet that assists the PET-CT staff with determining if an inpatient can safely be transported and scanned:

## 10. PET-CT image data distribution

Once the PET-CT image data has been acquired and processed, a convenient, rapid, and reliable system must exist to archive the image data. The historical arc of image archiving has spanned from hard-copy radiographic film systems to present day systems that permit viewing digital soft-copies of PET-CT images in Picture Archiving and Communication Systems (PACS). In most radiology and medical imaging settings, PACS has emerged as the preferred archival strategy although there continues to be a diversity of images rendered in the varied hospital and imaging center environments across the United States and globally.

PACS has been configured to support the extensive tomographic image production which is the result of torso axial coverage in the typical PET-CT. This has been especially important as multi-detector CT associated with PET has advanced and resulted in thinner and increased number of slices. It is not unusual for the combined PET-CT image set to contain in excess of 2000 image slices that require rapid transfer to the PACS server and corresponding distribution to image review workstations. Image transfer rates and efficiency will be a function of the bandwidth available throughout the hospital or imaging system network. Rate of image transfer is central to availability of image data on centralized and remote workstations. System slow-downs will also impact the performance of the PET-CT acquisitions if the processed data cannot be rapidly transferred to the PACS. This phenomenon is both vendor and system topology dependant but best practices require that an entire study be transmitted in under 5 minutes for a busy PET-CT imaging center. Figure

http://dx.doi.org/10.5772/57119

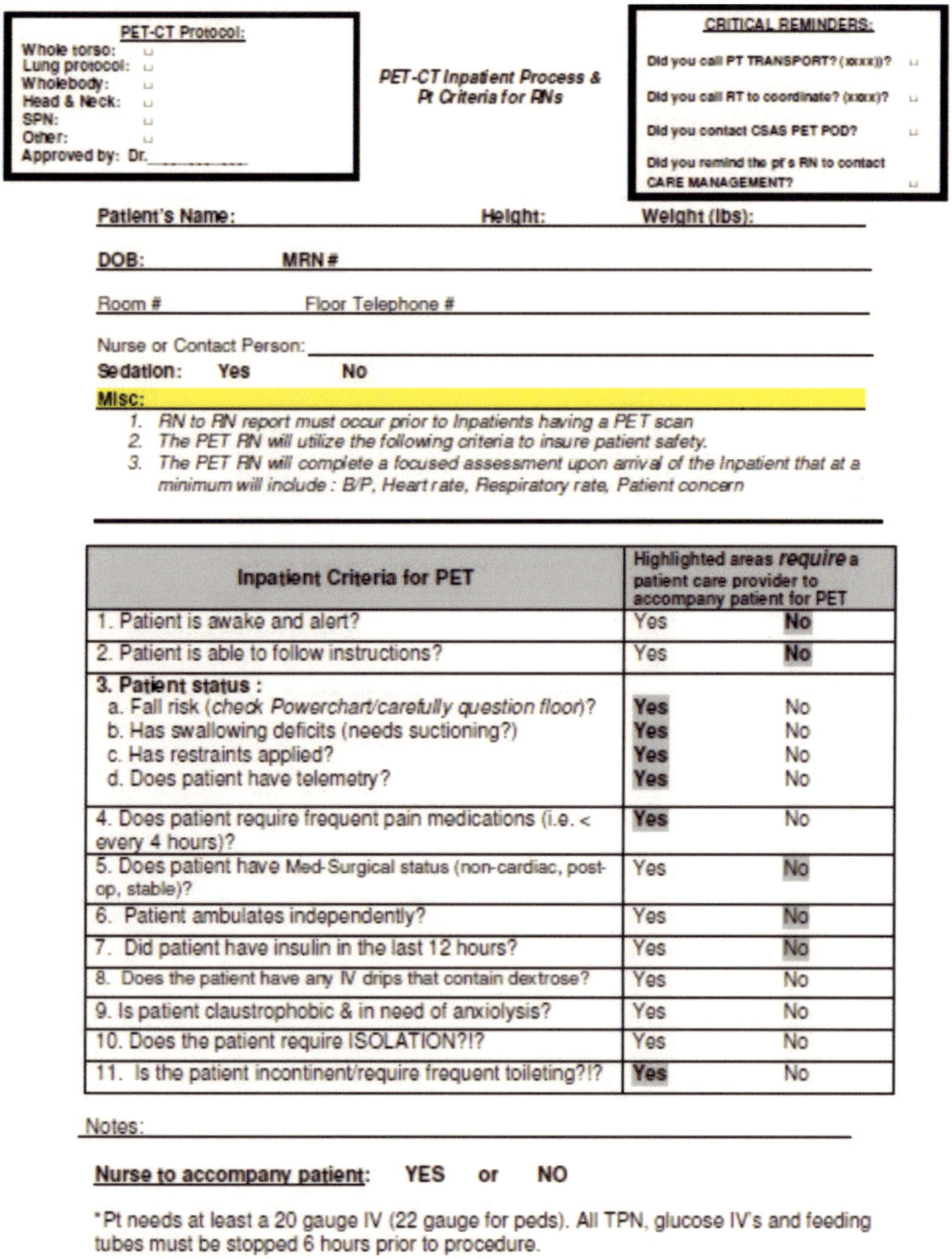

**PET-CT Protocol:**
Whole torso: ☐
Lung protocol: ☐
Wholebody: ☐
Head & Neck: ☐
SPN: ☐
Other: ☐
Approved by: Dr.____________

***PET-CT Inpatient Process & Pt Criteria for RNs***

**CRITICAL REMINDERS:**
Did you call PT TRANSPORT? (xxxxx)? ☐
Did you call RT to coordinate? (xxxx)? ☐
Did you contact CSAS PET POD? ☐
Did you remind the pt's RN to contact CARE MANAGEMENT? ☐

**Patient's Name:** ______ **Height:** ______ **Weight (lbs):** ______

**DOB:** ______ **MRN #** ______

Room # ______ Floor Telephone # ______

Nurse or Contact Person: ______

**Sedation: Yes No**

**Misc:**

1. *RN to RN report must occur prior to Inpatients having a PET scan*
2. *The PET RN will utilize the following criteria to insure patient safety.*
3. *The PET RN will complete a focused assessment upon arrival of the Inpatient that at a minimum will include : B/P, Heart rate, Respiratory rate, Patient concern*

| **Inpatient Criteria for PET** | **Highlighted areas *require* a patient care provider to accompany patient for PET** | |
|---|---|---|
| 1. Patient is awake and alert? | Yes | **No** |
| 2. Patient is able to follow instructions? | Yes | **No** |
| **3. Patient status :** | | |
| a. Fall risk (*check Powerchart/carefully question floor*)? | **Yes** | No |
| b. Has swallowing deficits (needs suctioning?) | **Yes** | No |
| c. Has restraints applied? | **Yes** | No |
| d. Does patient have telemetry? | **Yes** | No |
| 4. Does patient require frequent pain medications (i.e. < every 4 hours)? | **Yes** | No |
| 5. Does patient have Med-Surgical status (non-cardiac, post-op, stable)? | Yes | **No** |
| 6. Patient ambulates independently? | Yes | **No** |
| 7. Did patient have insulin in the last 12 hours? | Yes | **No** |
| 8. Does the patient have any IV drips that contain dextrose? | Yes | No |
| 9. Is patient claustrophobic & in need of anxiolysis? | Yes | No |
| 10. Does the patient require ISOLATION?!? | Yes | No |
| 11. Is the patient incontinent/require frequent toileting?!? | **Yes** | No |

Notes: ______

**Nurse to accompany patient: YES or NO**

*Pt needs at least a 20 gauge IV (22 gauge for peds). All TPN, glucose IV's and feeding tubes must be stopped 6 hours prior to procedure.

**Figure 15.** Inpatient criteria sheet example

16 graphically depicts the relationship between image data transfer rate and transfer time. There is a clear exponential relationship which is quickly realized within the imaging

workflow because transfer rate and time delays can cause backlogs and impair overall PET-CT system performance.

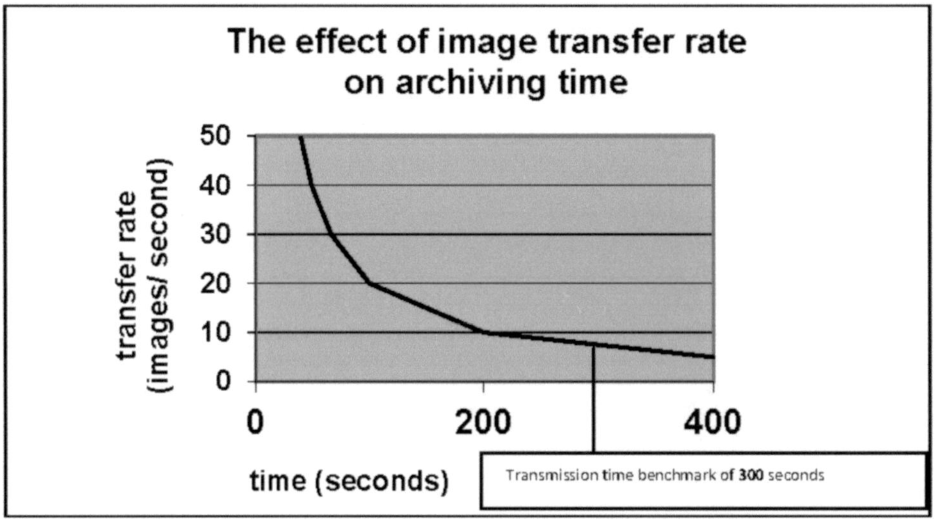


**Figure 16.** Relationship between rate of image transfer and archival time:

Given the opportunity, PET-CT, medical informatics professions, and information technology professionals should begin to collaborate early in the process of configuring PET-CT operations. This working relationship has become an imperative as image acquisition and corresponding PET-CT report turn-around-time have become an important metric in quantifying standard-of-care. The shape and layout of the network and nodes (topology) should be considered both before and during the establishing of the PET-CT infrastructure. For large hospital systems with multiple sites and remote viewing requirements, having a scalable network with very high bandwidth and redundancies will be paramount. This becomes a complicated and expensive undertaking as network cabling, switches, servers, and all manner of information technology infrastructure will need to be considered, purchased, deployed, and maintained over the course of many years. Figure17 illustrates an example of the configuration of a typical PET-CT system topology and interconnectivity. A clear understanding of the connectivity, dependence, and relationship of both hardware and software items is vital to initial troubleshooting during system failure. Many issues such as physical disconnection between devices due to lose cabling or locating of devices requiring a reboot can be identified simply by knowing the system topology and understanding the interrelationship of system components.

http://dx.doi.org/10.5772/57119

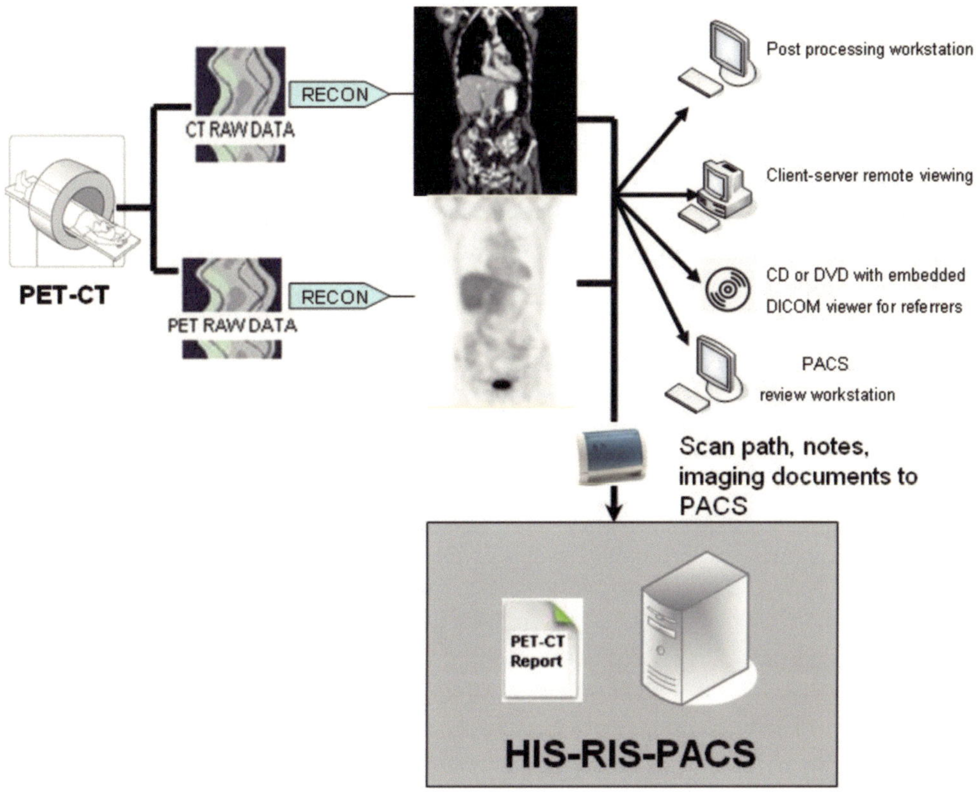


**Figure 17.** Example PET-CT system topology

# 11. PET-CT image archiving and retrieval

## 11.1. PACS workflows

A consistent, reproducible, and accessible PACS workflow should be conceived and followed by the PET-CT staff who generate the images. In particular, it will be important to consider ancillary information that the radiologist requires to read the images and the accessibility of said materials [1, 38]. The PET-CT images are certainly the centerpiece of the exam but additional information such as pathology reports, consults, and imaging reports augment the interpretation process. There are three approaches to incorporating this information into the PACS workflow effectively. The first option will be to simply printout and provide the radiologist with any ancillary clinical information that will be used to render the report. This is the least desirable method because it involves a substantial shuffling of paper and usage of printer resources. However, many institutions still use the standard paper method because of the imaging culture of the institution. The 2nd option will be to forego any printing of documents and deliver these to the radiologist in a purely "paperless" or soft format. This will require a favorable and convenient adjacency of the Health Information System/Radiology Information System (HIS/RIS) to the PACS workstation. It also requires support staff to scan in any documents that are not native to the hospital or imaging center. The third option that occurs in highly integrated healthcare environments is a merger of PACS, HIS, & RIS all within the PACS environment. This requires maximum collaboration and cooperation of Radiology and Medical Informatics as well as appropriately planned monitor and screen real estate. In a well-planned and executed fully integrated PACS/HIS/RIS, the radiologist can readily navigate and among the aforementioned applications with minimal paper waste and stream lined workflow. Figure 18 shows a fully functional PACS/HIS/RIS configuration.

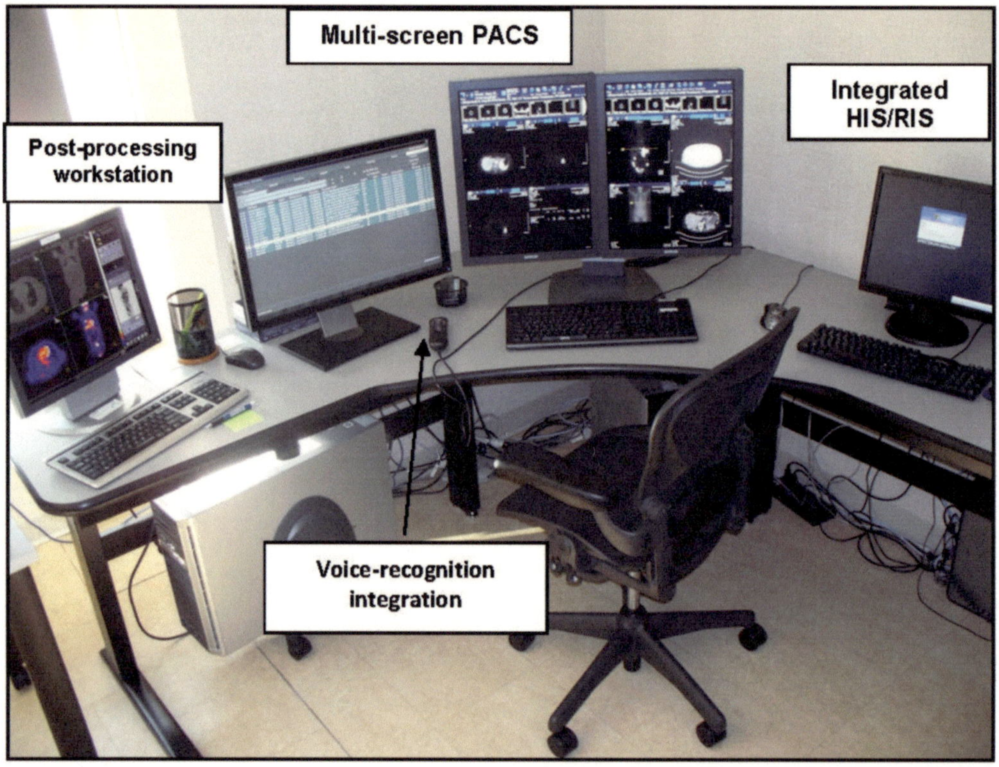


**Figure 18.** Fully-integrated PACS together with HIS & RIS. Note that full voice recognition transcription functionality has also been incorporated into the process for the most optimized report turn-around-time.

### 11.2. Non-PACS image distribution methodologies

In addition to PACS-based image viewing systems, it is inevitably necessary to view PET-CT images in other venues where PACS may not be available. Given that all data is DICOM-based, the best solution is to obtain the images on a solid-state media such as compact disk (CD) or digital video disk (DVD) and upload the data to PACS for viewing. This option also has the advantage of being executed on the user's computer regardless of bandwidth limitations.

Hospital or imaging centers with virtual private networking (VPN) capability may use file transfer protocol (FTP) as a means of securely and reliably transferring image data. With contemporary firewall systems, this often becomes a challenging undertaking fraught with information technology issues that will require an advanced user with administrative system access capabilities. Invariably, however, many institutions lack a full PACS or means of securely transmitting image data via ftp. This includes many surgical suites outside of the hospital or imaging center where the PET-CT originated, as well as community-based oncology groups, and virtually any location beyond the reach of native PACS. For such situations, the next best option for viewing images will be client-server based viewing capabilities. This will involve providing the remote user with a username and password to authenticate with the PACS server and then streaming data to the remote user's monitor. The distinct disadvantage of this method is that almost no PC-based client server monitors possess the appropriate resolution inherent to a PACS monitor that has true DICOM gray scale standard rendering [50, 51].

## 12. Internal archival methods

There are instances in which PACS does not provide a desirable location for storage. This is particularly true in instances whereby raw data sets such as PET or CT sinograms must be stored. This situation will commonly occur and be an imperative for research protocols that require the original raw data to be available in perpetuity. Sending the PET and/or CT sinograms across the network from the modality to PACS invariably results in raw data corruption resulting either in transmission failure or unusable data. Offline storage devices such as Redundant Arrays of Independent Disks (RAID) or terabyte hard drives are viable solutions in these cases. The compatibility of these options must first be vetted with the PET-CT scanner vendor to ensure long-term stability and recoverability of the raw data. These systems do have the advantage of being scalable as additional disk space can be added both to RAID and other types of offline hard drive systems [1, 38, 40].

## 13. Conclusion

From PET's primary research-oriented imaging in the 1970s and 1980s to contemporary PET-CT routinely used for oncology and neurology, PET continues to play an important role in the management of and characterization of a wide variety of disease processes. PET-CT as practiced today remains one of the most challenging and complex type of imaging studies performed in most hospital or imaging center environment. This derives largely from the integration of 2 somewhat divergent modalities along with the multifaceted diagnostic requirements of patients in oncology and neurology. An understanding of the acquisition, processing, and archiving of PET-CT data is central to sustaining a safe, patient-centered and high-quality PET-CT image product.

## Acknowledgements

The author wishes to thank Dr. Paul Shreve and the staff of the Spectrum Health Lemmen Holton PET-CT Cancer Pavilion for their insight and support in writing this chapter.

## Author details

Todd Faasse*

Address all correspondence to: todd.faasse@spectrumhealth.org

Spectrum Health, Grand Rapids, Michigan, USA

## References

[1] Faasse T. and Shreve, P., Positron Emission Tomography-Computed Tomography Patient Management and Workflow. Sem. in Ultrasound CT MR. 29(4):277-82, 2008

[2] Shreve P., Establishing a PET-CT Practice. AJR 184(5):146-151, 2005.

[3] Townsend D. Combined PET/CT: A Historical Perspective. Sem. in Ultrasound CT MR. 29(4): 232–235, 2008.

[4] Bendriem B., Townsend, D. editor-The Theory and Practice of 3D PET. Kluwer Academic Publishers, 26-38

[5] Bacharach, Stephen. PET/CT Attenuation Correction: Breathing Lessons. J. Nucl. Med. 48(5): 677-679, 2007

[6] Kinehan P. Quantitative Attenuation Correction for PET/CT Using Iterative Reconstruction of Low-Dose Dual-Energy CT. Institute of Electrical and Electronics Engineers (IEEE). http://web.eecs.umich.edu/~fessler/papers/files/proc/04/web/kinahan-04-qac.pdf (accessed 20 August 2012).

[7] Moses W. Nucl. Instrum. Methods Phys. Res. A. 648(1): 236–240, 2011 http://www.ncbi.nlm.nih.gov/pmc/articles/PMC3144741/ (accessed 29 August 2012).

[8] Moses W. Recent Advances and Future Advances in PET Time-of-Flight. Nucl. Instrum. Methods Phys. Res. A. 580(2): 919–924, 2007 http://www.ncbi.nlm.nih.gov/pmc/articles/PMC2084388/ (accessed 29 August 2012).

[9] Karp J. Benefit of Time-of-Flight in PET: Experimental and Clinical Results. J. Nucl. Med. 49(3): 462-470. http://jnm.snmjournals.org/content/49/3/462.full

[10] Melcher C. Scintillation Crystals for PET. J. Nucl. Med. 2000 Jun;41(6):1051-1055

[11] Kinehan P., Positron Emission Tomography-Computed Tomography Standardized Uptake Values in Clinical Practice and Assessing Response to Therapy. Sem. in Ultrasound CT MR. 31(6) 496-505, 2010

[12] Buchs M, Value of contrast-enhanced 18F-fluorodeoxyglucose positron emission tomography/computed tomography in detection and presurgical assessment of pancreatic cancer: A prospective study. Journal of Gastroenterology and Hepatology 26(4) 657-662, 2011 http://onlinelibrary.wiley.com/doi/10.1111/j.1440-1746.2010.06525.x/abstract (accessed on 29 August 2012)

[13] Wechalekar K., PET/CT in Oncology-a major advance. Clinical Radiology 60, 1143–1155, 2005 http://www.ectsia.org/radac/jc28020602.pdf (accessed 29 August 2012)

[14] Nehmeh SA. Correction for oral contrast artifacts in CT attenuation-corrected PET images obtained by combined PET/CT. J Nucl. Med. 44(12):1940-1944, 2003

[15] Antoch G. Focal Tracer Uptake: A Potential Artifact in Contrast-Enhanced Dual-Modality PET/CT Scans. J. Nucl. Med. 43(10):1339–1342, 2002

[16] Wiley G. Disruptive Technolology: The Conflict Over PET/CT. Imaging Economics. http://www.imagingeconomics.com/issues/articles/2005-06_02.asp (accessed 30 August 2012)

[17] Wong T., Practical Approach to Diagnostic CT Combined with PET. AJR.188(3) 622-629, 2007

[18] Wang C, Frequency, Management, and Outcome of Extravasation of Nonionic Iodinated Contrast Medium in 69 657 Intravenous Injections. Radiology, 243(1), 80-87, 2007

[19] Solomon R., The role of osmolality in the incidence of contrast-induced nephropathy: a systematic review of angiographic contrast media in high risk patients. Kidney Int. 68(5):2256-63, 2005.

[20] American College of Radiology Manual on Contrast Media: Treatment of Contrast Reactions: http://www.acr.org/Quality-Safety/Resources/Contrast-Manual (accessed 31 August 2012)

[21] Gleeson T., Contrast Induced Nephropathy. AJR 183(6) 1673-168, 2004.

[22] American College of Radiology: Practice Guideline for the Use of Intravascular Contrast Media. http://www.acr.org/~/media/ACR/Documents/PGTS/guidelines/IV_Contrast.pdf (accessed 31 August 2012)

[23] Gustav K., Integrated PET/CT: Current Applications and Future Directions. Radiology, 238(2), 405-422, 2006.

[24] Antoch G., Whole Body Positron Emission Tomography-CT-Optimized CT Using Oral And IV Contrast Materials, AJR 179(6):1555-1560, 2002.

[25] Computers in Radiology Series: PACS, RIS/HIS, DR/CR (Part 2) http://www.ceessentials.net/article10.html (accessed 31 August 2012).

[26] Deficit Reduction Act. http://www.cms.gov/Regulations-and- Guidance/Legislation/DeficitReductionAct/index.html?redirect=/deficitreductionact/ (accessed 31 August 2012).

[27] Renard S., A bigger bang: DRA sending shock waves, 'reduction without proper representation' to radiology, oncology communities. http://radiology-services.com/pdf/Bay_area_oncology_news_12-06.pdf (accessed on 31 August 2012).

[28] Timmerman R. editor. Image-Guided and Adaptive Radiation Therapy, Lippincott, Williams, and Wilkins, 2009, 4-10.

[29] Walsh B., PET/CT: Charting the Treatment Course. http://www.healthimaging.com/index.php?option=com_articles&view=article&id=6589 (accessed 31 August 2012).

[30] IMV Medical PET Benchmark report. http://www.imvinfo.com/index.aspx?sec=pet&sub=def (accessed 31 August 2012).

[31] Nadel H., Pediatric Positron Emission Tomography–Computed Tomography Protocol Considerations. Seminars in Ultrasound, CT and MRI. 29(4) 271-276, 2008

[32] Fahey FH. Dosimetry of Pediatric PET/CT. J Nucl. Med. 50(9):1483-1491. http://jnm.snmjournals.org/content/50/9/1483.full.pdf. (accessed 31 August 2012).

[33] McQuattie S. Pediatric PET/CT Imaging: Tips and Techniques. J. Nucl. Med. Technol.; 36:171–178, 2008.

[34] What are the Radiation Risks from CT? http://www.fda.gov/radiation-emittingproducts/radiationemittingproductsandprocedures/medicalimaging/medicalx-rays/ucm115329.htm, (accessed 31 August 2012).

[35] The Alliance for Radiation Safety in Pediatric Imaging-Image Gently. http://www.pedrad.org/associations/5364/ig/. (accessed 31 August 2012).

[36] Blodgett T., Best Practices: Consensus on Performing Positron Emission Tomography-Computed Tomography for Radiation Therapy Planning and for Therapy Response Assessment. Sem. in Ultrasound CT MR. 31(6):506-515, 2010

[37] Yoo D., The Role of Adaptive and Functional Imaging Modalities in Radiation Therapy: Approach and Application from a Radiation Oncology Perspective. Sem. in Ultrasound CT MR. 31(6):444-461, 2010

[38] Faasse T., Patient and Image Data Management in Positron Emission Tomography-Computed Tomography for Radiation Therapy and Therapy Response Assessment. Sem. in Ultrasound CT MR. 31(6):480-489, 2010

[39] Segall G., Therapy Response Evaluation with Positron Emission Tomography-Computed Tomography. Sem. in Ultrasound CT MR. 31(6):490-495, 2010.

[40] Shreve P., Positron Emission Tomography-Computed Tomography Protocols for Radiation Therapy Planning and Therapy Response Assessment. Sem. in Ultrasound CT MR. 31(6):468-479, 2010.

[41] Gray-Micelli D. Preventing falls in acute care. Evidence-based geriatric nursing protocols for best practice. 3rd ed. New York (NY): Springer Publishing Company; 2008. p. 161-98, 2008.

[42] Degelau J, Belz M, Bungum L, Flavin PL, Harper C, Leys K, Lundquist L, Webb B, Institute for Clinical Systems Improvement (ICSI). Prevention of falls (acute care). Health care protocol. Bloomington (MN): Institute for Clinical Systems Improvement (ICSI); 2012 Apr. 43 p.

[43] Nadzam D., Preventing Falls-Patient Safety and Quality Care. Joint Commission Resources. http://www.jcrinc.com/Preventing-Patient-Falls/ (accessed 1 September 2012).

[44] Joint Commission National Patient Safety Goals. http://www.jointcommission.org/standards_information/npsgs.aspx (accessed 1 September 2012).

[45] Shreve P., Clinical PET-CT in Oncology. New York. Springer: 2008.

[46] Murray BE., Vancomycin-resistant enterococcal infections. N. Engl. J Med. 342:710–21, 2000.

[47] Rice LB., Antimicrobial resistance in gram-positive bacteria. Am. J. Infect Control 34(5 Suppl. 1):11-9; discussion 64-73. 2000.

[48] David, M., Community-Associated Methicillin-Resistant Staphylococcus aureus: Epidemiology and Clinical Consequences of an Emerging Epidemics. Clin. Microbiol. Rev. 23(3) 616-687, 2010.

[49] Lipp MJ, The impact of hospital-acquired Clostridium difficile. J. Gastroenterol. Hepatol. 2012 Jul 31.

[50] Lowe J., Variations in Performance of LCDs Are Still Evident After DICOM Gray-Scale Standard Display Calibration. AJR 195(1): 181-187, 2010.

[51] Indrajit R., Monitor Displays in Radiology: Part 2. Indian J. Radiol. Imaging. 19(2): 94–98, 2010.

Chapter 3

# Basic PET Data Analysis Techniques

Karmen K. Yoder

Additional information is available at the end of the chapter

http://dx.doi.org/10.5772/57126

## 1. Introduction

### 1.1. Purpose of chapter

In many neuroscience-based PET research labs, procedures for data analyses are developed in-house and passed along as students, staff and post-doctoral fellows transition through training cycles. Although image processing and data analysis techniques are quite similar across many groups, there has not been any formal information available to the general scientific public. This becomes problematic from an instructional standpoint, as the increasingly cross-disciplinary nature of neuroimaging attracts researchers with vastly diverse backgrounds. It is not uncommon to find behavioral pharmacologists, bench neuroscientists, neuropsychologists, and neuroradiologists interested in using neuroimaging techniques for their research. However, often these individuals cannot pursue formal training in PET because of time constraints from other job demands. Although it is easy for seasoned PET researchers to quickly train someone in a laboratory-codified stream of image processing, the "why" of the steps may not get communicated sufficiently, which is a clear disservice to the trainees. This chapter was designed to remedy this problem. The intent of this chapter is to provide a broad foundation of the concepts behind basic PET image processing and data analyses, using data and images from several neuroligands to illustrate key points.

The reader is expected to have a basic working understanding of positron emission, gamma ray generation, and photon detection by the PET scanner.

### 1.2. Importance of study planning

First and foremost, the scientific question at hand should drive the research process. The first question to answer should be: does your institution have the capability to synthesize or obtain the ligand you need to answer your burning question about neuroscience? If the answer is yes, then the next step is in-depth consultation with the research PET experts at the institution, so

INTECH
open science | open minds

© 2013 Yoder; licensee InTech. This is a paper distributed under the terms of the Creative Commons Attribution License (http://creativecommons.org/licenses/by/3.0), which permits unrestricted use, distribution, and reproduction in any medium, provided the original work is properly cited.

that the study design and data analysis pathway(s) are clearly defined from the outset. The study design, data acquisition protocols, image processing stream, and analysis will differ from study to study, and will depend heavily on both the radioligand and the neurophysiological phenomenon of interest. Types of questions that need to be addressed include (but are not limited to) the following:

*What types of data analyses are available/accepted for the tracer?* In the clinic, non-quantitative (i.e., visual inspection) of PET images is perfectly acceptable- is the lesion still there? Getting larger? Shrinking? However, in research, there is a requirement for numerical characterization of the dependent variable. For most neuroligand tracers, extensive work has been done to determine what the best and most appropriate approaches are for generating the endpoint of interest. These can range from relatively simple, semi-quantitative methods, to conceptually complex and mathematically rigorous processes that may require additional invasive procedures (arterial cannulation), as well as computational expertise for implementation. Ultimately, the success of a neuroligand PET study will depend on understanding what the field accepts as reasonable outcome measures for a given tracer, and ensuring that the proper infrastructure exists to provide this information.

*What type of effect size is expected?* This is relevant for determining the number of subjects needed for the study – which, given the great expense of PET, is a nontrivial concern. If possible, it is helpful to know the test-retest reliability of a particular ligand, and to have a general idea of whether your effect of interest is expected to rise above this inherent background noise in the data. In the absence of this, relative variance could be ascertained from previously published data. If no previous documentation exists on the ligand in the species/population of interest, then caution should be used to not over-reach with study design in the beginning. Small pilot studies are very useful at providing initial data on anticipated effect sizes of group, treatment, and/or condition. Study design is a key component of arriving at a sample size: Are the tests to be single measurements between groups (for example, relative receptor availability between healthy normals and a disease condition), or multiple measurements within subjects? Is the tracer known for having either poor or stellar signal-to-noise ratio? All these factors- and others- will affect the ability to detect significant differences.

Group size is not the only consideration- knowledge of the expected spatial extent of the effect is also important. The newer-generation human PET scanners (and most small animal PET scanners) have excellent spatial resolution (1-2 $mm^3$), but excitement about this technological progress may be mitigated if your hypothesis is restricted to the CA3 region of the hippocampus in humans, or even the whole hippocampus in a mouse. Additionally, the spatial extent of the effect in question will affect the decision to use a region-of-interest based approach versus a voxel-wise analysis (see below).

At this point, hopefully the reader is now familiar with the importance of understanding the type of data that will result from the study, even before the study begins. Although study design is critically important, a thorough discussion of this topic is beyond the scope of this chapter. The remainder of the text will focus on defining concepts and outlining processes for preparing and analyzing neuroligand PET data. Within each subsection, the descriptions will

http://dx.doi.org/10.5772/57126

be presented in a linear fashion. However, the ultimate choices an investigator makes regarding a processing/analysis scheme will depend on multiple factors.

It is important to note that it is not the author's intent to endorse any one particular product or software platform. Examples used here are based primarily on the author's experience, and it is highly likely that many excellent programs are not mentioned. Choices of hardware and software should be made based on investigator preference and availability of individual and/ or institutional licenses.

## 2. Types of PET data – Definitions and purpose

*Dynamic acquisitions*: The term "dynamic data" refers to acquiring data in such a manner so that we may observe the long-term behavior of the tracer in tissue. Image acquisition begins immediately upon tracer injection, and the tracer's radioactivity is monitored continuously or near-continuously during the course of the scan. Dynamic data generates "time-activity curves" (TACs) of the tissue concentration of radioactivity (e.g., Bq/mL) over time. Dynamic data acquisition is the only way to obtain truly quantitative measurements of the system of interest. Said another way, "quantitative" measurements are operationally defined by pharmacokinetic and pharmacodynamic properties of a system (for example, $B_{max}$, $K_D$). The behavior of the tracer in the system (the TACs) can be described by sets of differential equations; the solutions to these equations yield quantitative outcome parameters. Common parameters of interest include terms such as "volume of distribution" and "binding potential." An excellent review of the definition and derivation of quantitative outcome variables can be found in Innis et al. (2007). In most cases, quantitative outcomes are preferable to semi-quantitative measures (see below). However, quantitative data requires information about the tracer in either arterial plasma of interest, or in a tissue that contains little or no targets of the ligand ("reference region").

Dynamic data can be acquired in two ways. One is by pre-specifying "frame times" for the acquisition, usually of increasing duration (for example, 6 frames at 10 seconds, 12 frames at 20 seconds, 5x60s, 5x120s, 4x300s, 2x600s). The scanner records all the coincidence events that occur during each specified time frame, and the reconstructed image consists of the average amount of radioactivity detected at each voxel during each time frame. The other method is "listmode acquisition", where the scanner records all the coincidence events continuously over time. After acquisition, the investigator specifies how the data should be binned into time frames during reconstruction. Listmode acquisition offers more flexibility for the investigator, especially when the ideal time frame sequence has not been identified. The capability for listmode acquisition varies across scanner platforms.

*"Static" Acquisition*: In the strictest sense, this refers to specifying one time frame over the course of scan acquisition. The result is a single frame that represents the average amount of radioactivity during the scan period. Only semi-quantitative information can be derived from static acquisitions, the most common of which is Standardized Uptake Value (SUV). SUV is the amount of radioactivity in the tissue (e.g., kBq/mL) divided by the injected dose per body-

weight (e.g., MBq/kg). Static acquisitions are often preceded by a tracer uptake period outside of the scanner environment. Some "static" protocols incorporate a "dynamic" component to facilitate motion-correction (see below), for instance, a 30-minute uptake period followed by five, five-minute frames. Even though multiple time frames are specified, because no image information is captured during the uptake period, this protocol is not considered to be truly "dynamic" data. The intensity values from the acquired frames are typically averaged to generate the mean radioactivity concentration during the scan – the functional equivalent of a "static" scan.

When deciding upon a static versus dynamic protocol, it should be kept in mind that capturing dynamic data leaves open the possibility for quantitative metrics (if the proper methods are available); static acquisition does not. Static images can always be created from dynamic data by calculating the weighted average of radioactivity over a specified set of time frames. However, static data cannot be "undone" into dynamic data.

## 3. Image processing algorithms – Qualitative description and functions

The advantage of PET imaging is that it provides unique information about the chemistry and physiology of the brain. However, even with high-resolution scanners, PET data often do not contain sufficient neuroanatomic information for identification of specific structures within the brain. The solution to this apparent conundrum is to collect an anatomic Magnetic Resonance Image (MRI) sequence (often an "T1-weighted" sequence) in the same subjects that underwent PET imaging. Having the MRI data confers many advantages to the PET image processing stream, as will be evident below. However, the PET images and MRI images, fresh off the scanner and reconstruction queues, will not be automatically matched up in image space. This is caused by many factors, but the biggest one is differences in final voxel dimensions and final image volume. One of the major objectives of post-processing of PET images is to move the PET and MRI images from the same subject into the same three-dimensional space.

A second main objective of post-processing is motion correction of the PET data. PET acquisitions typically require the subject to try and lay still for as little as 15 minutes, or for up to 90 minutes at a time. It is not uncommon for subjects to move their heads- from coughing, talking, or falling asleep (singing subjects have also been observed). In some protocols, subjects are allowed to get up for a break during the scan acquisition – which automatically means that the PET data will not be in the same exact place in the scanner. Some institutions have developed sophisticated motion-detection and correction systems that work at the level of the reconstruction; however, most investigators do not have access to this technology. Here, we describe a post-hoc method for motion correction after the image has been generated. Because the brain is encased by the skull, there is little concern about movement of the brain within its external bony boundaries. Therefore, the concept of using temporal gating to correct for organ motion, which is a major concern for cardiac and pulmonary imaging, will not be addressed here.

Finally, certain types of data analysis – specifically, voxel-wise analyses – require that all subjects brains be in the same coordinate space. We describe the process that "spatially normalizes" MRI images so that data can be sampled objectively and equivalently across subjects. The processing stream described herein has the goal of translating the PET image(s) into MRI space, so that spatial normalization parameters derived for the MRI likewise can be applied to the PET data.

A wealth of literature and scholarly work has been published on the mathematical basis for algorithms that shift, realign, warp, and reslice three-dimensional images from different modalities so they align correctly. The purpose of this section is to provide a basic, qualitative description of some of these algorithms in context of why they are useful for PET data.

Note: some image processing programs use the terms like "realign" and "co-register" to designate a very specific series of algorithm implementations. To avoid confusion, we will use these terms generically, without attaching any algorithmic meaning to either. We leave it to the reader to investigate the semantics and procedural implementations of a particular program.

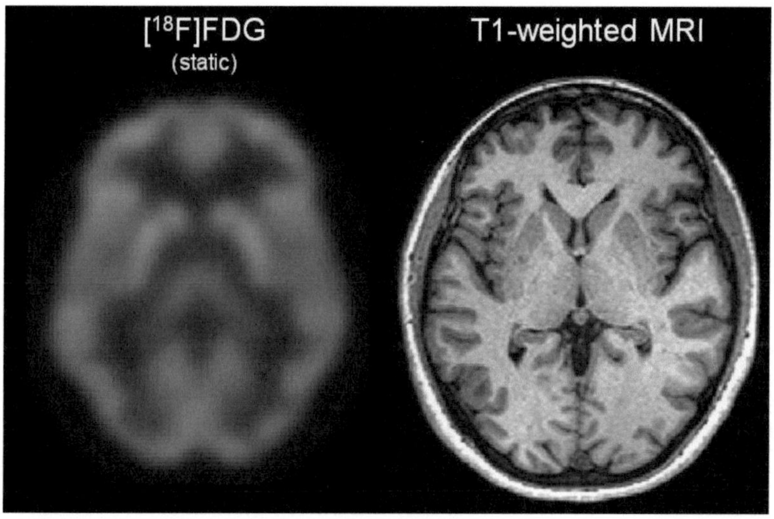


**Figure 1.** Representative examples of spatially normalized, co-registered images from a healthy subject. Images are axial slices at the level of the striatum and thalamus. Left, a "static" PET image of [$^{18}$F]flurodeoxyglucose (FDG) Right, the corresponding anatomic T1-weighted MRI. Note that the FDG image contains a high degree of anatomic information that is shared with the MRI (cohesive brain outline and subcortical structure delineation).

*Rigid body transformations.* Algorithms that perform rigid body transformations are based on the assumption that the rigid bodies (in our case, the PET and MRI image volumes of the same brain) are roughly the same size and geometry. Rigid body transforms only perform translations within object space, they do not allow for "stretching" or "shrinking". To move one object in space to match another's orientation, six parameters are required. Three translations are made along the $x$, $y$, and $z$ axes (typically considered right-left, superior-inferior, and anterior-posterior axes, respectively). Rotations are also made around the three axes; these are called pitch, roll, and yaw.

Rigid body algorithms typically "converge" (that is, come to the final, ostensibly correct answer) fairly quickly, and most co-registrations of PET and MRI are successful. However, the algorithms typically rely on the PET and MRI to share a sufficient amount of contrast and outline among anatomic structures for the alignment to work. In cases in which the PET data "looks" sufficiently similar to the structural MR (Figure 1), the registration process is straightforward, and the PET and MR can be aligned without additional steps. However, in the case of dynamic data, the tracer distribution and resulting structural information changes significantly over time. Additionally, different tracers will provide varying degrees of structural information (Figure 2). Because of the lack of similarity to the MRI, attempts to co-register individual early or late-time images will likely fail. Here, an intermediate strategy is often successful: create a PET image that shares sufficient features with *both* the MRI and *all* dynamic PET images so that the co-registration algorithm is successful. The general idea is as follows: (1) Create an average or summed image of early PET frames that will share properties with the MR (structural outlines/contrasts) and early and late-time PET data (Figure 3). At this time, performing an alignment or co-registration of the selected subset of PET frames to the first frame is helpful for eliminating spatial variance introduced by motion. The final balance of images to include will be unique to each tracer and frame sequence. Empirical testing is the best way to determine what will be an acceptable combination. For all tracers, early time images are dominated by "blood flow kinetics", or the extraction of tracer from the blood into the tissue. Thus, the early images will trace the general outline of the brain. In the case of tracers like [$^{11}$C]raclopride and [$^{18}$F]fallypride, mid-and late time images will be dominated by binding in the striatum, and the brain outline becomes diffuse (e.g., Figure 2a). Inclusion of too many of these striatal images will skew the registration process and should be avoided. For tracers that may not necessarily have a lot of tracer retention (e.g., amyloid in the example of [$^{11}$C]PiB, inflammation for [$^{11}$C]PBR28), the entire set of dynamic images may be needed to generate a sufficiently robust brain PET image. (2) Co-register the mean PET to the native-space structural MRI. Make sure the transformation parameters have been saved in the header files of the resliced PET. (3) Co-register all the dynamic PET frames to the co-registered mean PET (which is now in native MR space). Because all the frames are being registered to the same target, this step has the convenient function of also providing a robust method for motion correction. Additional refinements for motion-correction may be needed in cases in which the motion may be too severe to be corrected by a rigid-body algorithm alone. Occasionally, "manual" repositioning of a timeframe (meaning, the user specifies the translations to change the orientation) can be used to provide the registration algorithm with a better "initial guess." It is our experience that manually adjusting the position of a poorly aligned timeframe and re-running the algorithm can result in a successful motion correction. Representative time-activity curves from before and after manual manipulation of two errant time frames are given in Figure 4.

http://dx.doi.org/10.5772/57126

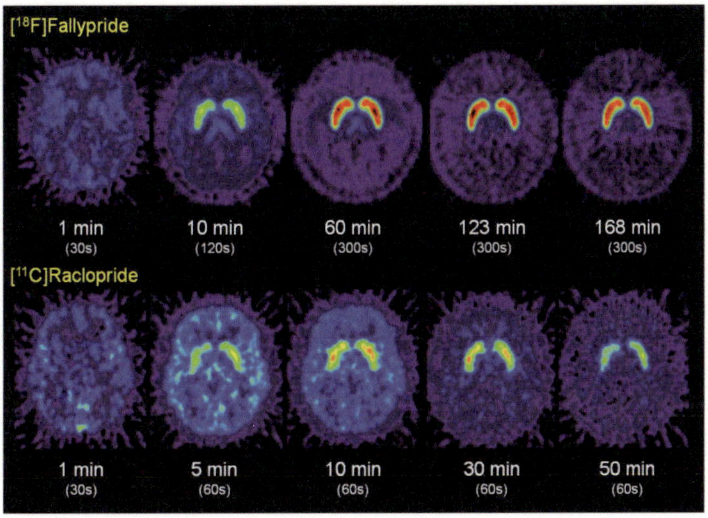


(a)

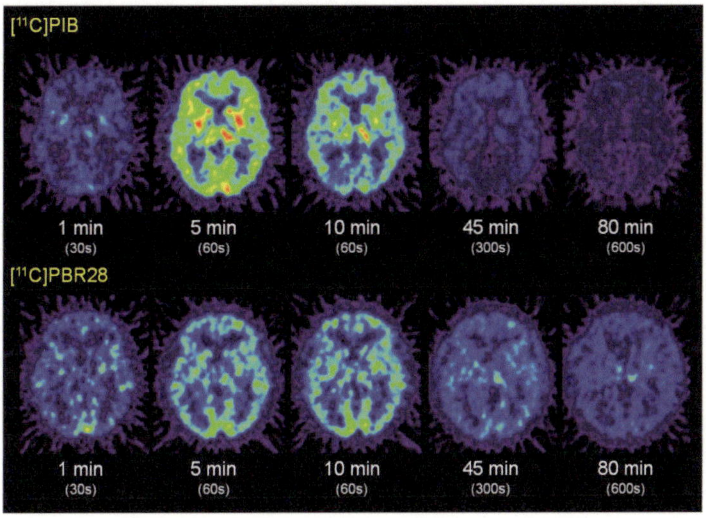


(b)

**Figure 2. (a)** Differential behavior of tracers over time. Multi-panel figure of early, mid, and late time frames from [$^{18}$F]fallypride (top panels) and [$^{11}$C]raclopride (bottom panels). Both tracers are dopamine $D_2/D_3$ antagonists; each has different kinetic and signal-to-noise properties. Underneath each panel: start time of each frame relative to tracer injection (min), and duration of each frame (s). **(b)** Differential behavior of tracers over time. Multi-panel figure of early, mid, and late time frames from [$^{11}$C]PiB in an Alzheimer's Disease subject (top panels) and [$^{11}$C]PBR28 in a healthy elderly control (bottom panels). [$^{11}$C]PiB binds to β-amyloid plaques, one of the primary pathological hallmarks of Alzheimer's Disease. The majority of healthy elderly subjects have no discernable [$^{11}$C]PiB uptake. [$^{11}$C]PBR28 binds to the Translocator Protein 18kDa, a mitochondrial marker associated with inflammation. There is some degree of consistent [$^{11}$C]PBR28 brain uptake in healthy subjects; the pathological patterns of [$^{11}$C]PBR28 in neurological and psychiatric disease are not yet well-understood. Underneath each panel: start time of each frame relative to tracer injection (min), and duration of each frame (s).

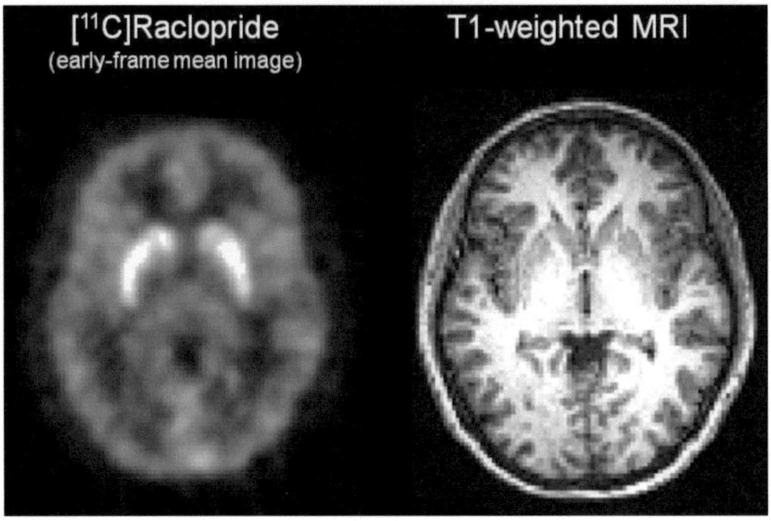


**Figure 3.** Example of how a mean dynamic image can be used to facilitate successful co-registration with an anatomic MRI. Left, spatially normalized "early" mean PET, consisting of the first ~10 minutes of dynamic [$^{11}$C]raclopride data. The number of frames required to achieve a balance of flow/binding for co-registration with the MRI depends heavily on the individual tracer kinetics, and must be determined empirically by each investigator for the particular tracer and acquisition sequence. This particular combination happens to work well for [$^{11}$C]raclopride. Note the general similarity to the FDG scan in Figure 2. Right, corresponding spatially normalized MRI from the same subject.

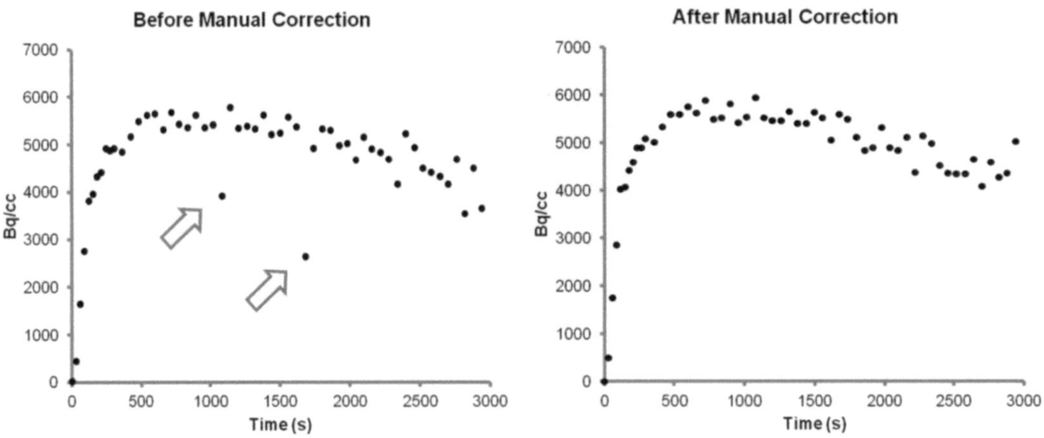


**Figure 4.** Time-activity curves (TACs) from a [$^{11}$C]raclopride scan with and without manual motion correction. Left: TAC from the right putamen of a subject after initial automated motion correction was conducted. Subject motion was severe enough that at least two frames could not be corrected by the algorithm (arrows). Right: resultant TACs after several frames were re-oriented manually and the co-registration algorithm was re-run. The improved initial guesses given by the manual manipulation resulted in better convergence for the algorithm and much smoother curves. This illustrates the need for use of TACs to check for motion in addition to the use of cine loops. It also illustrates the advantage of shorter time frames for capturing motion artifacts.

*Nonlinear transformations*. Nonlinear transforms are most commonly used to "warp" anatomic MRI brain images into a common stereotaxic coordinate space. This is necessary when a "voxel-wise" approach for data analysis is desired (see below). Typically, each individual subject brain is "warped" to a canonical template brain, typically supplied by the program that hosts the spatial transformation algorithm. However, canonical templates may not be the best representation of a given population sample, especially in patient populations that have unique structural disorders. Many investigators prefer to generate study-specific unique templates; this is definitely desirable in animal studies. Approaches to creating templates range from simple averaging of MRI (or PET) data across a sample to more sophisticated approaches that carefully map subject brains onto an existing defined coordinate system (e.g., Schweinhardt et al., 2003). It is up to the investigator to determine the optimal approach for their respective study.

If the investigator intends to rely on region-of-interest (ROI) analysis based on subject-specific ROIs from native-space MRIs, then this step may not be needed. Our laboratory uses a combined approach for ROI analysis (see below).

It should be noted that while the working assumption is that the deformations applied to subject data will render the brain totally "warped" to the template, not all individual variation in anatomy is lost. This should be taken into consideration when interpreting voxel-wise analyses (see below), or using template or group-averaged normalized MRs as starting points for ROIs.

## 4. Partial volume effects and partial volume correction

The term "partial volume effect" (PVE) and "partial volume correction" have become general terms in neuroimaging. However, it can mean very different things to MRI and PET experts. Even in PET, there can be confusion about between PVE and "spill-out/spill-in" effects. Therefore, definitions are warranted to prevent confusion.

**Spatial Resolution Effect:** This is often what is referred to as PVE. However, the term "spatial resolution effect" is more accurate. PET does not provide a spatially pristine representation of the radioactivity in the tissue – it is a "fuzzy" picture of the true concentration of radioactivity. This can be especially problematic when attempting to measure radioactivity in very small or very thin structures that are smaller than the inherent resolution of the scanner. For example, imagine a very small, very " hot" object (like a 1 mm sphere) that is surrounded by tissue that contains no radioactivity. If the intrinsic resolution of the scanner is e.g., 5 mm (please see Phelps (2006) and Bailey (2005) for details on how resolution is defined and specified), the geometry and properties of the scanner will inevitably blur the apparent concentration of radioactivity, effectively assigning spatial location of the radioactivity that originated from the object to the surrounding tissue. The amount of radioactivity measured in the object will be underestimated (from "spill-out"), and surrounding tissue will appear to have radioactivity ("spill-in"; please refer to Morris et al., 2004, for an excellent illustration and mathematical explanation of this phenomenon). Several strategies exist to correct for spatial resolution problems. They typically are both computationally and labor-intensive, and require a very detailed anatomic MRI image and robust a priori knowledge of the tracer distribution (Mawlawi et al., 2001; Morris et al., 2004). In deciding on whether or not to apply correction for spatial resolution, the key question is: How important is absolute quantitation? Does having absolute certainty of radioactivity concentration increase the ability to detect differences between groups or conditions? In many cases, it may be reasonable to assume that variability contributed by spatial resolution effects is homogenous across/within subjects, and therefore spatial resolution correction is not warranted. However, in cases where "spill-out" drastically reduces the dynamic range of signal, or interferes with the ability to detect signal above background (such as in small structures, especially in rodent PET studies), spatial resolution correction may be an important option to consider.

**Partial Volume Effect:** True PVE actually is a problem of tissue heterogeneity within a "volume." A volume could be a voxel, or a large region of interest that spans many different tissue types (e.g., a brain lesion). Even with MRI's superior spatial resolution, MRI voxels that sit on the borders between gray matter (GM), white matter (WM), and cerebrospinal fluid (CSF) may actually contain components of more than one type of signal. In MRI, this problem is addressed (in part) with probabilistic "segmentation" algorithms that assign voxels to either GM, WM, or CSF. These algorithms create tissue-specific maps, which are useful for many purposes, including creation of anatomic masks which can be used to restrict spatial extent of voxel-wise statistical analyses. Gray matter maps are also a good starting point for generation of subject-specific ROIs.

The source of concern of PVE in PET focuses mainly on quantitative analyses. Regardless of tracer, GM, WM, and CSF will have inherently different kinetics (although CSF does not have "kinetics" per se). This heterogeneity would necessitate accounting for multiple sets of tracer behaviors, complicating and potentially confounding quantitation via mathematical modeling. However, tissue heterogeneity in neuroligand PET data is typically not addressed. This is in part because scanner resolution has improved significantly, and in part because PET processing and analyses rely heavily on structural information from the MRI, which helps restrict the analyses to specific structures/tissue types.

## 5. Data analyses

So, the PET studies have been designed and data have been collected. Now what?

*Quantitative Analyses.* If dynamic data were acquired, it is possible to get quantitative information about the ligand in the brain- provided that an "input function" and software implementation of the proper tracer kinetic models are available. The two most common parameters of interest are "Volume of Distribution" ($V_T$) and "Binding Potential" (BP), both of which provide physiologically relevant data regarding tracer retention. Input functions are necessary to drive the tracer kinetic modeling procedures – they provide key information about free tracer concentration in the plasma (or parameters related to it). There are three main types of input functions: arterial plasma, reference region, and image-derived (for example, information from the carotid artery, left ventricle of the heart, or even lungs). Obtaining quantitative endpoints with tracer kinetic modeling and arterial plasma input functions is the "gold standard." The choice of either reference region and image-derived inputs must be substantiated by the literature and validated by extensive testing by kinetic modeling experts. Once time-activity curves (TACs) from both your input function and tissue of interest are at hand, the parameter estimation can begin. Explanation of the types of kinetic models, the assumptions of each, the parameters they yield, and advantages/disadvantages of each are beyond the intent of the present text. Regardless, the investigator should be aware that different model implementations may behave differently with different tracers. Consult with your local PET modeling expert to determine which methods are most appropriate and most convenient.

*Semi-quantitative.* This discussion refers to "static" images (see above). The voxel values within the PET image are in values of tissue radioactivity concentration, such as Bq/cc or kBq/mL. However, taken in isolation, these values are not meaningful and cannot be used as the final endpoint for analysis. Too many factors affect the radioactivity concentration, including the total dose injected, and the body weight of the individual. At a minimum, the data must be normalized to account for injected tracer dose.

The most common method used for data normalization is the index of "Standardized Uptake Value" (SUV), in which the radioactivity concentration is divided by injected dose per body weight (e.g., MBq/kg). This index comes with one major assumption, which is that the tracer has been distributed equally across the entire body- that is, all tissues have had an equal opportunity to be exposed to the tracer. If a "sink" for the tracer exists outside the target of interest, such that a great amount of tracer is sequestered during first pass circulation, then the tracer is not being distributed equally across the body. The whole-body distribution assumption has then been violated, and body weight is no longer the proper denominator. In this case, SUV measurements are rendered incorrect, and become unreliable as a dependent variable. Another type of normalization with SUV is "SUVR", which is the ratio of SUV from tissue that has specific binding of the tracer to tissue that does not (a reference region). This method was proposed for [$^{11}$C]PiB, and was evaluated thoroughly for this tracer against arterial and reference region kinetic approaches (Lopresti et al., 2005). If investigators are using a relatively new neuroligand and seek to use SUV or SUVR as endpoints, it is highly recommended the stability of the semi-quantitative index be assessed against either $V_T$ or BP, either with real data or via simulation studies.

*What kind of analysis do you want? Region-of-Interest versus Voxel-Wise.*

### Anatomic ROI Analyses

Broadly speaking, a region-of-interest (ROI) refers to a user-defined set of voxels (or voxel) on an image, from which PET data are extracted. First, we will address anatomically-defined ROIs.

Using anatomically-defined ROIs remains a popular approach for analyzing neuroligand PET data. Typically, anatomic ROIs are defined on a subject's MRI, and then transferred to the dynamic PET data (which is in register with the MRI). An average time-activity curve for the ROI is generated (that is, the time-activity curves of all voxels within the ROI are averaged), and the TAC is fed into a model for estimation of $V_T$ or BP.

**Pros:** The anatomic ROI approach is a good choice when the study hypothesis anticipates that the effect of group (or condition) with be consistent across the entire anatomic extent of the structure (that is, the ROI is chemically and/or functionally homogeneous). Additionally, if the ROIs are reasonably sized, the TACs are usually smooth. This results in more robust parameter estimates (noisy time-activity curves typically induce a negative bias, or lower values) (see below, and Figure 5).

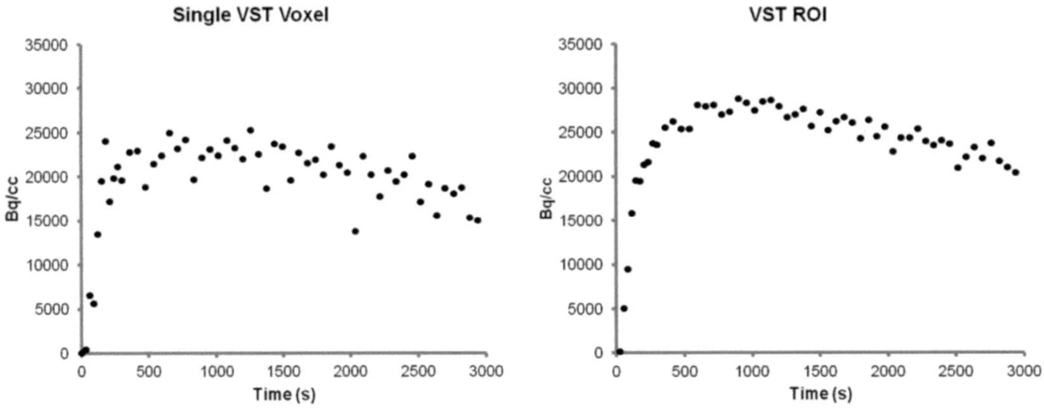


**Figure 5.** Time-activity curves (TACs) of [$^{11}$C]raclopride from, Left: a single voxel in the left ventral striatum ($BP_{ND}$ = 2.09) and Right: from the whole left ventral striatum region-of-interest (ROI) ($BP_{ND}$ = 2.74). $BP_{ND}$ values were estimated with MRTM (Ichise et al., 2003), using the same cerebellar input function. Note that the average TAC from the whole ROI is much smoother than the single voxel TAC. The slight difference in intensity scale of the single voxel could be attributed to its location in the more ventral aspect of the striatum, close to the base of the brain, which makes it more susceptible to "spillout" artifact.

**Cons:** ROI analyses may miss subtle effects that are spatially constrained to a small area within the larger ROI. If an effect is only present in a subset of voxels, then this may get lost (smoothed out) when all the TACs from all voxels are averaged together.

There are many ways to generate anatomic ROIs. Often, ROIs are painstakingly drawn by hand, which is labor- and time-intensive (and fairly boring for the individual charged with this task). This also has the risk of inducing subjective bias to the ROI definition, with the ensuing possibility data may not be completely comparable across institutions. However, adherence to strict and consistent anatomic definitions based on accepted atlas(es) (e.g., Martinez et al., 2003; Mawlawi et al., 2001) helps mitigate any investigator-induced bias. There are many software programs that offer sets of pre-defined ROIs, which are often defined from a single-subject MR. In our experience, these ROIs are not very representative and do not match well to our subject samples. We have also found that ROIs drawn by our lab on "canonical" average multi-subject T1 templates (again, available in many software packages) do not conform well to our subject samples. Yet another option is to utilize sophisticated software that automatically extract hundreds of ROIs by parcellation of a subjects' MRI. Our laboratory uses a combined approach, in which we start with an individual subjects' spatially normalized gray matter map and a template ROI (e.g., ventral striatum) generated from an average MR from our subject sample. These two sources are combined to generate a "starting point" MRI, which is then edited to explicitly conform to an individual's subject anatomy. Regardless of chosen method, the investigator should take care to ensure that the anatomic ROIs are spatially appropriate for each individual subject.

Choice of statistical analysis of ROIs depends on the study design: independent t-tests, paired t-tests, one-way ANOVA, mixed effects models, ANCOVA, correlations, etc. Regardless of the test, when multiple ROIs are being tested for between-group or between-condition effects, or for correlations with e.g., a particular subject characteristic, there is always the question of whether the results need to be corrected for multiple comparisons. This is a relevant but somewhat controversial issue. It is indeed the case that multiple comparisons can lead to false positive results (Type I error), and results that survive statistical adjustments for the multiple tests (e.g., a Bonferroni correction) can help assure the investigator that the effects are real. However, arguments have been made that in pilot studies and/or with exploratory data, such corrections are overtly stringent and unwarranted (Perneger, 1998). Investigators should be prepared to justify omission of correction for multiple comparisons based on the exploratory nature of the study and/or sample size.

**Voxel-Wise Analyses (voxels are ROIs, too)**

Technically speaking, a voxel is the smallest ROI that is possible within an image. Voxel-wise analyses assume that all subject brain data are in the same coordinate space (see above). Voxel-wise studies demand "parametric images", that is, voxels cannot be in units of radioactivity concentration, but must be converted to either a quantitative (e.g., $V_T$ or BP) or semi-quantitative (e.g., SUV) value. (In this context, "parametric" simply carries the general meaning of a uniformly normalized or an explicit physiologically descriptive value, and should not be confused with "parameter estimation" used to describe the process of kinetic modeling). In the case of quantitative values, the parameter of interest is generated based on the time-activity curve for each voxel (the input function is the same for all voxels). Taking a page from MRI processing procedures, many investigators will spatially smooth the parametric images to remove any spuriously high or low voxel values. The smoothing kernel should be roughly the size of the practical resolution of the PET scanner (not the ideal, intrinsic resolution). Statistical models are specified based on study design, and statistical testing is performed at each voxel. Most image analysis packages include the flexibility to specify different statistical thresholds, which allows investigators to interrogate the data for subthreshold effects. They also have the capacity to apply stringent corrections for a true multiple comparisons problem: performing statistical tests at tens of thousands of voxels across the brain simultaneously. Areas of significant results are shown as "clusters" (groups of contiguous voxels).

Although first-pass voxel-wise analyses does not necessarily have to correct for multiple comparisons, there may be logical reasons to spatially restrict the initial voxel-wise analyses. If the tracer is only anticipated to have specific binding in gray matter, use of an average gray matter mask (derived from the sample) would be appropriate to exclude WM and CSF voxels. [$^{11}$C]raclopride (a dopamine $D_2/D_3$ antagonist) is another good example- the signal-to-noise properties of this tracer are such that it cannot be used to quantitate $D_2/D_3$ receptor binding in areas outside the striatum (which has the highest concentration of $D_2/D_3$ in the brain). In our laboratory, we use a striatal mask to restrict the search area to the striatum. However, with tracers that can bind to processes that are not restricted to gray or white matter, whole-brain sampling would be more appropriate (unless the investigator has an a priori hypothesis that targets a specific region). An example of this would be [$^{11}$C]PBR28, which is a marker of neuroinflammatory processes. Additionally, if the investigator has specific a priori hypotheses about a structure of interest, it is reasonable to use an anatomic ROI to restrict analysis to a particular nucleus or cortical area. By now, the reader should appreciate that the distinctions between voxel-wise and ROI analyses begin to blur a bit.

**Pros:** Voxel-based analyses have two main advantages over ROI analyses. First, they sample the entire brain (or a spatially restricted region) objectively. Second, a voxel-wise approach they can pick up spatially discrete areas of effect that may be "washed away" by an ROI approach.

**Cons:** TACs at the voxel level can be extremely noisy (Figure 5). In many kinetic models, noise can cause underestimation of the quantitative parameters. However, if subjects have received approximately the same dose of tracer, then the noise at the voxel level should be uniform across subjects. Gray-matter voxels that share boundaries with CSF, air (sinuses), or white matter are especially subject to spatial resolution problems (see above); results that seem to outline "edges" of ventricles or other structures near white matter should be considered with caution. Also, even including one or two subjects with severe atrophy not corrected for by spatial normalization can skew voxel-wise results. Again, this brings to light the care an investigator must take with understanding the data (see QC section, below).

**Congratulations, you've got statistically significant results with a voxel-wise analysis. Now what?**

The output of most voxel-wise analyses is a series of parametric maps with *t*-statistic values at each voxel where there was a statistically significantly effect at a given *p*-threshold. However, the programs typically don't give you direct information about the actual effect size you are detecting. In addition to the statistical results, investigators should report the quantitative description of the data such as what the percent change was between groups/conditions, what the nature of the correlation was, etc.

Many analysis programs will allow you to save out a cluster of significant voxels as an ROI; single voxels may even be used as ROIs (this would be useful for characterizing peak effects). You may also choose to use a predefined anatomic ROI, especially when the effect of interest spans areas of interest, or the region was part of an *a priori* hypothesis. Once the ROI has been designated, there are two main methods for extracting the data. The ROIs can be applied to all subject's parametric images, and then the mean values (e.g., $V_T$, BP, SUV) for the ROI can be compiled across groups, conditions, etc. Alternatively, the ROIs can be applied directly to the dynamic data to extract the average TAC from the ROI, which is then fed into a modeling program to estimate the parameter of interest (as described above).

http://dx.doi.org/10.5772/57126

# 6. Quality control and automation

Many of the processes discussed here involve computer-based procedures. However, it is unwise to assume that the algorithms will work perfectly and that the data will always be robust. In order to assure the quality of the study, quality control by real humans is required- at every point along the processing and analysis stream. Simple visual checks can be made to determine the success of the co-registration, motion correction, and normalization steps. Here is a sample checklist:

1. MR-PET co-registration: Is the mean/summed PET in the same space as the native MR? Multiple anatomic landmarks should be assessed- from outer cortical layers to subcortical landmarks such as striatal boundaries, ventricles, and corpus callosum. Cortical landmarks may be the best visual assessment for PET studies that do not contain much subcortical binding (for example, [$^{11}$C]PiB in healthy controls)

2. MR normalization. The "warping" of the native space MR to the target coordinate space should be checked against the coordinate template. This step does not always converge appropriately, and some very strange brains can result from incorrect convergence of the spatial normalization algorithm. A helpful step to ensure successful normalization is to first perform a rigid-body co-registration between the subject native space MR and the canonical template, then perform the spatial normalization step.

3. PET normalization. To perform this QC step, create a mean or summed PET from all the spatially normalized dynamic PET frames (or spatially normalized single static frame), and compare it to both the subject's normalized MR and the template MR. If the MR normalization step was successful, then in most cases the PET normalization will be fine – but this should never be taken for granted.

4. Motion-correction. Programs that read in multiple 3D volumes in a cine loop are extremely useful for visually detecting motion. Make sure that the program can read in the numerical convention of sequential mages (i.e., decimal or hexadecimal). Investigators must learn to distinguish between true anatomic subject motion and the random noise inherent in PET images- which can create an optical illusion of motion.

5. Anatomic regions of interest. This QC should be done during the generation of the regions of interest, but is still a crucial trouble-shooting step, especially if a subject's data appears to be a high or low outlier relative to the sample. It is extremely important to check the overlay of the ROIs on the PET data. Reslicing of the PET data during the motion correction and spatial normalization can result in "chopping off" of brain regions, especially cerebellum and frontal cortex. It is very important to make sure the anatomic ROIs are not sampling image "air". This is especially important for quantitative analyses that utilize BP with a "reference regions" (see above). If the reference region is corrupted by white matter, CSF, or "air", then the BP estimate of the target region (or voxel) will be corrupted.

6. Time-activity curves. Even if the investigator intends to only run a voxel-wise analysis, it is always a good idea to visually check the TACs from at least one, if not several, anatomic

regions of interest. This may help identify motion that needs to be corrected, or may shed light on other data quality problems that should be addressed.

7. Parametric images. Regardless of outcome variable (e.g., SUV $V_T$, BP), the parametric images should be examined to make sure the values are reasonable. If outlying values are observed, then more intensive investigation is warranted to identify the source of the (apparently) aberrant data.

Executing all the image processing steps individually can be time-consuming and labor-intensive. With many programs, it is possible to automate, or "batch", many steps together through the use of scripts. In fact, automation is often implemented at the level of multiple subjects at once. The degree of automation implemented must be up to the discretion of the laboratory and what works best with the current laboratory culture, which encompasses both available manpower and study completion rate. Some labs may run hundreds of subjects, then perform QC steps for each step in batches for each QC point. Other labs may choose to implement QC for each individual subject as those data come through. Workload distribution of QC is ultimately up to each investigator, based on their needs.

## 7. Small animal PET considerations (especially rodent)

In general, the same principles described above regarding types of data (semi-quantitative, quantitative) and analyses (ROI, voxel-wise) apply to PET imaging in small animals. Having said that, some special concerns need to be addressed (or alleviated). In most studies, animals will be anesthetized during imaging. If the animal is restrained by a device that prohibits head motion (e.g., for neuroimaging, a stereotaxic head-holder), then motion correction for the dynamic PET data may not be needed. (Again, gating acquisition methods for thoracic and abdominal imaging are beyond the scope of this discussion). If the animal's skull is not explicitly restrained, then head motion may occur from breathing, and motion-correction algorithms may be warranted.

If one acquires parallel data in other modalities for the purposes of co-registration, the nature of the PET data must be considered within the context of aligning one modality to another. Tracer kinetics in rodents can be vastly different than what is observed in humans. Some tracers may have very little apparent brain uptake, and therefore the outline of the brain may not be obvious. If there is little information about brain shape in the PET data, a co-registration algorithm may not work accurately, or may even crash. If alternate modality images are acquired and needed for co-registration (e.g., CT for attenuation correction; MR for anatomic localization of anatomic structures), then image editing may be required for successful co-registration between the PET data and MRI and/or CT. For example, if the lack of a coherent brain outline in the PET image data is problematic, it may be useful to edit out the skull in CT or MR images. On the other hand, in rodents, tracers with high uptake areas (e.g., dopaminergic ligands in the striatum) may not register well to a rodent MR, which will not have clear delineation between subcortical nuclei in rodents. In this case, an early-time PET image may be useful for registration. Finally, if the animal is restrained with a headholder, the extra image information from the headholder material may need to be edited out to render a more purely anatomic image and facilitate co-registration with the PET (which will not show the presence of the holder). Again, there is no "set" approach, and it is up to the investigator to empirically determine what is most appropriate for their particular imaging system.

Regardless if an ROI or voxel-wise approach is used for small animal PET data analysis, it is important that the investigator appreciate the practical resolution limitations of the imaging modality. Even with the most advanced small animal PET scanners, it is difficult to resolve structures below a ~1mm$^3$ volume. This is true even if high-resolution anatomic MR data are available. Two key concepts are worth emphasizing:

1. The presence of micron resolution in an MR image co-registered to a PET image does not guarantee micron resolution in the PET dataset (see above section for discussion on partial voluming artifacts).

2. The voxel size in a PET image does not necessarily correspond to the practical resolution of the scanner. Images can be resliced almost infinitely to very small voxels by relatively simple interpolation of the original PET data. However, this does not change the actual resolution of the scanner. If the final PET voxel size is one 0.25mm x 0.25mm x 0.25mm, and the practical scanner resolution is 1mm x 1mm x 1mm, then the resolution is still 1mm x 1mm x 1mm. Information is not gained by voxel sizes that are smaller than the intrinsic scanner resolution. Check with your local PET expert to determine what the resolution of the small animal scanner is.

Voxel-wise studies in small animal PET data require careful consideration with respect to how spatial normalization will be achieved, especially with rodent data. Brain structure between rodent strains is likely to be quite different; it should not be assumed that one-rat (or mouse) brain-fits-all. Additional factors like gender, age, and weight of the animal also influence brain shape and structure. Of particular note is that brain development and growth in rodents is nonlinear across structures (Sullivan et al., 2006), and therefore a younger brain should not simply be scaled up to the size of an older rodent brain. Three-dimensional templates and atlases of mice and rat brains are becoming more common. However, when possible, the investigator should consider generating an in-house brain template specific to the strain, age, gender, and weight of the sample being studied.

## 8. Summary

Image processing and data analysis of neuroligand PET data requires multiple steps. There are an almost infinite number of possible iterations and refinements to data processing streams. Hopefully, this chapter has provided a useful overview of the key concepts investigators need to consider when working with these expensive and often complex datasets. Regardless of the exact sequence of processing procedures selected, a thorough working knowledge of the rationale behind each step will help ensure the fidelity and quality of the laboratory's datasets.

## Acknowledgements

The author would like to thank Daniel Albrecht and Dr. Shannon Risacher for processing the PET data presented in this report, and for providing data for the figures.

## Author details

Karmen K. Yoder

Indiana University School of Medicine, Department of Radiology and Imaging Sciences, Indiana Institute for Biomedical Imaging Sciences, Center for Neuroimaging, Indianapolis, Indiana, USA

## References

[1] Bailey DL. 2005. Data acquisition and performance characterization in PET. In: Bailey DL, Townsend DW, Valk PE, Maisey MN, editors. Positron emission tomography: Basic sciences. London: Springer-Verlag. p. 41-62.

[2] Ichise M, Liow JS, Lu JQ, Takano A, Model K, Toyama H, Suhara T, Suzuki K, Innis RB, Carson RE. 2003. Linearized reference tissue parametric imaging methods: application to [11C]DASB positron emission tomography studies of the serotonin transporter in human brain. J Cereb Blood Flow Metab 23(9):1096-1112.

[3] Innis RB, Cunningham VJ, Delforge J, Fujita M, Gjedde A, Gunn RN, Holden J, Houle S, Huang SC, Ichise M, Iida H, Ito H, Kimura Y, Koeppe RA, Knudsen GM, Knuuti J, Lammertsma AA, Laruelle M, Logan J, Maguire RP, Mintun MA, Morris ED, Parsey R, Price JC, Slifstein M, Sossi V, Suhara T, Votaw JR, Wong DF, Carson RE. 2007. Consensus nomenclature for in vivo imaging of reversibly binding radioligands. J Cereb Blood Flow Metab 27(9):1533-1539.

[4] Lopresti BJ, Klunk WE, Mathis CA, Hoge JA, Ziolko SK, Lu X, Meltzer CC, Schimmel K, Tsopelas ND, DeKosky ST, Price JC. 2005. Simplified quantification of Pittsburgh Compound B amyloid imaging PET studies: a comparative analysis. J Nucl Med 46(12):1959-1972.

[5] Martinez D, Slifstein M, Broft A, Mawlawi O, Hwang DR, Huang Y, Cooper T, Kegeles L, Zarahn E, Abi-Dargham A, Haber SN, Laruelle M. 2003. Imaging human mesolimbic dopamine transmission with positron emission tomography. Part II: amphetamine-induced dopamine release in the functional subdivisions of the striatum. J Cereb Blood Flow Metab 23(3):285-300.

[6] Mawlawi O, Martinez D, Slifstein M, Broft A, Chatterjee R, Hwang DR, Huang Y, Simpson N, Ngo K, Van Heertum R, Laruelle M. 2001. Imaging human mesolimbic dopamine transmission with positron emission tomography: I. Accuracy and precision of D(2) receptor parameter measurements in ventral striatum. J Cereb Blood Flow Metab 21(9):1034-1057.

[7] Morris ED, Endres CJ, Schmidt KC, Christian BT, Muzik Jr. RF, Fisher RE. 2004. Kinetic modeling in positron emission tomography. In: Wernick MN, Aarsvold JN, editors. Emission tomography: the fundamentals of PET and SPECT: Elsevier. p. 499-540.

[8] Perneger TV. 1998. What's wrong with Bonferroni adjustments. BMJ 316(7139): 1236-1238.

[9] Phelps ME, editor. 2006. PET: Physics, instrumentation, and scanners. New York: Springer.

[10] Schweinhardt P, Fransson P, Olson L, Spenger C, Andersson JL. 2003. A template for spatial normalisation of MR images of the rat brain. J Neurosci Methods 129(2): 105-113.

[11] Sullivan EV, Adalsteinsson E, Sood R, Mayer D, Bell R, McBride W, Li TK, Pfefferbaum A. 2006. Longitudinal brain magnetic resonance imaging study of the alcohol-preferring rat. Part I: adult brain growth. Alcohol Clin Exp Res 30(7):1234-1247.

Section 2

# PET Applications in Neurological and Behavioral Research

Chapter 4

# Functional Imaging Studies of Human Cognition Using Positron Emission Tomography

Sandro Misciagna

Additional information is available at the end of the chapter

http://dx.doi.org/10.5772/57124

## 1. Introduction

In past times behavioural neurologists have shown how discrete brain lesions provoked different types of cognitive disorders such as language, praxic, gnostic, spatial or memory domain.

They interpreted these anatomo-clinical associations conjecturing that the normal brain function (impaired by brain damage) was localized within the lesioned region (lesional hypothesis) and had been impaired from brain damage (Marshall & Fink, 2003). They also hypothesized that cognitive impairments could arise from lesions that spared the functional centers but disconnected them from other centers (disconnectional hypothesis). According this argument "basic psychological functions" are localized in a punctate fashion and complex psychological functions are constituted from many such basic functions joined together in distributed circuits. It follows that the symptoms may have arisen from a reconfiguration of the entire circuit in response to cerebral damage.

During the late 19th century, the advent of structural brain imaging, first the computed tomography (CT) and later the magnetic resonance imaging (MRI), gave the possibility to study anatomical localization of the cognitive deficits that were manifest after brain injury. Since then neuroimaging studies have helped medical doctors in clinical practice to identify cerebral damage caused by spaced-occupying lesions, strokes or degenerative processes.

During the 20th century other instrumental techniques such as single photon computed tomography (SPECT), positron emission tomography (PET), functional magnetic resonance imaging (f-MRI) or magnetoencephalography (MEG) started to be used for evaluation of cognitive activation not only in patients with cerebral lesions, but also in living normal brains and localize mental faculties in different regions of the brain. Further, functional techniques

INTECH
open science | open minds

© 2013 Misciagna; licensee InTech. This is a paper distributed under the terms of the Creative Commons Attribution License (http://creativecommons.org/licenses/by/3.0), which permits unrestricted use, distribution, and reproduction in any medium, provided the original work is properly cited.

and both can be thought as originating from imaging and functional technologies: neuroelectrical (MEG and electroencephalography), and hemodynamic (PET, SPECT, fMRI, optical).

These advances in medical technology have led to study structural brain imaging early in patients, explore relationship between structure and function or hypothesize brain cognitive functioning also in normal subjects.

For example Positron Emission Tomography has been used in healthy volunteers to study brain activation during specific goal-directed behaviours (Raichle et al., 2001) such as arithmetical computation (Dehaene et al., 1996), memory tasks, visuoconstructive abilities or specific language tasks.

Since then various neuroimaging technologies have also been applied to identify and measure a range of biological processes that occur along neurological disease associated with cognitive impairment as in neurodegenerative conditions.

In this chapter we will review some applications of PET in understanding the cognitive functions in normal subjects, in patients with cognitive deficits during normal aging or following vascular or degenerative damage.

We will also discuss how PET scanning of glucose metabolism, could be used to differentiate Alzheimer's disease from other forms of dementia such as Vascular dementia, Lewy boby dementia or Frontotemporal dementia, which helps to guide clinicians in symptomatic treatment strategies.

We will also expose how PET exam could be useful to identify potential risk of developing dementia in persons with mild cognitive impairment (MCI) resulting useful in predicting further cognitive decline.

## 2. Pet study of human cognitive functions

The human brain is an extremely complex organ. The energy required for this complex structure is almost exclusively covered by oxidative metabolism of glucose (Clarke and Sokoloff, 1999). Since PET is a technology based on study of glucose metabolism has great impact on research in study of human cerebral activity.

PET has been adopted in normal subject to study cognitive functions in a particular case of functional connectivity that is the so-called default mode or "**resting state connectivity**", successively extended with fMRI studies. It quantified the spatial correlation of brain activity in the absence of a specific cognitive task. Typically, this is performed by having the subject fixate a visual cue in the absence of a cognitive task (Raichle and Mintun, 2006). The baseline activity of the resting state has spatial correlations that involve the same prefrontal, medial temporal lobe and parietal lobe systems involved in some memory tasks. It could be hypothesized that memory system, especially the declarative memory system, might be activated in the resting state (Vincent et al., 2006).

http://dx.doi.org/10.5772/57124

"**Functional effective connectivity**" consists in the measure of correlation of connectivity among brain regions or better the influence of brain nodes on each other. PET studies have been applied to quantify causal interactions between brain regions (McIntosh et al., 1994; Horwitz et al., 2005). This measure estimates the strength of connectivity between cerebral areas and statistically infers a causal effect of connectivity. For example a PET study of human working memory for faces has suggested that the network for underlying activity changes as the task requirements change (McIntosh et al., 1996). Models of connectivity have been explored with PET in the study dynamic neural networks underlying **language processing** using specific tasks such as word generation (Warburton et al., 1996) or reading (Price and Friston, 1997). PET studies have also been applied to demonstrate **hemispheric dominance of language**. The laterality of language is usually achieved by activating language areas and comparing the relative strength of activation between the right and the left hemispheres (Stippich et al., 2003; Lohmann et al., 2004). Studies on multiple groups have reported a strong correlation with PET or fMRI compared with intraoperative mapping techniques and the results of classical Wada test (Roux et al., 2003; Woermann et al., 2003; Atlas et al., 1996).

PET or task-activated fMRI can locate, with a high spatial resolution, both receptive and productive language areas. One practical application of PET for language localization consists in the presurgical evaluation of epileptic or brain tumor patients. This PET neurosurgical application makes possible a precise **localization of essential language** areas in individual patient rather then participating areas. Essential language areas are ones that when removed result in a language deficit; while participating areas are ones that are activated during language paradigms, but do not result in a post-operative language deficit after surgical resection, because these are areas of redundant processing or because other areas learn to take over the same function. Currently, there is no way to distinguish essential from participating areas with non-invasive imaging and improving the detection of essential areas is a major goal of clinical functional imaging. Language areas found to be lateralized in left hemisphere with a variety of language tasks are essentials four: prefrontal cortex (inferior frontal gyrus, superior frontal gyrus and the anterior cingulate), angular gyrus (excluding the supramarginal gyrus), ventrolateral temporal lobe (superior temporal, middle temporal, inferior temporal and fusiform gyri) and retrosplenial cortex. This means that studies on patients with lesion of anterior lateral prefrontal cortex (known as Broca's area) overemphasize the role of these cerebral areas in onset of language disorder (Broca's aphasia) as confirmed by patients with isolated lesions of "Broca's areas" having only apraxis deficits of articulation rather then aphasia. On the other hands a real and permanent Broca's aphasia requires more extensive cerebral lesions involving anterior frontal gyrus, middle frontal gyrus and peri-central gyri. These functional studies suggest that a wide area of left frontal lobe participate in language processing outside the classical confines of Broca's area, as confirmed by clinical cases of people with large frontal stroke and receptive aphasia which later may evolve into a so-called expressive aphasia. Task activated fMRI provide evidence of cortical reorganization of language areas, do to tumoral lesions or after a surgical resection.

PET, fMRI, MEG and EEG have been used in numerous studies to **investigate the cerebral sites of declarative memory** (for a review see Gazzaniga, 2004) that consists in explicit memory for facts and events. Declarative memory has often been studied using the so-called "subsequent memory effect" that is brain activity during encoding of items that are subsequently forgotten. On the other way the retrieval of declarative memory has been studied with the "old/new effect" that consists is the comparison of brain activity recorded during correctly recognized old items versus correctly identified new items. Memory for events involves processing in the medial temporal lobes (Milner et al., 1998) and in the prefrontal cortex. Frontal lobe activity is related to both encoding and retrieval of memory events for both long-term and short-term memory.

Functional memory localization has been applied in presurgical evaluation of epileptic (Detre, 2004) or brain tumor patients and predicts post-surgical memory deficits following temporal lobectomy (Rabin et al., 2004).

Episodic (conscious memory of events) and semantic memory (memory concerned with ideas, meanings, and concepts which are not related to personal experiences) might recruit different brain areas (Tulving and Markowitsch, 1998). In fact, amnesic patients with specific episodic memory impairment (intact priming, category learning, learning of artificial grammars) have temporal lobe damage, while patients with semantic deficits show dysfunction in prefrontal cortex. In particular left prefrontal cortex increases activity during semantic encoding while right prefrontal cortex increases activity during retrieval task. Recent neuroimaging studies implicate also the parietal lobe in episodic memory (Wagner et al., 2005).

Functional studies on **working memory** (memory that makes possible the temporary retention of information) suggest an overlapping of brain mechanism with attention (Jha, 2002) and associative learning in prefrontal cortex (Fuster et al., 2000). This association has also been demonstrated on behavioural studies (Sheth and Shimojo, 2003). Many of the changes in cerebral activation studied with PET during working memory tests are task specific. PET studies executed during Wisconsin Card sorting Test, which depends heavily on working memory, has demonstrated reduction of activation with age in the dorsolateral prefrontal cortex. On the other hand PET executed during Raven's Progressive Matrices, which also has a working memory component, but depends more on visuospatial processing, has demonstrated reduction of activation with age in in portions of the inferolateral temporal cortex more involved in visuo-spatial processing (Esposito ed al., 1999).

Recent PET studies of brain activation during tasks of **visuospatial processing** have reported that age-related cognitive changes are accompanied by altered cerebral activation in temporo-occipital and extrastriate regions (Grady et al., 1994). Increased prefrontal activation was found both during face and location processing (Grady et al., 1994) and during memory recall (Cabeza et al., 1997a), while reduced prefrontal activation was reported during memory encoding (Grady et al., 1995; Cabeza et al., 1997b).

Temporal resolution of hemodynamic techniques such as PET or fMRI can be improved combining the activation maps from these imaging modalities with high-temporal resolution information obtained by other sources such as EEG/MEG or information on tissue oxygenation obtained from diffusion optical tomography. Recent methods of statistical combination of

http://dx.doi.org/10.5772/57124

these techniques may provide benefits especially to neurosurgeon (Fischl et al., 2001; Dale et al., 2000).

## 3. Pet study of cognitive functions in cerebrovascular disease

Cerebrovascular disease affects prominently elderly persons through alterations in brain structure and metabolism that produce cognitive decline. Cognitive deficit revealed in cerebrovascular disease regards especially the domains of executive functions (Starkstein et al., 1996), attention, language (Powell et al., 1998) and less prominent memory deficits (Villardita, 1993; Tierney et al., 2001). Vascular cognitive disorders may be caused by multiple neuropathological substrates, including multi-infarct encephalopathy, single infarcts in strategic areas, lacunas and lacunar states, Biswanger's leukoencephalopathy and leukoarariosis, hippocampal sclerosis, watershed infarcts and neuronal loss/atrophy due to diffuse hypoperfusion (Ferrer, 2010). These substrates can be a consequence of different vascular diseases including atherosclerosis, small vessel disease, hypertensive angiopathy, inflammatory disease of blood vessels, inherited vascular disorders such as amyloid angiopathy and CADASIL (central autonomic dominant arteriopathy with subcortical infarcts and leukoencephalopathy) or the consequence of single or multiple cerebral hemorrhages.

Despite the considerable degree of accuracy in diagnosing Alzheimer's disease (AD), the clinical differentiation with Vascular cognitive impairment (cognitive impairment in absence of dementia) and mixed dementia (Alzheimer's disease plus cerebrovascular disease) remains a matter of controversial opinions and one of the most challenging diagnostic issues (Misciagna et al., 2005). Dementia in older adults is frequently caused by the combined conditions of Alzheimer disease and cerebrovascular disease (mixed disease) since frequently occur together in overlap presentations (such as vascular lesions in Alzheimer Disease or cerebral atrophic condition in Cerebrovascular Disease). Nevertheless, there is evidence that they contribute separately to the development of cognitive impairment and dementia (Snowdon et al., 1997; Bennett, 2001).

The differential diagnosis between Alzheimer disease and dementia in cerebrovascular disease known as Vascular Dementia (VaD) is based on presence of vascular risk factors (such as hypertension, atrial fibrillation, obstructive arteriopathy, previous strokes or transitory ischemic attacks), clinical features (such as acute onset, stepwise progression, emotional lability) (Hachinski et al., 1974) and is supported by results of neuropsychological tests and neuroimaging. Whereas computed tomography or magnetic resonance are able to detect morphological lesions related to vascular disease, these modalities cannot determine functional impairment. PET allows imaging of the localized and/or diffuse metabolic disturbances responsible for cognitive impairment and dementia and is effective in differentiating vascular from degenerative dementia (Heiss and Zimmermann-Meinzingen, 2012). In particular PET can differentiate areas of focal cortical and subcortical hypometabolism that differ from the typical metabolic pattern seen in AD characterized by marked hypometabolism in association areas (Benson et al., 1983). In patients with severe Vascular Dementia, PET reveals a significative reduction of metabolism in widespread cerebral regions as middle frontal cortex, temporoparietal cortex, basal ganglia, cerebellum and brainstem (Mielke et al., 1992). Hypometabolism is more marked than AD in subcortical areas and primary sensorimotor cortex, while it is less affected in the association areas.

The metabolic ratio, which reflects the pattern of metabolic pathology in AD, is generally higher in VaD than in AD. Both in VaD and AD there is a parallel decline of the metabolic ratio with increasing dementia severity suggesting equal ability to discriminate VaD and AD in early and advanced stages of the disease. The volume of functional loss detected with PET is also important since it includes the effects of incompletely infarcted tissue and morphologically intact but deafferented cortex. Diagnostic accuracy for classification of patients in VaD versus AD is clearly superior for FDG PET even in patients with mild cognitive impairment (Mielke et al., 1994).

In a study on 153 subjects PET differentiated VaD from AD demonstrating lower metabolism in deep gray nucley, cerebellum, primary cortices, middle temporal gyrus and anterior cingulate cortex in VaD, whereas in AD showed lower metabolism in hippocampal region, orbitofrontal, posterior cingulate and posterior parietal cortices (Kerrouche et al., 2006).

PET can also detect vascular inflammatory changes (Mehta et al., 2012) and their interaction with amyloid depositions for development of mixed dementias after stroke (Heiss & Zimmermann-Meinzingen, 2012). Microglia activation that occurs in patients with mild cognitive deficits is not proven to be correlated with amyloid deposition as imaged by 11C-PIB (Okello et al., 2009). However, in animal models, the inflammation due to an infarct is exacerbated in the presence of amyloid; compared to animals without amyloid deposition the infarcts induced in presence of amyloid grew over time (Whitehead et al., 2007). The interaction of inflammatory reaction and amyloid deposition can be relevant for development of dementia in cerebrovascular disease as studied by multitracer PET with PK 11195 and PIB (Mok et al., 2010).

Episodic memory decline and hippocampal cerebral volume (typically associated with Alzhemier disease) are related to temporo-parietal hypometabolism (Desgranges, Chételat and Eustache, 2004) while executive dysfunction and white matters hyperintensities (typical of cerebrovascular disease) correlate with frontal lobe hypometabolism (Tullberg et al 2004). On the bases of this hypothesis a fluorodeoxyglucose-PET longitudinal study on 38 subjects ranging from normal condition to dementia in a follow up of 2 years have demonstrated a different pattern of metabolic decline in condition of dementia in Alzheimer disease or in cerebrovascular disease. In fact low baseline hippocampal volume can predict development of medial temporal hypometabolism; on the other hand white matter hyperintensities can predict hypometabolism over time in the fronto-parietal regions (Kuczynski et al., 2008). These studies suggest that pattern of cognitive decline studied with neuropsychological test batteries, anatomic changes and study of cerebral metabolism are useful in defining etiology of dementia in cerebrovascular disease and understand future evolution of cognitive deficits.

http://dx.doi.org/10.5772/57124

# 4. Pet study of cognitive functions in normal ageing, mild cognitive impairment and degenerative dementias

With normal aging neocortical neurons are lost in specific regions (Morrison, 1997), dendridic trees undergo progressive regression and axons degenerate leading to an age-related axonal loss. This process leads to a decrease of myelinated nerve fibers of 45% from the age of 20 to 80 years (Marner et al., 2003) and a reduction of the number of synapses by 15 to 50% (Pannese, 2011). The cerebral morphological changes that occur during normal ageing develop cognitive changes in particular about memory that could be considered age-related and a physiological process. These cognitive changes are related to physiological age-related brain atrophy with concomitant ventricular enlargement (Rusinek et al., 2003) and to a diffuse and frontally accentuated degrease of glucose metabolism as revealed with PET (Pawlik et al., 1989). The condition of "age associated memory impairment" is characterized by self perception of memory loss and standardised memory test score that shows low performances in memory tasks compared with younger adults. By contrast, "mild cognitive impairment" (MCI) is considered a transitional state between normal ageing and dementia (Petersen, 2004). Subjects with MCI are indipendent in activity daily living even if suffer with cognitive deficits in particular in the area of memory (in the amnestic form of MCI) typically in delayed recall, althought non-memory cognitive domains might also be impaired (in non-amnestic form of MCI). Patients with the amnestic subtype of MCI frequently progress to Alzheimer disease (AD) (Petersen et al., 2006) so that MCI is associated with an increased risk of developing dementia. When cognitive impairment concerns not only memory, but also other cognitive domains (such as abstract reasoning, judgment capabilities, language, praxic, gnostic or spatial function) dementia is often diagnosed (American Psychiatric Association, 2000). Alzheimer Disease is the most common cause of progressive form dementia in which cognitive decline interferes significantly with activities of daily living. Other causes of common degenerative dementia include dementia with Lewy bodies (characterized by fluctuating consciousness, parkinsonian symptoms and progressive decline in visuospatial, visuoperceptual, literacy and praxic skills, including visual allucinations) and Frontotemporal dementia (characterized by executive dysfunction, changes in personality and behaviour, semantic deficits and progressive aphasia). Secondary forms of dementia include depression (pseudo-depressive dementia), drug toxic effects or other medical conditions.

Many of brain changes that occur in neurodegenerative disease can be evidenced by neuroimaging technologies designed to identify alterations of cerebral biological processes. The main brain change consists in focal or diffuse cerebral atrophy induced from neuronal synaptic degeneration and loss of neurons. Some forms of dementia have a particular pattern of athophy (Josephs et al., 2007). For example, widespread atrophy or medial temporal atrophy points toward a pathologic diagnosis of Alzheimer Disease, fronto-temporal loss suggest a diagnosis of Frontotemporal Dementia (Neary et al., 2005), more focal atrophy predominantly involving the premotor and supplemental motor area suggests Corticobasal Degeneration (CBD) or Progressive Supranuclear Palsy (PSP) (Whitwell et al., 2010); on the contrary Lewy bodies disease is characterised by posterior cortical atrophy (Crutch et al., 2012). Other cerebral anomalies observed in auptoptical studies conducted in middle-aged adults (Price & Morris, 1999), patients with MCI (Petersen et al., 2006) or Alzheimer Disease (Braak & Braak, 1991) consist in presence of plaques of amyloid ß and neurofibrillary tangles of tau protein.

Neurofibrillary tangles have been observed in the hippocampus and temporal regions in MCI, in neocortical areas (frontal and parietal cortex) as MCI progress to AD. Patients with autoptical diagnosis of Alzheimer disease have a hight number of both amyloid plaques and neurofibrillary tangles (McKhann et al., 1984).

Cerebrospinal fluids (CSF) studies conducted on patients with AD (Sidoryk-Wegrzynowicz et al., 2011) or post-mortem (Reinikainen et al., 1990) have documented alterations in cholinergic, serotonergic, dopaminergic, somatostatinergic, noradrenergic and glutamatergic neurotransmitters. These and other pathogenetic mechanism as insulin resistance (Craft, 2006) contribute to compromise cerebral regional glucose metabolism studied in PET techniques.

Studies conducted on patients with AD often use the radiolabelled glucose analogue FDG (**[18]FDG-PET**) to measure cerebral glucose metabolism, which indicates the levels of neurosynaptic activity. PET studies have demonstrated that Alzheimer's disease is characterized by regional impairment of cerebral glucose metabolism in neocortical association areas (posterior cingulate, temporoparietal and frontal multimodal association cortex), whereas the primary visual and sensorimotor cortex, basal ganglia, and cerebellum are relatively well preserved (for a review see Herholz, 2003).

An automated voxel-based analysis of FDG-PET images can distinct AD from controls with 93% sensitivity and 93% specificity as dimonstrated in a multicentre study comprising 10 PET centers (Herholz et al., 2002).

These studies have shown that cortical brain alterations begin in the posterior cingulate regions and spread to the temporal and prefrontal cortices. This pattern of brain metabolism is useful to differentiate patients with AD from other forms of dementia and from cognetively health people (Silverman et al., 2001).

Regional cortical hypometabolism also correlates with greater cognitive losses so that [18]FDG-PET can differentiate patients with MCI from others with AD or normal subjects (Small et al., 2006).

When [18]FDG-PET is added to standard clinical assessment, diagnostic accuracy for dementia of Alzheimer type increases sensitivity and specificity (Jagust et al., 2007). [18]FDG-PET is important in helping differential diagnosis between AD and Frontotemporal Dementia since the latter dementia do not seem to respond well to currently available symptomatic treatments.

Longitudinal studies of patients with MCI have found that if baseline assessment with [18]FDG-PET scan suggests an AD-like pattern, the probability of conversion in AD within several years is extremely hight (Drzezga et al., 2005; Chételat et al., 2003). Therefore in these MCI patients pharmacological treatment with specific anti-dementia drugs could be achieved, so that might be modified the trend of the desease and reduce social costs of illness.

[18]FDG-PET assists the diagnosis of AD when combined with specific genetic assessment. In fact hypomethabolism in posterior cingulate, parietal, prefrontal, entorhinal and temporal

regions have been found to predict future cognitive decline in older APOE ε4 carriers than non-carriers (Small et al., 2000). Moreover several [18]FDG-PET studies have shown that patients with MCI and AD-like metabolic pattern are hightly predictive of conversion to AD within several years, in particular in patiens that are APOE ε4 carriers (Mosconi et al., 2004).

[18]FDG-PET scans, when combined with Magnetic Resonance imaging and other biomarkers, are likely to improve diagnostic accuracy (Mueller et al., 2005) and might be used to monitor treatment that affect cerebral blood flow, metabolism, or neuronal dysfunction.

Characteristic patterns of regional hypometabolism are also seen in other degenerative dementia (Bohnen et al., 2012). Frontotemporal dementia is identified by distinct frontal or frontotemporal metabolic impairment that are typically quite asymmetrically centered in the frontolateral cortex and the anterior pole of temporal lobe. Dementia with Lewy bodies shows reduction of glucose metabolism in primary visual cortex in addition to that in posterior association areas. Other degenerative disorders show typical hypomethabolism in the specifically affected brain structures: the putamen and cortex in corticobasal degeneration, the caudate nucleus in Huntington's chorea, the frontal cortex and midbrain in progressive supranuclear palsy, pons and cerebellum in olivopontocerebellar atrophy.

In recent years different small molecule probes have been developed for use with PET to measure deposits of amyloid- ß plaques and tau tangles in vivo (Klunk et al., 2004; Kudo et al., 2007). The most studied amyloid-binding radiotracer is **[$^{11}$C]PIB** ([$^{11}$C]-labelled Pittsburg Compound B) which is a derivative of thioflavin-T amyloid dye that binds specifically amyloid-ß plaques but not neurofibrillary tangles. Studies using [$^{11}$C]PIB-PET have demonstrated cortical retention in patients with AD compared with normal subjects (Klunk et al., 2004). Studies of MCI patients have showed that [$^{11}$C]PIB uptake is increased in approximately 50% of them (Kemppainen et al., 2007). [$^{11}$C]PIB-PET could potentially be used to diagnose cerebral amyloid angiopathy since it also detects cerebrovascular amyloid (Johnson et al., 2007). PET studies with [$^{11}$C]PIB is useful in differential diagnosis of degenerative type of dementia, since patients with Lewy bodies dementia show lower binding than in AD, while patients affected with Fronto-temporal dementia show no cortical binding (Rowe et al., 2007).

Recently several $^{18}$F labelled amyloid tracers are commercially available permitting large scale clinical use (Rowe and Villemagne, 2011).

**[$^{18}$F]-BAY94-9172-PET,** based on amyloid legand florine-18, could be used to discriminate patients with AD from frontotemporal dementia and healthy controls (Rowe et al., 2008).

Tau deposition in neurofibrillary tangles together with amyloid can be specifically detect by the tracer **[$^{18}$F]-FDDNP**, providing additional insight in AD pathology (Small et al., 2008).

Other PET legands have been used in research to measure functionality of many neurotransmitter systems such as serotoninergic, cholinerdic and dopaminergic. The neurotrasmitters systems are impaired in various types of dementia and may help in differential diagnosis and in the definition of pathophysiological process. **MPPF** (4-[$^{18}$F]-fluoro-N-piperazynil-N-2-methoxy-phenyl-pyridinil benzamide) is a molecular imaging probe for 5-$HT_{1A}$ receptors which density correlates with the number of pyramidal neurons of the hippocampus (Kepe et al., 2006). Patients with AD show diminished hippocampal signal, while patients with MCI show binding values intermediate between controls and Alzheimer's disease patients (Kepe et al., 2006). Since MPPF binding correlates with neuronal losses in the hippocampus, therefore it can be used as an early diagnostic measure in the continuum between MCI and dementia conversion, before onset of symptoms of dementia. PET radioligands used to visualize cholinergic nicotinic receptors correlate with cognitive measure of attention in Alzheimer's disease (Kadir et al., 2006). PET measures of cholinergic system with $^{11}$**C-nicotine** can be used to assess nicotine binding sites in the brain before and after treatment with anti-cholinesterase drugs (Kadir et al., 2007).

**[$^{11}$C]ß-CFT** ([$^{11}$C]2ß-carbomethoxy-3ß-4fluorophenyl tropane) is a molecular dopamine reuptake ligand used to study the cerebral dopaminergic system. Striatal uptake of [$^{11}$C]ß-CFT is reduced in patients with AD (Rinne et al., 1998). The ligand **[$^{11}$C]-PK11195** has been used in other PET research to measure microglial activation as response to neuronal degeneration in patients with Alzheimer Disease (Cagnin et al., 2001). Microglial activation seems to be an inflammatory reaction to amyloid deposition that might increase the formation of pathological protein deposits.

## 5. Conclusions

An enormous progress has been made in the science of human cognition using neuroimaging and integration with neuropsychological assessment, multimodal structural and functional imaging technologies based on study of cerebral glucose metabolism as in Positron Emission Tomography. PET exam has led to a revolution in understanding of the basic neuroscience principles involved in where and how the brain processes information both in normal subjects and in patients with cerebral lesions.

Different PET methodologies in combination with traditional neuroimaging techniques are more and more used to accurately localize and characterize cognition not invasively.

The current clinical applications of using PET or other functional neuroimaging to mapping cognitive function include lateralization and presurgical mapping of language and memory mapping (Stufflebeam and Rosen, 2007). The development of advanced techniques and the combination of imaging technologies is further expanding the understanding of cognitive processing and is extending the clinical applications of functional neuroimaging into new areas.

With recent advances in neuroimaging technology novel PET applications are developing to measure various biological processes or to study cognitive alterations in patients with diseases that affect central nervous system. Combining PET procedures with other neuroimaging studies, genetic risk measures and other biomarkers measures from other tissues it might increase diagnostic sensitivity and specificity in particular in differential diagnosis of dementia, in the early stages of vascular or degenerative dementia, since presence of different PET pattern (neocortical association areas in AD, frontolateral cortex and anterior pole of temporal lobe in FTD, posterior association areas in LBD).

http://dx.doi.org/10.5772/57124

PET investigations will increase understanding and monitor pathophysiological process of many neurological diseases, track the biological effects of treatments in clinical trials and assist in identifying responders to specific treatments (Reiman et al., 2001). Several of the neuroimaging technologies in development promise in proving measurement of potential biomarkers but further research is necessary to validate their use. In fact many of these methods are still used in research settings and require further studies to better understand their clinical usefulness. Another limitation to the adoption of PET techniques is the relatively high cost and lack of wide availability, but when compared costs to the high diagnostic accuracy of PET, these benefits incurred high costs (McMahon et al., 2003). In future, with more extensive use of these new PET technology, costs will also decline and improvement of diagnostic accuracy will lead to cost saving. For example healthy adults with risk factors for cognitive decline (e.g. age, previous head trauma, familiar history) might undergo a PET check scan for measures of cognitive decline risk and physicians will use medications or other interventions to prevent or delay onset of disease or avoid future cognitive losses.

## Author details

Sandro Misciagna*

Don Gnocchi Foundation, Rome, Italy

## References

[1] American Psychiatric Association. Diagnostic and statistical manual of mental disorders (IV-Tr) 4th edn—text revised. Washington, DC: American Psychiatric Association; 2000.

[2] Atlas SW, Howard RS, Maldjian J, Alsop D, Detre JA, Listerud J, et al. Functional magnetic resonance imaging of regional brain activity in patients with intracerebral gliomas: findings and implications for clinical management. Neurosurgery. 1996 Feb; 38(2):329–338.

[3] Bennett D. Public health importance of vascular dementia and Alzheimer's disease with cerebrovascular disease. Int J Clin Pract Suppl. 2001 May;(120):41–48.

[4] Benson DF, Kuhl DE, Hawkins RA, Phelps ME, Cummings JL, Tsai SY. The fluorodeoxyglucose 18F scan in Alzheimer's disease and multi-infarct dementia. Arch Neurol 11 1983;40(12):711-4.

[5] Bohnen NI, Djang DS, Herholz K, Anzai Y, Minoshima S. Effectiveness and safety of 18F-FDG PET in the evaluation of dementia: a review of the recent literature. J Nucl Med Jan 2012;53(1):59-71.

[6] Braak H, Braak E. Neuropathological staging of Alzheimer-related changes. Acta Neuropathol. 1991;82:239–259.

[7] Cabeza R, Grady CL, Nyberg L, McIntosh AR, Tulving E, Kapur S, et al. Age-related differences in neural activity during memory encoding and retrieval: a positron emission tomography study. J Neurosci 1997a; 17: 391–400.

[8] Cabeza R, McIntosh AR, Tulving E, Nyberg L, Grady CL. Agerelated differences in effective neural connectivity during encoding and recall. Neuroreport 1997b; 8: 3479–83.

[9] Cagnin A, Brooks DJ, Kennedy AM, et al. In-vivo measurement of activated microglia in dementia. Lancet. 2001;358:461–467.

[10] Chételat G, Desgranges B, de la Sayette V, et al. Mild cognitive impairment: can FDG-PET predict who is to rapidly convert to Alzheimer's disease? Neurology. 2003;60:1374–1377.

[11] Clarke DD, Sokoloff L. Circulation and energy metabolism of the brain. In: Siegel G, Agranoff B, Albers RW, Fisher S, editors. Basic neurochemistry: molecular, cellular, and medical aspects. 6th ed. Philadelphia: Lippincott-Raven; 1999. p. 637-69.

[12] Craft S. Insulin resistance syndrome and Alzheimer disease: pathophysiologic mechanisms and therapeutic implications. Alzheim Dis Assoc Disord. 2006;20:298–301.

[13] Crutch SJ, Lehmann M, Schott JM, Rabinovici GD, Rossor MN, Fox NC. Posterior cortical atrophy. Lancet Neurol. 2012 Feb;11(2):170-8. Review.

[14] Dale AM, Liu AK, Fischl BR, Buckner RL, Belliveau JW, Lewine JD, et al. Dynamic statistical parametric mapping: combining fMRI and MEG for high-resolution imaging of cortical activity. Neuron. 2000 Apr;26(1):55–67.

[15] Dehaene S, Tzourio N, Frak V, Raynaud L, Cohen L, Mehler J, Mazoyer B, 1996. Cerebral activations during number multiplication and comparison: a PET study. Neuropsychologia 34, 1097–1106.

[16] Desgranges B, Chételat G, Eustache F. Brain substrates of episodic memory disorders in Alzheimer's disease. Rev Neurol (Paris). 2004 Apr;160(4 Pt 2):S44-54.

[17] Detre JA. fMRI: applications in epilepsy. Epilepsia. 2004;45 4:26–31.

[18] Drzezga A, Grimmer T, Riemenschneider M, et al. Prediction of individual clinical outcome in MCI by means of genetic assessment and (18)F-FDG PET. J Nucl Med. 2005;46:1625–1632.

[19] Esposito G, Kirkby BS, Van Horn JD, Ellmore TM, Berman KF. Context-dependent, neural system-specific neurophysiological concomitants of ageing: mapping PET correlates during cognitive activation. Brain. 1999 May;122 ( Pt 5):963-79.

[20] Ferrer I. Cognitive impairment of vascular origin: neuropathology of cognitive impairment of vascular origin. J Neurol Sci Dec 2010;299:139-49.

[21] Fischl B, Liu A, Dale AM. Automated manifold surgery: constructing geometrically accurate and topologically correct models of the human cerebral cortex. IEEE Trans Med Imaging. 2001 Jan;20(1):70–80.

[22] Fuster JM, Bodner M, Kroger JK. Cross-modal and cross-temporal association in neurons of frontal cortex. Nature. 2000 May 18;405(6784):347–351.

[23] Gazzaniga MS, editor. The cognitive neurosciences. 3rd. Cambridge, Mass: MIT Press; 2004.

[24] Grady CL, Maisog JM, Horwitz B, Ungerleider LG, Mentis MJ, Salerno JA, et al. Age-related changes in cortical blood flow activation during visual processing of faces and location. J Neurosc 1994; 14: 1450–62.

[25] Grady CL, McIntosh AR, Horwitz B, Maisog JM, Ungerleider LG, Mentis MJ, et al. Age-related reductions in human recognition memory due to impaired encoding. Science 1995; 269: 218–21.

[26] Hachinski VC, Lassen NA, Marshall J. Multi-infarct dementia. A cause of mental deterioration in the elderly. Lancet 07/27/1974;2(7874):207-10.

[27] Heiss WD, Zimmermann-Meinzingen S. PET imaging in the differential diagnosis of vascular dementia. J Neurol Sci. 2012 Nov 15;322(1-2):268-73. doi: 10.1016/j.jns.2012.09.023. Epub 2012 Oct 6.

[28] Herholz K, Salmon E, Perani D, Baron JC, Holthoff V, Frölich L, et al. Discrimination between Alzheimer dementia and controls by automated analysis of multicenter FDG PET. Neuroimage 2002;17:302-26.

[29] Herholz K. PET studies in dementia. Ann Nucl Med Apr 2003;17(2):79-89.

[30] Horwitz B, Warner B, Fitzer J, Tagamets MA, Husain FT, Long TW. Investigating the neural basis for functional and effective connectivity. Application to fMRI. Philos Trans R Soc Lond B Biol Sci. 2005 May 29;360(1457):1093–1108.

[31] Jagust W, Reed B, Mungas D, Ellis W, DeCarli C. What does fluorodeoxyglucose PET imaging add to a clinical diagnosis of dementia? Neurology. 2007;69:871–877.

[32] Jha AP. Tracking the time-course of attentional involvement in spatial working memory: an event-related potential investigation. Brain Res Cogn Brain Res. 2002 Dec; 15(1):61–69.

[33] Johnson KA, Gregas M, Becker JA, et al. Imaging of amyloid burden and distribution in cerebral amyloid angiopathy. Ann Neurol. 2007;62:229–234.

[34] Josephs KA, Whitwell JL, Ahmed Z, et al. Beta-amyloid burden is not associated with rates of brain atrophy. Ann Neurol. 2007 published online Sept 25.

[35] Kadir A, Almkvist O, Wall A, Långström B, Nordberg A. PET imaging of cortical $^{11}$C-nicotine binding correlates with the cognitive function of attention in Alzheimer's disease. Psychopharmacol. 2006;188:509–520.

[36] Kadir A, Darreh-Shori T, Almkvist O, Wall A, Långström B, Nordberg A. Changes in brain $^{11}$C-nicotine binding sites in patients with mild Alzheimer's disease following rivastigmine treatment as assessed by PET. Psychopharmacol. 2007;191:1005–1014.

[37] Kemppainen NM, Aalto S, Wilson IA, et al. PET amyloid ligand [$^{11}$C]PIB uptake is increased in mild cognitive impairment. Neurology. 2007;68:1603–1606.

[38] Kepe V, Barrio JR, Huang S-C, et al. Serotonin 1A receptors in the living brain of Alzheimer's disease patients. Proc Natl Acad Sci USA. 2006;103:702–707.

[39] Kerrouche N, Herholz K, Mielke R, Holthoff V, Baron JC. 18FDG PET in vascular dementia: differentiation from Alzheimer's disease using voxel-based multivariate analysis. J Cereb Blood Flow Metab Sep 2006;26(9):1213-21.

[40] Klunk WE, Engler H, Nordberg A, et al. Imaging brain amyloid in Alzheimer's disease with Pittsburgh Compound-B. Ann Neurol. 2004;55:306–319.

[41] Kudo Y, Okamura N, Furumoto S, et al. 2-(2-[2-Dimethylaminothiazol-5-yl]ethenyl)-6-(2-[fluoro]ethoxy)benzoxazole: a novel PET agent for in vivo detection of dense amyloid plaques in Alzheimer's disease patients. J Nucl Med. 2007;48:553–561.

[42] Kuczynski B, Reed B, Mungas D, Weiner M, Chui H.C., Jagust W. Cognitive and Anatomic Contributions of metabolic decline in Alzheimer Disease and Cerebrovascular Disease. Arch Neurol. 2008 May;65(5):650-5.

[43] Lohmann H, Deppe M, Jansen A, Schwindt W, Knecht S. Task repetition can affect functional magnetic resonance imaging-based measures of language lateralization and lead to pseudoincreases in bilaterality. J Cereb Blood Flow Metab. 2004 Feb;24(2): 179–187.

[44] Marner L, Nyengaard JR, Tang Y, Pakkenberg B. Marked loss of myelinated nerve fibers in the human brain with age. J Comp Neurol Jul 21 2003;462(2):144-52.

[45] Marshall JC, Fink GR. Cerebral localization, then and now. Neuroimage 2003;20:S2-S7.

[46] McIntosh AR, Grady CL, Ungerleider LG, Haxby JV, Rapoport SI, Horwitz B. Network analysis of cortical visual pathways mapped with PET. J Neurosci. 1994 Feb; 14(2):655–666.

[47] McIntosh AR, Grady CL, Haxby JV, Ungerleider LG, Horwitz B. Changes in limbic and prefrontal functional interactions in a working memory task for faces. Cereb Cortex. 1996 Jul-Aug;6(4):571–584.

[48] McKhann G, Drachman D, Folstein M, et al. Clinical diagnosis of Alzheimer's disease —report of the NINCDS-ADRDA work group under the auspices of the Department

of Health and Human Services Task Force on Alzheimer's Disease. Neurology. 1984;34:939–944.

[49] McMahon PM, Araki SS, Sandberg EA, Neumann PJ, Gazelle GS. Cost-effectiveness of PET in the diagnosis of Alzheimer disease. Radiology. 2003;228:515–522.

[50] Mehta NN, Torigian DA, Gelfand JM, Saboury B, Alavi A. Quantification of atherosclerotic plaque activity and vascular inflammation using [18-F] fluorodeoxyglucose positron emission tomography/computed tomography (FDG-PET/CT). J Vis Exp. 2012 May 2;(63):e3777. doi: 10.3791/3777.

[51] Mielke R, Herholz K, Grond M, Kessler J, Heiss WD. Severity of vascular dementia is related to volume of metabolically impaired tissue. Arch Neurol 09 1992;49(9): 909-13.

[52] Mielke R, Pietrzyk U, Jacobs A, Fink GR, Ichimiya A, Kessler J, et al. HMPAO SPET and FDG PET in Alzheimer's disease and vascular dementia: comparison of perfusion and metabolic pattern. Eur J Nucl Med 10 1994;21(10):1052-60.

[53] Milner B, Squire LR, Kandel ER. Cognitive neuroscience and the study of memory. Neuron. 1998 Mar;20(3):445–468.

[54] Misciagna S, Masullo C, Giordano A, Silveri MC. Vascular dementia and Alzheimer's disease: the unsolved problem of clinical and neuropsychological differential diagnosis. Int J Neurosci. 2005 Dec;115(12):1657-67.

[55] Mok V, Leung EY, Chu W, Chen S, Wong A, Xiong Y, et al. Pittsburgh compound B binding in poststroke dementia. J Neurol Sci Mar 15 2010;290(1–2):135-7.

[56] Morrison JH, Hof PR. Life and death of neurons in the aging brain. Science Oct 17 1997;278(5337):412-9.

[57] Mosconi L, Perani D, Sorbi S, et al. MCI conversion to dementia and the APOE genotype: a prediction study with FDG-PET. Neurology. 2004;63:2332–2340.

[58] Mueller SG, Weiner MW, Thal LJ, et al. Ways toward an early diagnosis in Alzheimer's disease: the Alzheimer's Disease Neuroimaging Initiative (ADNI) Alzheim Dement. 2005;1:55–66.

[59] Neary D, Snowden J, Mann D. Frontotemporal dementia. Lancet Neurol. 2005;4:771–780.

[60] Okello A, Edison P, Archer HA, Turkheimer FE, Kennedy J, Bullock R, et al. Microglial activation and amyloid deposition in mild cognitive impairment: a PET study. Neurology Jan 6 2009;72(1):56-62.

[61] Pannese E. Morphological changes in nerve cells during normal aging. Brain Struct Funct Jun 2011;216(2):85-9.

[62] Pawlik G, Heiss WD. Positron emission tomography and neuropsychological function. In: Bigler ED, Yeo RA, Turkheimer E, editors. Neuropsychological function and brain imaging. New York: Plenum Publ. Corp.; 1989. p. 65–138.

[63] Petersen RC. Mild cognitive impairment as a diagnostic entity. J Intern Med. 2004 Sep;256(3):183-94. Review.

[64] Petersen RC, Parisi JE, Dickson DW, et al. Neuropathology of amnestic mild cognitive impairment. Arch Neurol. 2006;63:665–672.

[65] Powell, A. L., Cummings, J. L., Hill, M. A., & Benson, D. F. (1998). Speech and language alterations in multi-infarct dementia. Neurology, 38, 717–719.

[66] Price CJ, Friston KJ, 1997. The temporal dynamics of reading: a PET study. Proc. R. Soc. London Ser. B 264, 1785–1791.

[67] Price JL, Morris JC. Tangles and plaques in nondemented aging and "preclinical" Alzheimer's disease. Ann Neurol. 1999;45:358–368.

[68] Rabin ML, Narayan VM, Kimberg DY, Casasanto DJ, Glosser G, Tracy JI, et al. Functional MRI predicts post-surgical memory following temporal lobectomy. Brain. 2004 Oct;127(Pt 10):2286–2298.

[69] Raichle ME, MacLeod AM, Snyder AZ, Powers WJ, Gusnard DA, Shulman GL, 2001. A default mode of brain function. Proc. Nat. Acad. Sci. 98, 676–682.

[70] Raichle ME, Mintun MA. Brain work and brain imaging. Annu Rev Neurosci. 2006;29:449–476.

[71] Reinikainen KJ, Soininen H, Riekkinen PJ. Neurotransmitter changes in Alzheimer's disease: implications to diagnostics and therapy. J Neurosci Res. 1990;27:576–586.

[72] Reiman EM, Caselli RJ, Chen K, Alexander GE, Bandy D, Frost J. Declining brain activity in cognitively normal apolipoprotein E epsilon 4 heterozygotes: a foundation for using positron emission tomography to efficiently test treatments to prevent Alzheimer's disease. Proc Natl Acad Sci USA. 2001;98:3334–3339.

[73] Rinne JO, Sahlberg N, Ruottinen H, Nagren K, Lehikoinen P. Striatal uptake of the dopamine reuptake ligand [$^{11}$C]β-CFT is reduced in Alzheimer's disease assessed by positron emission tomography. Neurology. 1998;50:152–156.

[74] Roux FE, Boulanouar K, Lotterie JA, Mejdoubi M, LeSage JP, Berry I. Language functional magnetic resonance imaging in preoperative assessment of language areas: correlation with direct cortical stimulation. Neurosurgery. 2003 Jun;52(6):1335–1345. discussion 1345-1337.

[75] Rowe CC, Ng S, Ackermann U, et al. Imaging beta-amyloid burden in aging and dementia. Neurology. 2007;68:1718–1725.

[76] Rowe CC, Ackerman U, Browne W, et al. Imaging β-amyloid in Alzheimer's disease with 18F-BAY94-9172, a novel fluorine-18 labeled positron emission tomography tracer. Lancet Neurol. 2008;7:129–135.

[77] Rowe CC, Villemagne VL. Brain amyloid imaging. J Nucl Med Nov 2011;52(11): 1733-40.

[78] Rusinek H, De Santi S, Frid D, Tsui WH, Tarshish CY, Convit A, et al. Regional brain atrophy rate predicts future cognitive decline: 6-year longitudinal MR imaging study of normal aging. Radiology Dec 2003;229(3):691-6.

[79] Sidoryk-Wegrzynowicz M, Wegrzynowicz M, Lee E, Bowman AB, Aschner M. Role of astrocytes in brain function and disease. Toxicol Pathol. 2011 Jan;39(1):115-23. Epub 2010 Nov 12.

[80] Silverman DHS, Small GW, Chang CY, et al. Positron emission tomography in evaluation of dementia: regional brain metabolism and long-term clinical outcome. JAMA. 2001;286:2120–2127.

[81] Small GW, Ercoli LM, Silverman DHS, et al. Cerebral metabolic and cognitive decline in persons at genetic risk for Alzheimer's disease. Proc Natl Acad Sci USA. 2000;97:6037–6042.

[82] Small GW, Kepe V, Ercoli L, et al. PET of brain amyloid and tau in mild cognitive impairment. N Engl J Med. 2006;355:2652–2663.

[83] Small GW, Bookheimer SY, Thompson PM, Cole GM, Huang SC, Kepe V, et al. Current and future uses of neuroimaging for cognitively impaired patients. Lancet Neurol Feb 2008;7(2):161-72.

[84] Snowdon DA, Greiner LH, Mortimer JA, Riley KP, Greiner PA, Markesbery WR. Brain infarction and the clinical expression of Alzheimer disease: the Nun Study. JAMA. 1997;277(10):813–817.

[85] Starkstein, S. E., Sabe, L., Vazquez, S., Teson, A., Petracca, G., Chemerinski, E., Di Lorenzo, G., & Leiguarda, R. (1996). Neuropsychological., psychiatric, and cerebral blood flow findings in vascular dementia and Alzheimer's disease. Stroke, 27, 408–414.

[86] Sheth BR, Shimojo S. Signal strength determines the nature of the relationship between perception and working memory. J Cogn Neurosci. 2003 Feb 15;15(2):173–184.

[87] Stippich C, Mohammed J, Kress B, Hahnel S, Gunther J, Konrad F, et al. Robust localization and lateralization of human language function: an optimized clinical functional magnetic resonance imaging protocol. Neurosci Lett. 2003 Jul 31;346(12):109–113.

[88] Stufflebeam SM, Rosen BR. Mapping cognitive function. Neuroimaging Clin N Am. 2007 Nov;17(4):469-84, viii-ix. Review.

[89] Tierney M C, Black S E, Szalai J P, Snow W G, Fisher R H, Nadon G, & Chui H C. (2001). Recognition memory and verbal fluency differentiate probable Alzheimer disease from subcortical ischemic vascular dementia. Archives in Neurology, 58, 1654–1659.

[90] Tullberg M, Fletcher E, DeCarli C, et al. White matter lesions impair frontal lobe function regardless of their location. Neurology. 2004;63(2):246–253.

[91] Tulving E, Markowitsch HJ. Episodic and declarative memory: role of the hippocampus. Hippocampus. 1998;8(3):198–204.

[92] Villardita C. (1993). Alzheimer's disease compared with cerebrovascular dementia: Neuropsychological similarities and differences. Acta Neurol Scand., 87, 299–308.

[93] Vincent JL, Snyder AZ, Fox MD, Shannon BJ, Andrews JR, Raichle ME, et al. Coherent spontaneous activity identifies a hippocampal-parietal memory network. J Neurophysiol. 2006 Dec;96(6):3517–3531.

[94] Wagner AD, Shannon BJ, Kahn I, Buckner RL. Parietal lobe contributions to episodic memory retrieval. Trends Cogn Sci. 2005 Sep;9(9):445–453.

[95] Warburton E, Wise RJS, Price CJ, Weiller C, Hadar U, Ramsay S, Frakowiak RSJ, 1996. Noun and verb retrieval by normal subjects: studies with PET. Brain 119, 159–179.

[96] Whitehead SN, Bayona NA, Cheng G, Allen GV, Hachinski VC, Cechetto DF. Effects of triflusal and aspirin in a ratmodel of cerebral ischemia. Stroke Feb 2007;38(2):381-7.

[97] Whitwell JL, Jack CR Jr, Boeve BF, Parisi JE, Ahlskog JE, Drubach DA, Senjem ML, Knopman DS, Petersen RC, Dickson DW, et al. Imaging correlates of pathology in corticobasal syndrome. Neurology. 2010 Nov 23; 75(21):1879-87.

[98] Woermann FG, Jokeit H, Luerding R, Freitag H, Schulz R, Guertler S, et al. Language lateralization by Wada test and fMRI in 100 patients with epilepsy. Neurology. 2003 Sep 9;61(5):699–701.

# Chapter 5

# How to Study Smoking and Drinking with PET

Evan D. Morris, Molly V. Lucas and Kelly P. Cosgrove

Additional information is available at the end of the chapter

http://dx.doi.org/10.5772/57414

## 1. Introduction

### 1.1. Historical background

The era of imaging neuroreceptors in humans with PET was ushered in by Wagner et al. (1983) with a report in Science showing the first human brain scan of dopamine receptors (Wagner, 1983). The tracer was N-methylspiperone (NMSP) tagged with carbon-11. The brain that was scanned belonged to one of the authors. Ethical concerns notwithstanding, this act placed the researchers in the good company of famous scientists throughout history who had experimented on themselves. The publication of this paper excited the field and garnered some publicity as well (see Figure 1). Although the study did not employ the quantitative analysis techniques we describe below, it presaged some of the key concepts. Namely: (1) early images contain mostly blood flow information; (2) late images primarily reflect binding; (3) radioactive tracer in the target tissue can be "free" or "bound", which often necessitates the examination of a "reference region", which is devoid of receptor sites; (4) co-injection of radiolabelled tracer with an *excess* of unlabeled tracer can be used to prevent radiotracer from binding and thus measure unbound (aka, non-displaceable) signal by itself. Injection of excess unlabeled tracer is generally not performed in humans; in this case, it was done in baboons. As we discuss below, the ability to use PET to measure receptor number or some index thereof opens up additional measurement possibilities which take advantage of a key concept: competition. In the Wagner paper, the competition was between hot (labeled) and cold (unlabeled) tracer (Wagner, 1983). In another ground-breaking paper that followed it, the competition was between a radiotracer and an unlabeled neuroleptic drug (Farde et al., 1986). Farde and colleagues did what amounts to the first drug occupancy study with PET using the tracer, [$^{11}$C]raclopride, in 1986. Their paper was intended to examine the occupancy level of drugs for schizophrenia in treated schizophrenics by examining the degree of tracer blocking at the dopamine D2 receptor sites achieved by each patient's respective drug. Whereas Wagner et

INTECH
open science | open minds

© 2013 Morris et al.; licensee InTech. This is a paper distributed under the terms of the Creative Commons Attribution License (http://creativecommons.org/licenses/by/3.0), which permits unrestricted use, distribution, and reproduction in any medium, provided the original work is properly cited.

al. could examine the difference between a baboon at baseline and following a co-injection of tracer with an excess of cold NMSP (Wagner, 1983), Farde et al. did not ask their patients to go off medication to get a baseline measurement of tracer binding (Farde et al., 1986). So how did they make an assessment of drug occupancy, which requires at least two measurements? They extrapolated what baseline binding might have been in their schizophrenics from a cohort of control subjects. Provocatively, they found that three schizophrenics undergoing (successful) treatment with different drugs all had receptor occupancies of very similar levels. Their approach would likely not pass muster today, but at the time, the paper was highly innovative, and it foreshadowed one of the major usages of PET and neuroreceptor tracers: measuring target occupancy by drugs in people.

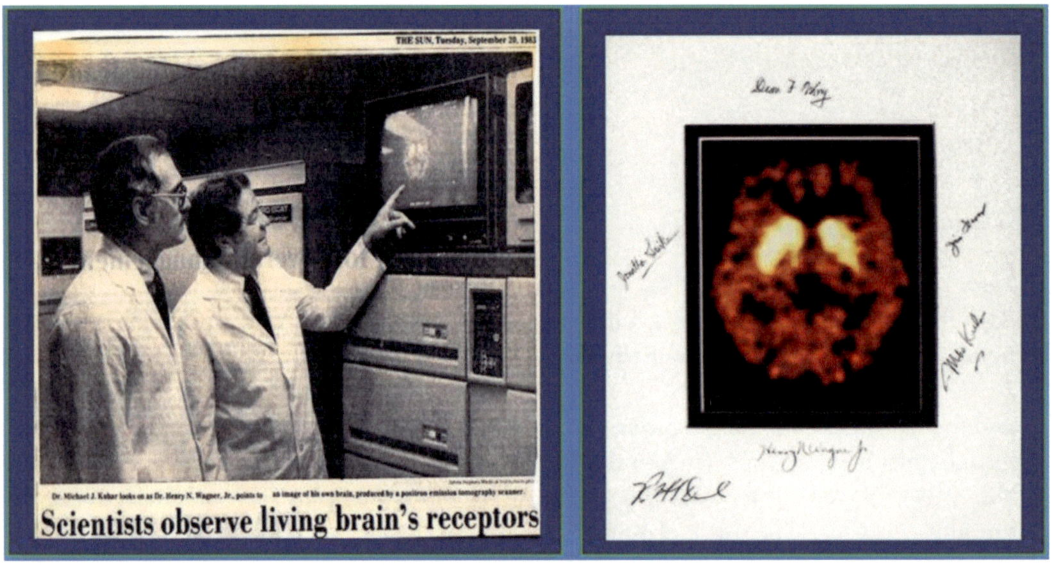


**Figure 1.** Left) Newspaper clipping from the Baltimore Sun, Sept 20, 1983, shows senior authors, Drs. Henry Wagner, Jr. and Mike Kuhar observing the first images of D2 receptors in a human brain, *in vivo*. (Right) A keepsake from the experiment adorns the offices of many of the landmark study's participants. Signatures, from the center bottom going clockwise, Wagner, Robert Dannals, Joanthan Links, Dean F. Wong, Jim Frost, and Kuhar. Photos care of M. Kuhar.

## 1.2. Basics

### *1.2.1. Molecular specificity*

PET is unique among medical imaging modalities for its exquisite molecular specificity. From this specificity, PET derives its unique ability to image highly selective biological *processes* – that is, to act as a *functional* imaging modality. In the brain (and everywhere in the body), different processes are facilitated by highly specialized molecules. Individual enzyme molecules exist to catalyze highly selective and uni-purpose biochemical reactions. Unique receptors and transporters exist to bind highly specialized endogenous ligands and carry out unique physiological functions. Some of the functions of interest that are controlled by

http://dx.doi.org/10.5772/57414

individual molecules and which we may want to image are shown in Figure 2. PET can image any of these molecular targets provided two obstacles have been overcome. First, a tracer molecule that binds or interacts with the target site must exist and be labeled with a positron emitting isotope (typically, carbon-11 or fluorine-18). Second, it must be possible to deliver the tracer to the target site. In brain imaging, the most likely cause of tracer failure is the inability of the tracer to cross the blood brain barrier to access the target.

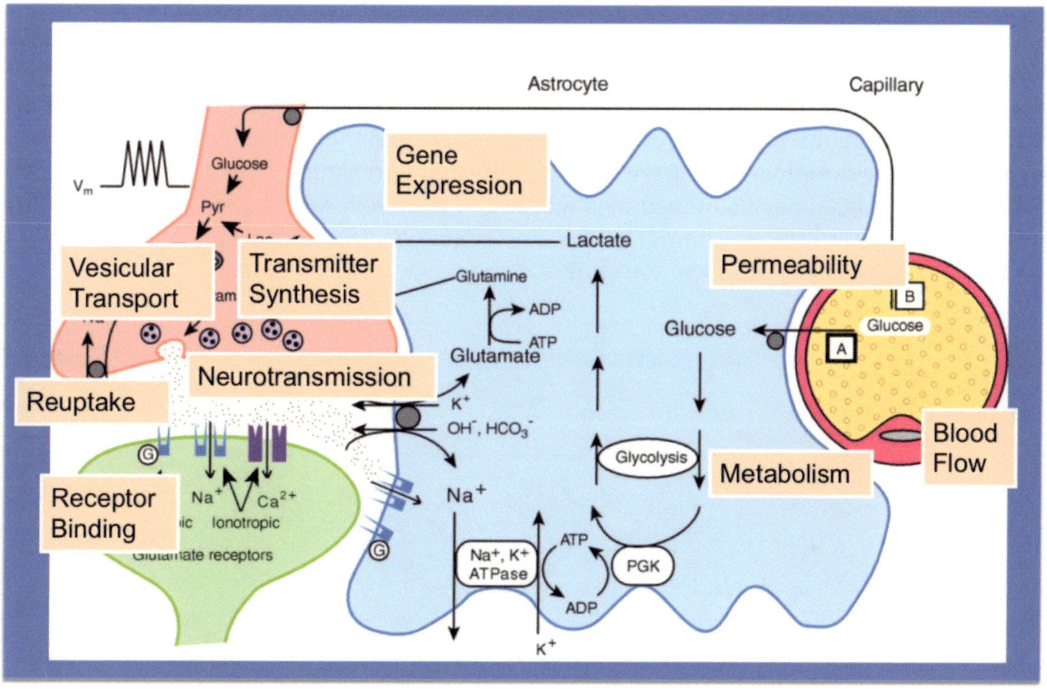


**Figure 2.** Molecular processes that can be imaged with the appropriate PET ligand. Figure modified (Pellerin et al., 1994).

### *1.2.2. Many tracers for many targets*

At this writing, there are tracers for many of the common neurotransmitter receptor sites: dopamine ($D_2$/$D_3$ and $D_1$), serotonin ($5HT_{1a}$, $5HT_{1b}$, $5HT_4$...), and transporter sites (DAT, SERT, NET...). Tracers generally arise through one of three pathways. (1) Radiolabeling of a dye or other molecule that is known to be selective for a particular target of interest (e.g., [$^{11}$C]PIB arose from the radiolabelling of thioflavin-T) (Mathis et al., 2002). (2) Radiolabeling of a candidate drug for the target molecule of interest. Such candidate compounds may have been failed drugs (adverse drug side-effects on patients, kinetics too rapid to sustain clinically useful levels in blood and tissue) but make good tracers (no adverse side-effects, because tracers are given in micro-dose amounts, favorably rapid kinetics). (3) De novo design of new PET tracer based on knowledge of the structure of the target molecule.

### *1.2.3. Specific binding vs. nonspecific background*

Tracers are administered to subjects intravenously and travel to the brain via the circulation. Once they traverse the blood brain barrier (typically by passive diffusion), they can follow three possible fates. Some tracer molecules remain free (unbound), eventually clear back to the vasculature and are removed from the organ. Other tracer molecules, once inside the tissue, may bind to the specific target of interest. Because no tracers are perfectly ideal in their behavior, some molecules are bound nonspecifically (nondisplaceably) before clearing from the tissue. Thus, in toto, radioactive emissions that are detected by the PET scanner are a (time-varying) sum of emissions of radio-isotopes on tracer molecules in all four different possible states: blood-borne, free in tissue, specifically bound to a receptor or other target molecule, or nonspecifically bound (Figure 3). The PET scanner records all of these emissions indiscriminately. Nothing about the photons that are emitted from an annihilation event in the blood or tissue makes their original state knowable from the detected signal. Thus, on any given *static* PET image (a single image summed over a time frame), the desired signal – i.e., the amount of specifically bound tracer – cannot be discerned easily because the signal is confounded by background activity coming from tracer in its three other possible states.

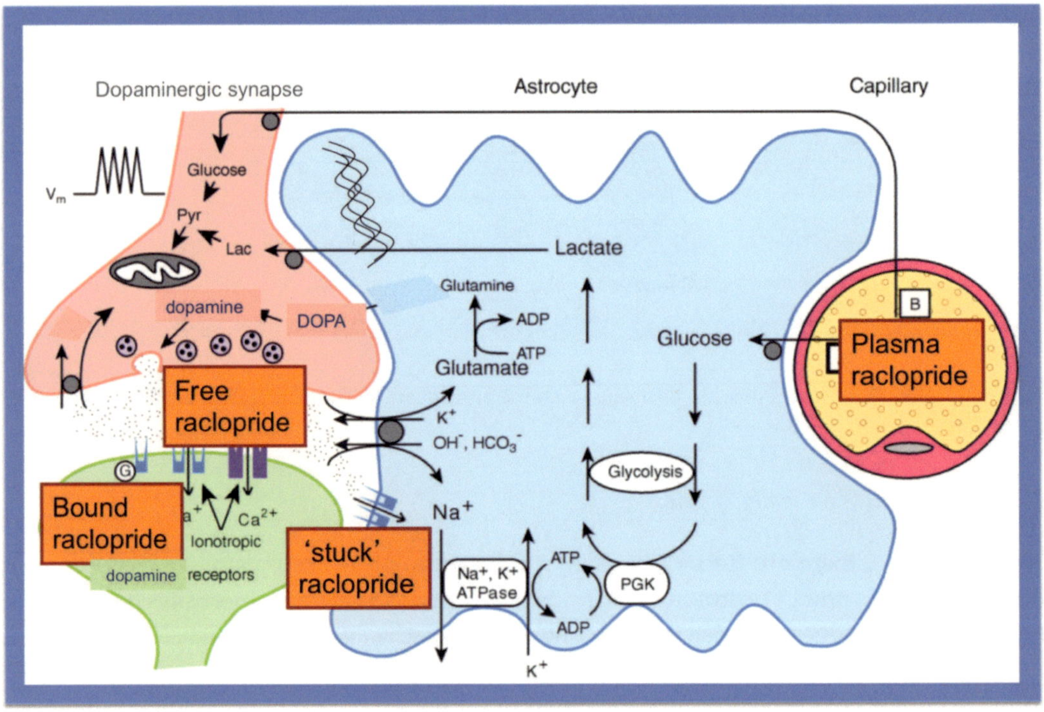


**Figure 3.** Possible states of an injected radiotracer. The states can be thought of as distinct, interconnected pools. Figure modified (Pellerin et al., 1994).

The one thing that allows us to differentiate the binding from the background is the difference in temporal behavior of the various tracer states. The persistence of activity (in a sense, the

http://dx.doi.org/10.5772/57414

residence time) in each of the plasma, free, bound, and nonspecific pools is different (see curves in Figure 4). Thus, to identify the specific binding component of the total PET signal (green curve on Fig. 4, also called a time-activity curve (TAC)), we must (a) acquire dynamic data (over many time frames), (b) identify an input function to the system (either plasma radioactivity or image-derived), and (c) apply a mathematical model to separate the dynamic data into its constituent parts.

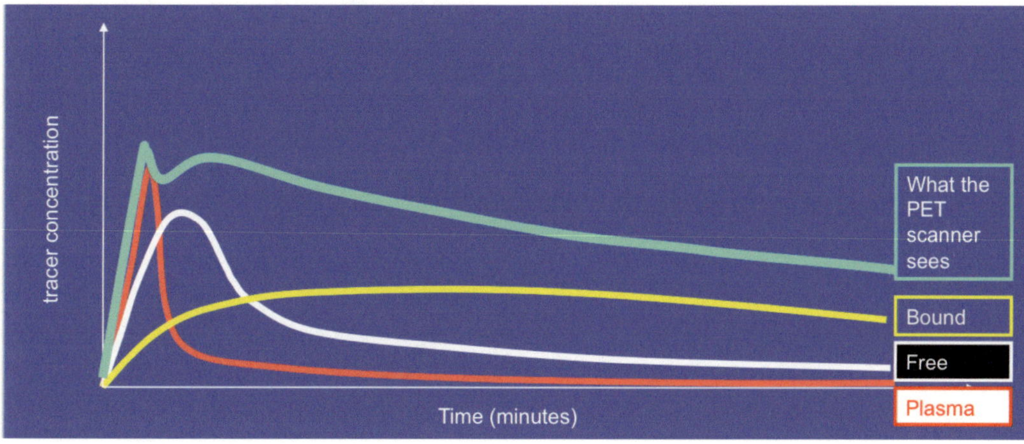


**Figure 4.** Different pools (compartments) of tracer activity are distinguishable by their different kinetics. Plasma activity (red) is cleared fastest. The free tracer pool (white) is slightly slower. The bound tracer pool (yellow) persists for longest. The PET scanner measures the sum of all the radiactivity (green).

### *1.2.4. Binding potential as endpoint*

The most common endpoint for imaging neuroreceptor or neurotransmitter targets with PET is the compound parameter, binding potential (BP). The term was first introduced by Mintun and is equivalent to the steady state ratio in the target tissue of specifically bound tracer to free tracer (Mintun et al., 1984). Binding potential is a "compound" parameter, because it is equivalent to the ratio of individual rate constants (specifically, the association and dissociation rate constants). The rate constants arise in the standard compartmental model used to describe a TAC measured in a region of interest in the dynamic PET images. Readers should be aware that there are a few variations on the definition of binding potential (Innis et al., 2007). The definitions differ by what data are used as the input function to drive the particular kinetic model and by what assumptions are made. Nevertheless, the general principle can be stated: BP can be estimated as the steady state ratio of bound to free tracer. BP is also proportional to the available binding sites and inversely proportional to the equilibrium dissociation constant, $K_D$, of the tracer for the binding site. The former concept is diagrammed in Figure 5. We see that there are four species of interest in imaging neuroreceptor targets. First, the receptor, second, the tracer molecule that binds to the target and emits a positron, third, the unlabeled tracer which also binds to the target but emits no positron, and fourth, the endogenous ligand that is also specific for the target but (naturally) emits no positron.

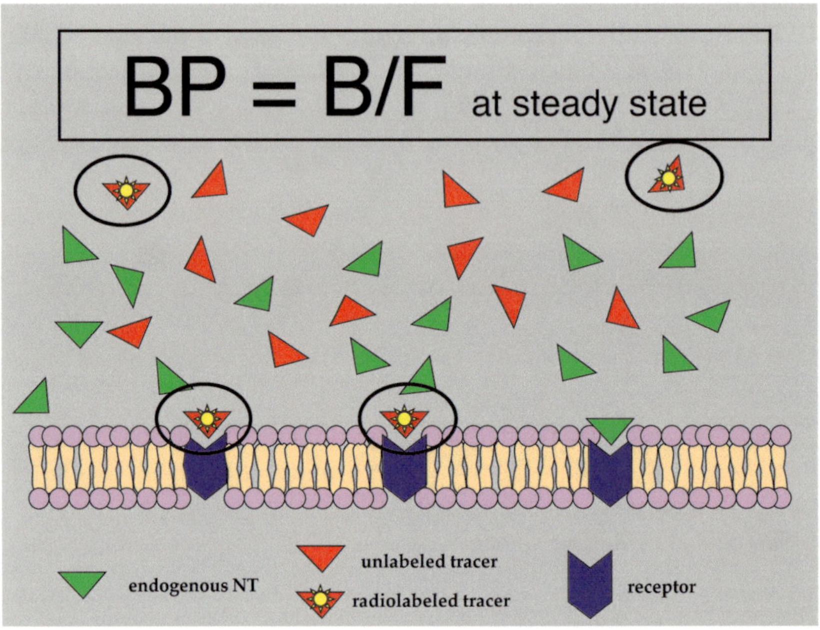


**Figure 5.** Binding potential depicted as bound over free tracer (red with star) at steady state. Receptor (or transporter) molecules (blue) may be embedded in a cell membrane. Two other species compete with tracer for limited binding sites: cold tracer (red), endogenous ligand (green).

*1.2.5. Changes in receptor number*

As previously stated, BP is proportional to number of available receptor binding sites and typically serves as a convenient surrogate for receptor density, provided the proportionality constant can be taken as a constant across the groups or conditions being compared. When BP is estimated from dynamic data using the arterial plasma concentration of tracer as the input function, the proportionality between BP and Bmax is simply $1/K_D$. (i.e., $BP = B_{max}/K_D$). Perhaps the most common use of BP as an endpoint is to assay receptor density (e.g., dopamine $D_2R$) in two groups of subjects (e.g., healthy controls and cocaine addicts) and compare them (Martinez et al., 2003; Volkow et al., 1997). In such a case, the density of receptors may be believed to have a direct functional role in a disease process. Alternatively, receptor number can be a surrogate marker for number of functioning neurons. Consider Parkinson's disease (PD), which involves loss of nigro-striatal connections. Because functioning nigro-striatal projections contain D2 receptors and dopamine transporters on their striatal terminals, absence of such sites in a PET scan is indicative of disease progression and attendant loss of neurons. Low dopamine receptors and low dopamine transporters have each been demonstrated with either [$^{11}$C]raclopride or [$^{11}$C]CFT, respectively, by comparing the BP for healthy controls to that of PD patients (Biju et al., 2009; Brooks et al., 1990). The schematic in Figure 6 represents the case of low BP caused by low receptors (Figure 6 should not be interpreted too literally. e.g., in the case of PD, the entire cell membrane along with the receptors might be missing).

http://dx.doi.org/10.5772/57414

*1.2.6. Changes in endogenous neurotransmitter*

Another popular use of BP is as a measure of steady state neurotransmitter level. Such measurements are typically made by comparing BP in the same subject at baseline and in a drug or treatment condition. This can be done via two paired bolus injections of tracer or via one bolus plus infusion of tracer (see section 1.2.10 below). Typically, a drug will be given prior to the PET scan. The drug (e.g., cocaine, methylphenidate, amphetamine) will cause elevation of endogenous neurotransmitter, which will in turn occupy more binding sites. As a result, fewer binding sites will remain available for binding by the labeled tracer, and the measured BP will be lower than at baseline. The fractional change in BP is the parameter that is most often reported as an indicator that there has been a prolonged change in neurotransmitter level (Here, "prolonged" simply means on the order of, or longer than, the scan duration). Figure 7 illustrates the principle using the same scheme as in Figures 5 and 6. Because specific binding sites exist in limited number, the approach to full binding will follow a saturation curve. That is, for greater and greater amounts of neurotransmitter release, we expect to see less and less incremental reduction of binding potential.

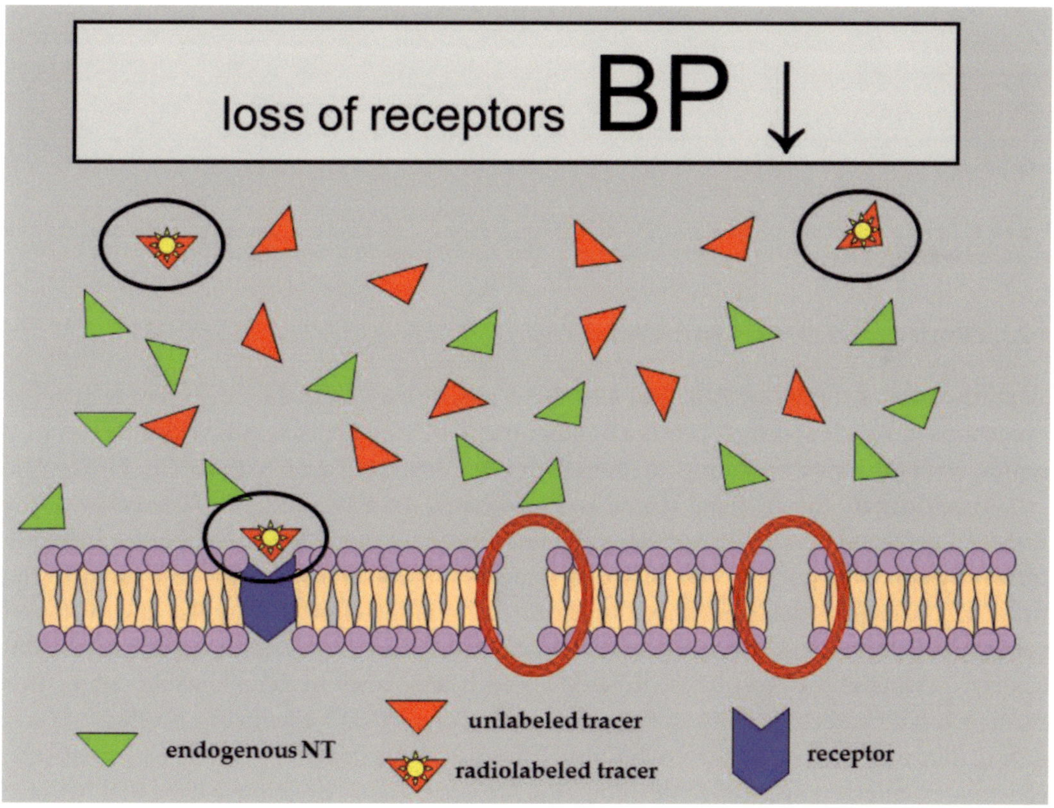


**Figure 6.** Lower Binding Potential reflects lower receptor density. (Compare to Figure 5).

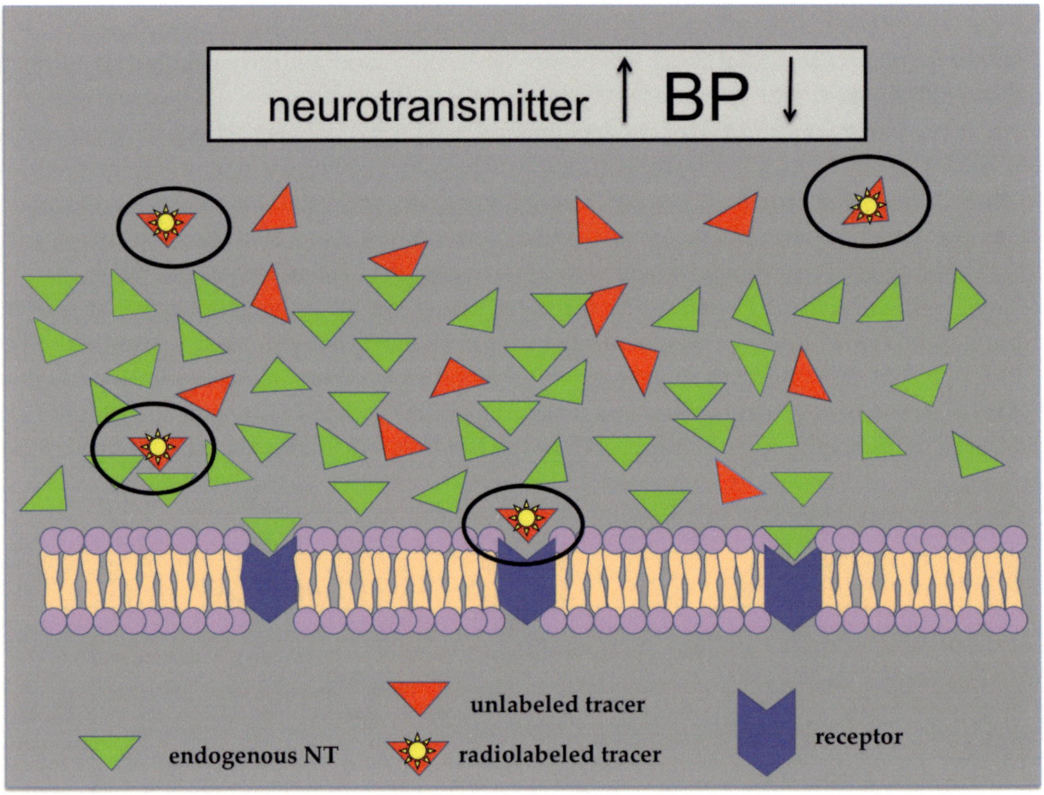


**Figure 7.** Elevation of endogenous neurotransmitter (green triangles) blocks available receptors and is detected as a reduction in BP.

### *1.2.7. Changes in occupancy by an exogenous drug*

A third common usage of PET and BP is for measuring occupancy of receptor sites by exogenous (unlabeled) drugs. This is a popular use of PET by pharmaceutical companies who typical want to know three things: (a) does their candidate drug get into the brain, (b) does the candidate drug hit the intended target, and (c) what is the relationship between dose of the drug and percentage occupancy of the available (target) receptors? When companies are ready for a drug-occupancy study with PET they usually already know the safe dose range of the drug (i.e., the range of doses that cause little to no adverse side-effects). They also have a desired occupancy level in mind that will produce the desired drug effects. The question that PET can answer is: what is the receptor occupancy for each dose level in the allowable range. This relationship is characterized by an $ED_{50}$ (drug dose at which 50% occupancy is achieved) and an $E_{max}$ (maximal achievable level of binding if there were no upper limit on dose). Just as with elevation of endogenous neurotransmitter, the presence of cold exogenous drug that binds to the same receptor as the tracer and reduces the concentration of available receptor sites can be imaged. This scenario is diagrammed in Figure 8. An essential element of occupancy studies is that there must exist a tracer that binds selectively to the desired drug target. On the other hand, the *drug* need not be selective. The change in binding of the PET tracer will reflect the occupancy of the drug only at the tracer's target. Again, occupancy of specific receptor binding sites is saturable and reduction in BP (i.e., increase in drug occupancy) increases less and less for given increases in drug as the concentration gets higher and higher. We typically define change in BP as a percentage change:

$\Delta BP = [1 - BP(\text{under a challenge condition}) / BP(\text{at baseline})] * 100.$

For the case of an exogenous drug binding to target sites, it turns out, Occupancy = $\Delta BP$.

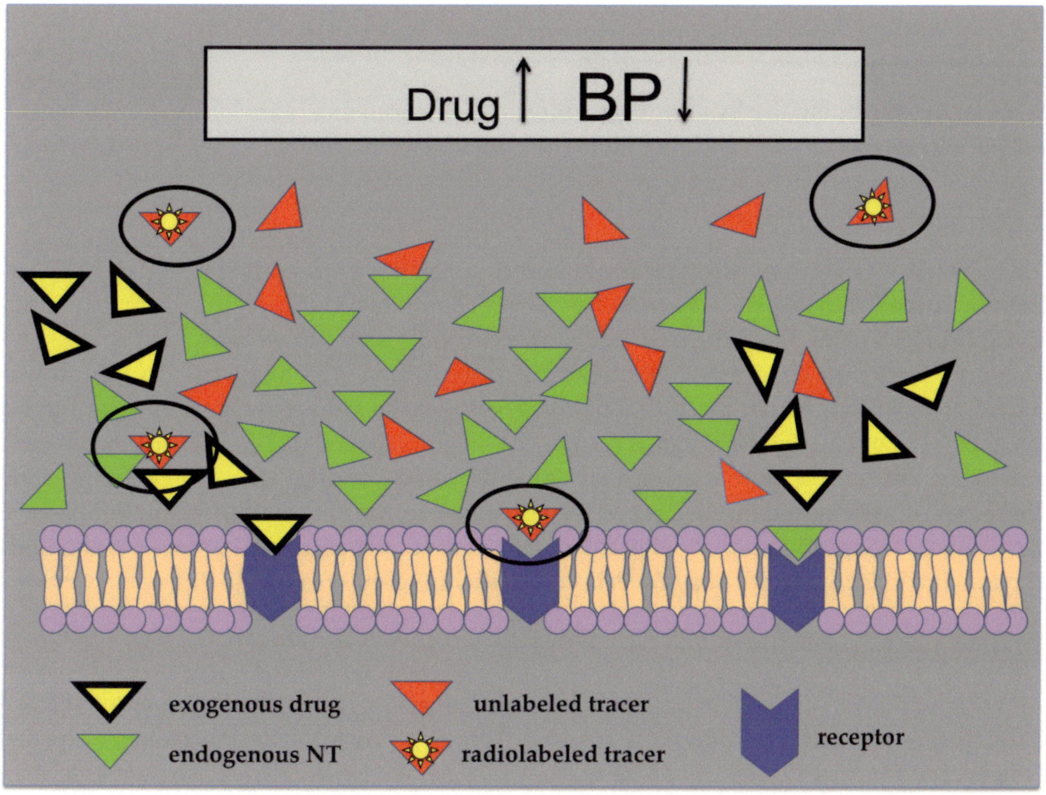


**Figure 8.** Effect of exogenous drug on binding potential. Drug (yellow triangles) occupies some receptor sites reducing available binding sites and then reducing BP.

### *1.2.8. Ambiguities in interpretation of PET data*

The flexibility of BP as an endpoint of PET studies with neuroreceptor ligands (as stated, one can measure receptors, transmitters, drugs) is also the source of potential ambiguity in interpretation. How can one tell the difference between lower receptor density under scan condition B vs. A from higher neurotransmitter level in scan condition B vs. A? These ambiguities are inherent in the compound parameter, BP. Generally, they can be resolved by considering the context of the measurement. If a stimulus was given just before the scan and the BP was lower than at baseline, we interpret this to mean that neurotransmitter levels rose due to the stimulus. We reject receptor up-regulation as the explanation, because it is a slower process than the time-scale of the PET scan (1-2 hours). On the other hand, if baseline scans are repeated on the same individuals after a year of psychotherapy and the average BP value is higher in the latter scan, we interpret this to mean that receptor number is increased by psychotherapy. (We must admit that long-term depression of baseline neurotransmitter level is also a valid interpretation.) Certainly we can say that "available receptor sites" were increased with therapy. In all cases, one must be alert to alternative interpretations of BP and ΔBP and try as best as possible to control for them via appropriate study designs.

*1.2.9. Common confounding conditions in PET experiments*

Some sources of ambiguity in the interpretation of BP measurements are inherent in the nature of PET data, but others can and should be controlled experimentally.

*1.2.9.1. Effect of age*

The densities of many neuroreceptors are known to decline with normal aging and this has been confirmed with PET (E. D. Morris et al., 1999). Thus, BP will be lower in a group of healthy control subjects with a higher mean age than a second group whose mean age is younger. Similarly, there may be no effect of a treatment or condition (e.g., long-term drug abuse) on the numbers of a particular receptor, but it might appear so if the drug abusers have a mean age that is older than the mean age of the healthy subjects to whom they are being compared. Any careful reading of journal articles reporting BP values for different cohorts must include checking to make sure that the ages of the respective groups are not different. Similarly, a longitudinal study examining the effect of long-term treatment on a single group of individuals should correct for aging of the subjects if the length of the study is considerable.

*1.2.9.2. Effect of mass*

As we saw above, an exogenous drug that occupies the target receptor reduces available binding sites for the tracer, and BP is reduced. This is the basis for drug occupancy studies. However, if the specific activity of the tracer (ratio of activity to mass) is low enough, then mass of cold tracer acts like any exogenous drug. This poses two problems. First, we normally do not want the tracer species to exert its own drug effects. Second, the mass of cold tracer – as with any exogenous ligand for the target site – will occupy an appreciable number of receptors and the measured BP will be lower than if the mass of tracer were negligible. Unwanted drug effects notwithstanding, poorly controlled mass of tracer has the potential to introduce a confound into an experiment. If a patient group is being compared to a control group but the patients receive a significantly higher mean tracer mass (i.e., lower specific activity for the same amount of radioactivity injected), then the patients will appear to have lower BP due to their disease, when in fact, the difference may be caused solely by a bias introduced by experimenters.

http://dx.doi.org/10.5772/57414

### *1.2.10. Experimental approaches to estimate binding potential*

There are generally two approaches to estimating BP and by extension, change in BP. Both approaches turn on recognizing that BP represents a steady state quantity: the ratio of bound to free tracer in the tissue at steady state – that is, when the ratio of these quantities is not changing on a macroscopic level. To make such a measurement, one can either perform an experiment that brings the pools of bound and free tracer to steady state or, if that is not possible or not desired, one can predict the steady state from non-steady measurements. If these ideas seem unintuitive, consider the two fun experiments depicted in Figure 9 for predicting the steady state (i.e., adult) height of one's daughters. Steady state approach: one can make a few measurements (greater reliability than a single measurement) once the child reaches her adult height (Figure 9, left). Non-steady approach: one can make periodic measurements throughout childhood and – given a model of growth patterns of women in the United States – *predict* the adult height of the child based on these non-steady measurements (right).

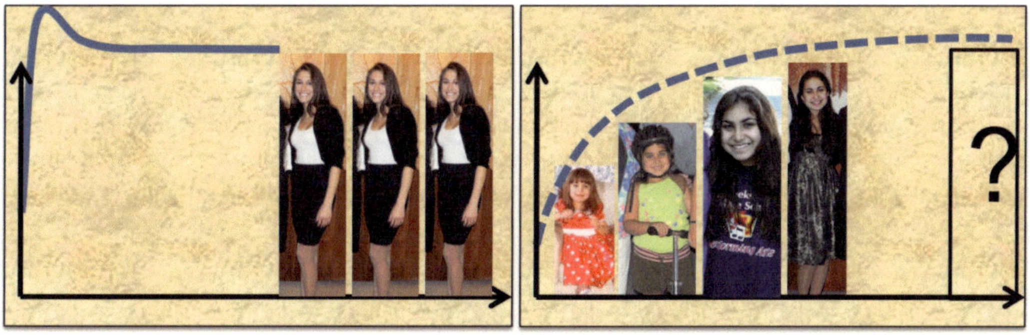


**Figure 9.** Schematic for (left) a type of steady state experiment for *measuring* height of a fully grown female child, as compared to (right) a type of non-steady experiment for *predicting* the adult height of the female children of one of the authors.

#### *1.2.10.1. Bolus plus constant infusion*

In PET, the steady state or equilibrium approach to measuring BP consists of administering the tracer as an initial bolus followed by a constant infusion of additional tracer for the duration of the experiment. If the bolus and infusion fractions of the tracer are balanced correctly, the TAC in the region(s) of interest will achieve a steady state in a minimal amount of time (Carson et al., 1993) at which point tracer concentrations in plasma, free and bound compartments will remain in constant proportions to each other. At said point, BP can be measured directly from the levels of the plasma and tissue curves without the need for a model or any curve-fitting. It must be pointed out that infusions are more taxing experimentally. An infusion pump is required. More tracer is required (as compared to a bolus injection), since some of it decays while sitting in the syringe waiting to be infused. Not all tissue regions are the same. Tissue regions with differing kinetics of tracer uptake will reach equilibrium at different times – or not at all. Not all subjects are the same. For a given injection protocol, one subject's tissue curves might reach equilibrium but another's might not.

*1.2.10.2. Bolus studies*

Alternatively, if an infusion experiment is impractical, a bolus administration of tracer is used. This approach includes a bolus injection of tracer, a dynamic acquisition of PET data, and a kinetic model to fit the data, estimate parameters, and calculate BP from the estimated model parameters. The parameters of the kinetic model are rate constants (they each have units of time$^{-1}$), but their ratio is an equilibrium (i.e., steady state) constant (BP is unitless).

Both experimental designs (bolus and bolus/infusion) can be used to measure the change in BP. In the case of the bolus administration, two separate injections are required to measure change in BP (ΔBP) – perhaps in response to a drug challenge. A single bolus plus infusion (B/I) study can suffice to measure ΔBP provided the drug challenge of interest acts rapidly enough and the tracer is sufficiently displaceable so that the effect can be detected during the duration of the scan. The two different paradigms for measuring ΔBP are diagrammed in Figure 10. Each paradigm has advantages and disadvantages that the investigator must consider carefully when planning a study (Table 1). The order of a paired bolus study (baseline vs. challenge condition) can be randomized; the B/I cannot. Both scans of a paired bolus studies with 18F-labelled tracers cannot both be performed on a single day. This may lead to greater variability in the data or even loss of some subjects who fail to return for a second scan. Equilibrium must be reached before the drug challenge in the B/I design. Unfortunately, there is no way of knowing that equilibrium has been achieved in a subject before giving the drug challenge, since PET data are not reconstructed and analyzed in real time. Finally, on the side of the B/I paradigm, the analysis of the data – provided equilibrium has been reached – is simple and requires no modeling and no curve fitting. For bolus studies, with some rare exceptions, one must use a kinetic model to describe the data in order to estimate BP.

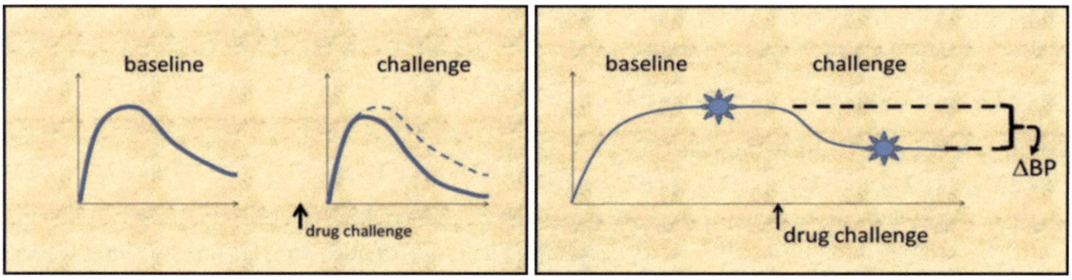


**Figure 10.** Two common schemes for measuring change in BP with PET. General appearance of data from a paired bolus study (left) compared to a single bolus plus infusion study (right). Stars on right indicate that only two static measurements are necessary to get change in BP from an equilibrium study

*1.2.11. Modeling basics (to get to binding potential via bolus or bolus + infusion)*

As we discussed in Section 1.2.3 and diagrammed in Figure 4, the PET signal consists of tracer molecules in different pools, only one of which is the specific binding we are most interested in. These pools or compartments differentiate themselves over time. They have different temporal characteristics based on their degree of retention of the tracer. The PET signal can be

| Paired Bolus design | Bolus plus Infusion design |
|---|---|
| order of conditions can be randomized: baseline/ challenge | requires no model-fitting to estimate BP, ΔBP |
| requires two successful syntheses | requires only one successful synthesis of tracer |
| studies with [18F]-labeled tracers require two separate scan days; more chance of physiological variability | requires computerized injection |
| | (high- and low-binding) regions don't all reach equilibrium at same time. |
| | requires that regions of interest reach equilibrium; data may be unusable if equilibrium is not achieved |
| | B/I scan needs more radioactivity than single bolus scan |

**Table 1.** Experimental Design. Some common advantages (blue) and disadvantages (red) of paired bolus and bolus plus infusion designs for measuring drug-induced changes in the neurotransmitter levels with PET.

dissected into its constituent parts with the use of a kinetic model that describes the processes of uptake and retention of the tracer, as well as the interconnectedness of the compartments.

#### *1.2.11.1. The modeling process*

The process of moving from some knowledge of the system of interest to a tracer kinetic model is diagrammed in Figure 11. One must first identify the organ(s) of interest. In the case of imaging drugs, the organ, naturally, is the brain. Next one must consider the relevant (neuro)chemistry of the selected organ and how it relates to the tracer to be used. In a simple conception of the brain, we must include the vasculature that delivers the tracer to the tissue. The blood brain barrier – how does the tracer traverse it? Once inside the tissue, are there receptors or transporters to (specifically) bind the tracer? If there are multiple possible specific binding sites, is there one site that is likely to dominate? Inevitably there will be nonspecific (i.e., non-displaceable) binding as well, because there are other entities in the tissue that appear to retain foreign molecules. Due to mathematical limitations (related to the limits of parameter identifiability), most models will treat the nonspecific binding pool as a sub-pool of the free, unbound tracer; nevertheless, we must keep in mind that such a process lurks under the surface even if it is not explicated in the model statement. Next, we must conceptualize the possible fates of the tracer into distinct pools or compartments of the model (all compartments are pools, but not all pools are compartments – see next section for explanation). Every route by which tracer can move from one compartment to another must be assigned a rate constant (designated by an arrow in Figure 11c). Finally, we turn a diagram of connected pools into a series of equations. Because what drives movement of tracer is mass action (diffusion from pools of high concentration to low), we must write mass balance equations for each compartment. Mass balance equations assert that the net accumulation of tracer over time is equal to the amount of tracer coming into the compartment per time, minus the amount of tracer leaving per time, plus tracer generated, minus tracer destroyed. Typically, generation does not apply – our bodies do not create exogenous compounds. These equations take the form of ordinary differential equations. The only dependent variable is time. The dependent, or "state", variables are the unknown concentrations in the respective compartments.

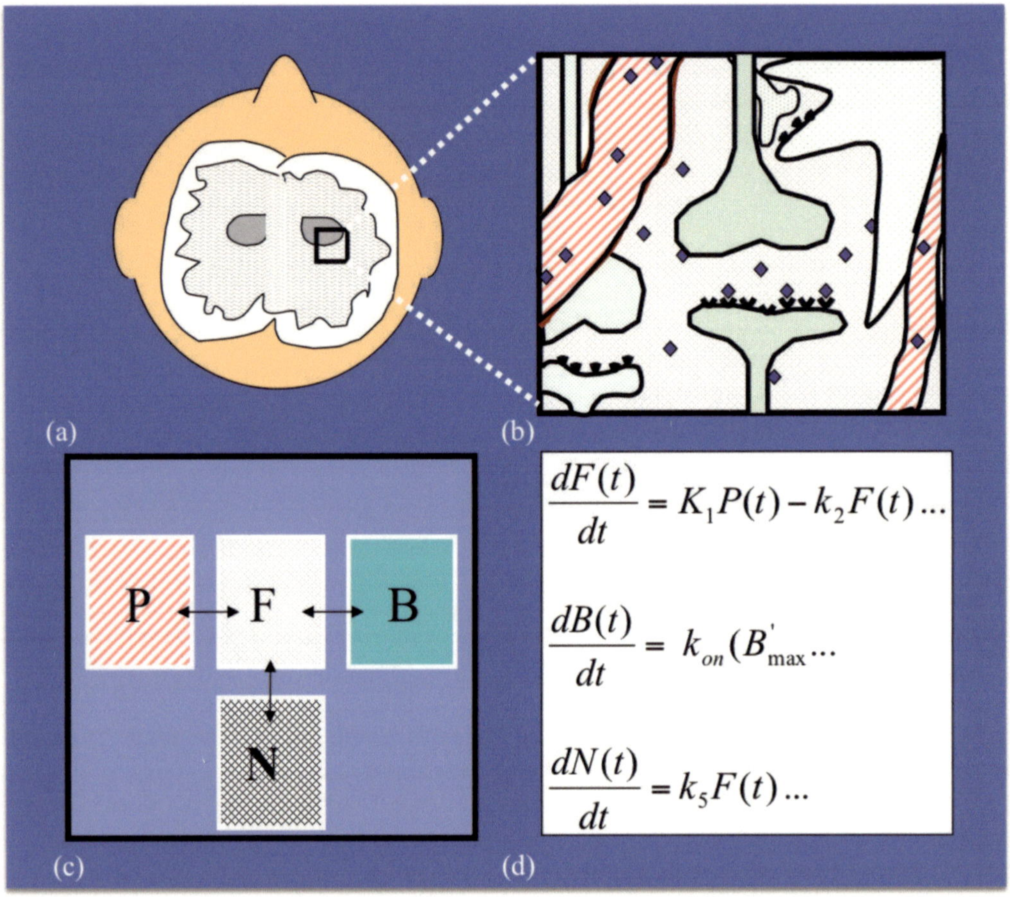


**Figure 11.** Schematic of the tracer kinetic modeling process. (a) Identify an organ of interest and a region of interest within it. (b) Consider the relevant physiology or biochemistry. (c) Abstract the tracer pools into connected compartments. (d) Write the mass balance equations

### *1.2.11.2. Compartmental models (1T, 2T)*

Compartments represent the unknown variables of a model (free tracer, F, bound tracer, B). These are sometimes referred to as "state" variables. Although in most circumstances plasma-borne tracer can be thought of as a distinct "pool", we typically do not assign it a compartment, because it is measured directly via an arterial catheter and therefore not an unknown. Rather, the plasma tracer concentration over time is an input to the system. That is the case for the two most common compartmental models used to describe PET tracers: the one-tissue compartment (1T) and the two-tissue compartment (2T) models (see Figure 12). Each of these models requires measurement of the arterial plasma concentration of tracer as the input function.

Arterial blood taken from the arm is considered a good representation of the tracer concentration in arterial blood reaching the brain at each moment in time. For tracers that are known to bind specifically to a target, it would seem natural to model them with the 2T model. However, the 2T model has 4 unknown parameters: $K_1$, $k_2$, $k_3$, $k_4$. By contrast, the 1T model has one variable, the concentration of tracer in the tissue and only 2 parameters, $K_1$ and $k_2^{1T}$. Note that the $k_2$ parameters have different meanings for each of the two models and so in this chapter, we give them different superscripts to distinguish between them (the reader is advised that this is typically not done in the PET literature). While the 2T model would seem the intuitive choice – especially if we know that specific binding of tracer to a target occurs - it is not always supported by the data. That is, the specific binding may be too fast to allow for reliable estimation of $k_3$ and $k_4$ or it represents only a small fraction of the total uptake or perhaps the signal to noise ratio of the data is poor. Whatever the reason, if we cannot uniquely identify all the parameters of the 2T model by fitting it to the data, the 1T model can be used and the total volume of distribution, $V_t = K_1/k_2^{1T}$, becomes the estimated endpoint. By contrast, $V_t$ as measured with the 2T model is defined as $V_t = K_1/k_2^{2T}(1+BP)$. If the $V_t$ is estimated from parameters of the 1T model, but specific binding exists, then $k_2^{1T}$ implicitly contains effects of the specific binding term, BP.

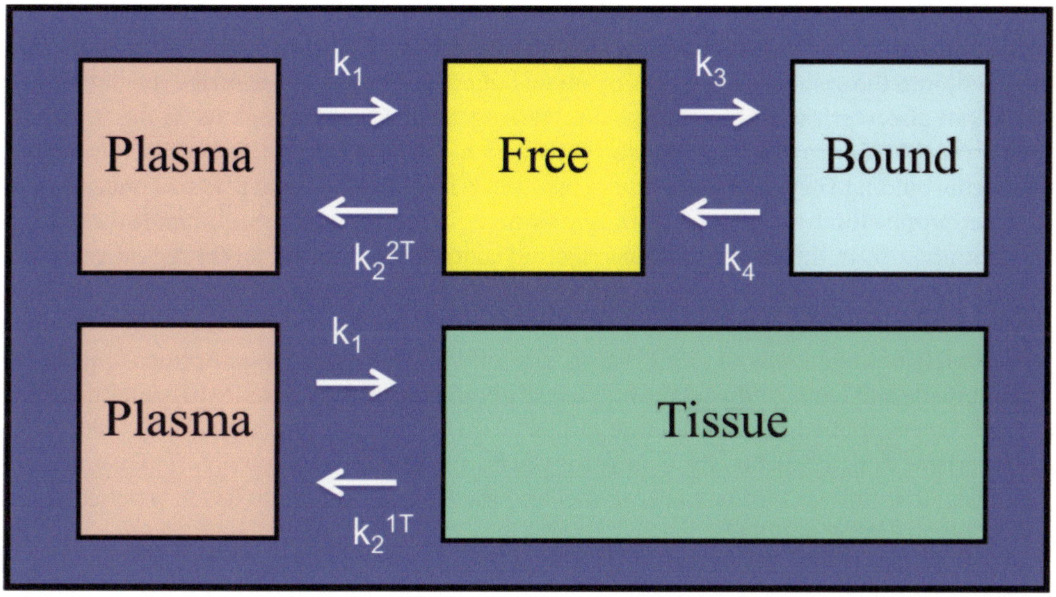


**Figure 12.** Common compartmental models used to analyze PET TACs. 2T model (top) has 2 unknown variables and 4 parameters (rate constants) to be estimated from the data. 1T model has only one variable (the tissue compartment) and 2 rate constants to be estimated.

*1.2.11.3. Graphical methods*

To fit TACs with the 1T or 2T models requires an iterative algorithm and some knowledge of numerical methods, parameter estimation, and computer programming. There is a popular alternative to iterative curve fitting that can be used in many circumstances. Collectively, these methods are based on rearrangements of the model equations to yield linear relationships between measured quantities (Ichise et al., 2003; Logan et al., 1996; Logan et al., 1990; Patlak et al., 1985; Patlak et al., 1983; Zhou et al., 2006). One can think about these methods as transformations akin to a logarithm that transforms an exponential relationship into a linear one. The Logan plot was the first linearization of the 2T model to be applied widely to reversibly bound tracers (e.g., [11C]raclopride). The slope of the original Logan plot is equivalent to the volume of distribution, $V_t$, the same parameter that can be estimated directly with either the 1T or 2T model (Logan et al., 1990). An advantage of using the Logan plot is it is possible to perform all the necessary calculations in a spreadsheet. Further, the estimate of $V_t$ via the Logan plot is highly robust. That is, it almost never fails to produce an estimate with high precision. A disadvantage of the Logan plot is that it is not unbiased. It has been shown to underestimate $V_t$ with increasing noise in the PET data (Slifstein et al., 2000). As with proper experimental design, one must be cognizant of potential biases that can be introduced into the analysis by the model or the model transform and guard against misinterpretation.

#### *1.2.11.4. Reference region methods*

From the diagrams in Figure 12, it would appear that one always needs a measured plasma input function to drive a kinetic model. On its face, this makes sense, since tracers enter (are inputted) into the system via the plasma. In fact, models designed to describe the data in the tissue can also work with input functions derived from reference regions in the image. A reference region is one that is essentially equivalent to the target region except that it is devoid of specific binding sites. By taking advantage of the fact that the same plasma concentration of tracer supplies both the target and the reference regions, it is possible to eliminate the plasma concentration from the model and describe the concentration in the target region compartments in terms of the reference region concentration. In effect, the reference region has become the input function. This concept was first applied to PET data by Farde et al. and by Cunningham et al. (Cunningham et al., 1991; Farde et al., 1989). Subsequent assumptions applied by Lammertsma and Hume reduced the number of parameters in the reference tissue model (thus named the "simplified reference tissue model" (SRTM)) (A. Lammertsma et al., 1996; A. A. Lammertsma et al., 1996). Finally, Gunn et al. devised an implementation of SRTM (using basis functions) that turned it into a linear model and thus almost as easy to use in practice as the Logan plot (Gunn et al., 1997).

### *1.2.12. Physics basics*

The spatial precision of PET is based on the concept of "electronic collimation". That is, radioactive decays lead to pairs of 511KeV photons being emitted in (nearly) opposite directions. When they are captured simultaneously by detectors in the PET scanner ring, a coincidence is recorded. Because of the co-linearity of the paths of the two photons, the direction from which they came is known and physical collimators (used to filter out photons approaching at various angles to the detector) are not needed. The sequence of coincidence detection is diagrammed in Figure 13. But there are certain common ways that electronic

http://dx.doi.org/10.5772/57414

collimation can be foiled and standard corrections must be applied to the raw data to assure that the emission images are quantitative and proportional to concentration of tracer. Some common artifacts that require correction are diagrammed in Figure 14 (counter-clockwise from top left).

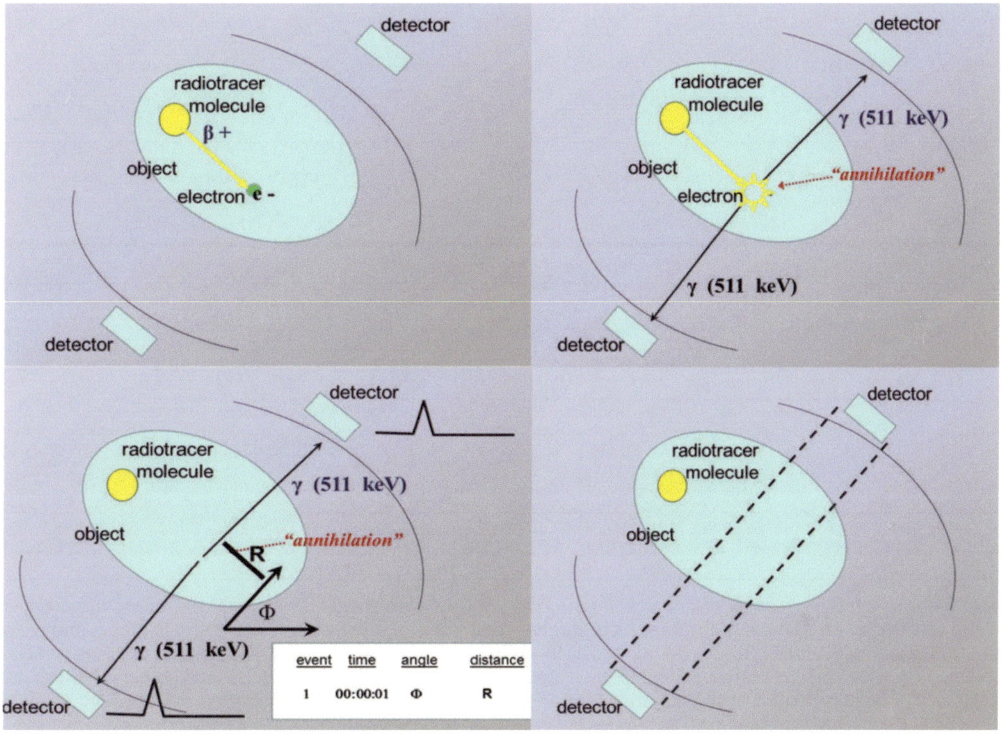


**Figure 13.** (top left) A positron emitter emits a beta particle. (top right) Beta particle annihilates with an electron and two photons are produced which exit the object in opposite directions. (bottom left) The two 511 KeV photons are detected by opposing detectors, leading to signals being recorded. Coincidence logic determines that the events happened within a pre-set time window. The time of the coincidence event and its unique angle, Φ, and distance, R, are recorded. (bottom right) Image reconstruction locates the original annihilation event along a line-of-response (within the dotted lines).

### *1.2.12.1. Scatter*

If either pair of photons emanating from a single annihilation event is deflected from its path but still detected simultaneously with the non-deflected photon, then the positioning of the line of response (between the two detectors) will be incorrect.

### *1.2.12.2. Randoms*

If one photon each from two separate annihilation events is lost to attenuation or scatter and the remaining photons (from different events) are detected simultaneously, the apparent coincidence event will be located improperly.

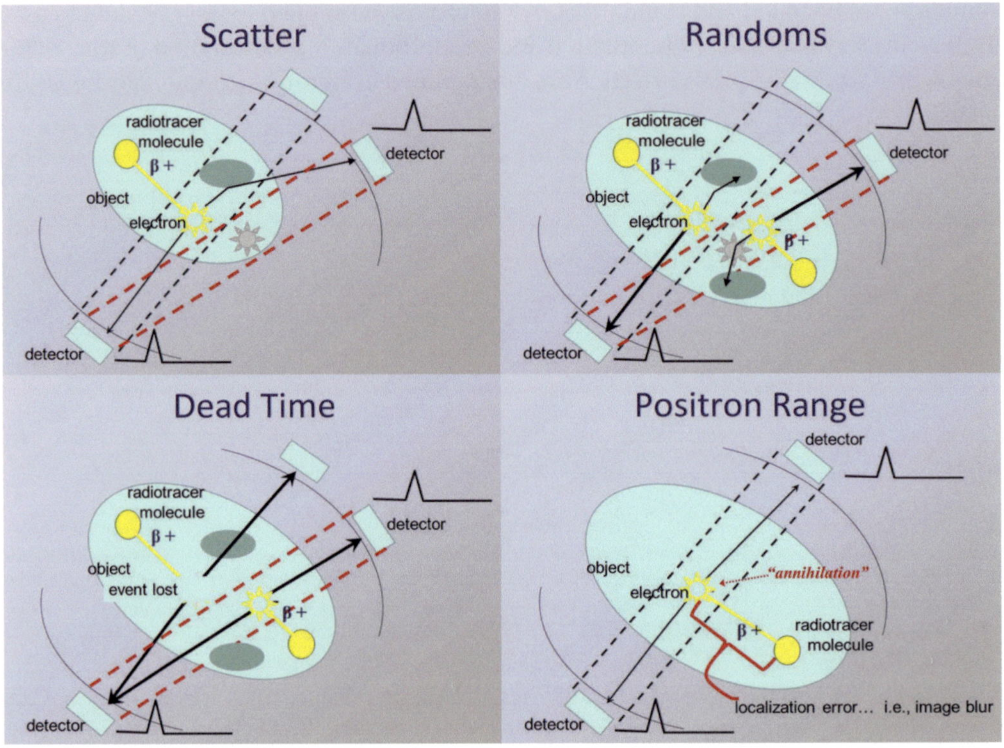


**Figure 14.** (a) Scatter: A collision of one of the daughter photons with scattering material disrupting the normal co-linearity of the photon paths but not their ultimate detection leads to a mis-placement of the line of response (grey start). (b) Randoms: if single photons are absorbed or otherwise not detected, unrelated pairs of photons can be detected as a coincidence leading to a mis-location of the originating event (grey star). (c) Dead Time: if too much radioactivity is in the object such that detectors cannot keep pace with decay events, then information is lost and radioactivity is no longer proportional to tracer concentration. (d) Positron Range: notice that the relocation along a line of response is never tied to the tracer molecule but rather the annihilation even though, in fact, we seek to locate tracer molecule itself. The positron range of a beta particle is inversely related to its energy and represents an unavoidable blurring of the image from ideality.

#### *1.2.12.3. Deadtime*

If the amount of radioactivity in the object is so great that the rate of annihilation events exceeds the capacity of the detectors to record them, then annihilation events will be lost. This condition threatens the quantitative value of PET. We assume that detected coincidences are proportional to concentration of radiotracer molecules in the object. If the detectors are "maxed out", then this desired linear relationship no longer holds and the images are no longer quantitative.

Commercial PET scanners typically come with reconstruction software that corrects for scatter, randoms, and deadtime.

#### *1.2.12.4. Positron range*

When a beta emitter ejects a beta particle, the particle travels some finite distance before annihilating with an electron. The two 511 KeV photons that result from the annihilation are

http://dx.doi.org/10.5772/57414

thus emitted from a location that is some distance from the location of the tracer molecule that we seek to localize. This distance, called the positron range, is an average distance that is dependent on the energy of the emitted beta (see Table 2). Positron range contributes uncertainty to the localization of the deposited radiotracer. Because it is not directional (equally likely for beta to travel in any direction), the positron range contributes a blur to the image.

| Nuclide | $T_{1/2}$ (min) | Photon Energy (keV) | Positron Energy (MeV) | Positron Range (mm in $H_20$) |
|---|---|---|---|---|
| $^{15}O$ | 2.1 | 511 | 1.70 | 1.5 |
| $^{13}N$ | 10.0 | 511 | 1.19 | 1.4 |
| $^{11}C$ | 20.3 | 511 | 0.96 | 1.1 |
| $^{18}F$ | 109 | 511 | 0.64 | 1.0 |

**Table 2.** Beta energies for common PET isotopes and their positron range

### *1.2.13. Attenuation correction*

Without attenuation correction, regions of an object near its outer surface would appear hotter than regions deep inside because photons emerging from within a body are more likely to be scattered or absorbed and not detected than those starting on or near the body's surface. Data from a CT scan or model can correct non-uniform attenuation in the brain.

#### *1.2.13.1. Attenuation correction artifacts*

A lot of work has gone into improving attenuation correction for whole body images. Consider PET images of the chest. There are large translations of the chest from the beginning to the end of the normal respiratory cycle. Unlike CT imaging which is very fast, we cannot ask subjects to hold their breath for 10 minutes while we acquire an FDG-PET scan of their torso. In fact, the development of PET/CT (two scanners integrated together) was driven in part by the need to have multiple attenuation scans for different phases of the respiratory cycle. Kinahan and colleagues have shown – quite persuasively – that failure to align the transmission scan to data from separate 'gates' (images acquired in different phases of breathing, gated -or triggered - by the respiratory signal) causes serious artifacts on images of the chest (Liu et al., 2009). These artifacts can be so serious that they can be mistaken for tumors (Liu et al., 2009) or as serious defects in cardiac perfusion (Alessio et al., 2007). Alessio et al. showed that perfusion was underestimated by 60% if the attenuation map was misaligned due to normal respiration (Alessio et al., 2007).

Generally, a skull does not expand and contract like a chest (due to respiration), so a single transmission scan taken at the beginning or end of a PET scan session is adequate for attenuation correction of brain images. However, this may not be the case for certain types of studies of drug taking (reviewed below). In these cases, the act of taking a subject out of the scanner and then re-positioning them following drug administration could potentially lead to a mismatch between the transmission scan (taken at start of session) and the PET images acquired after the re-positioning.

## 2. PET Imaging of drug challenge studies

Here, we discuss a series of parameters or conditions that make it challenging to use PET to image receptor changes and drug-induced changes in the human brain. These themes will be repeated throughout the remainder of the chapter as they arise in the discussions of the literature.

### 2.1. Novelty

Many different imaging groups measure drug-induced changes in dopamine release in the scanner or during the study day. However, dopamine is released in response not just to drugs of abuse but also to stress and to novelty. As the majority of subjects in these studies will not have been exposed to these experimental situations in their past, the experience will be novel to them. Suffice to say, it would not be helpful to be imaging novelty-induced dopamine release when one is trying to measure the effect of a drug. One way to avoid this common confound is to expose the subject to the study environment before their participation begins. In the case of our smoking-in-the-scanner studies, we have the subjects lie down in the scanner and simulate smoking at a session prior to a real scan session.

### 2.2. Order effects

Order effects can occur in any scientific study. In rodent studies of drug treatment when a placebo is compared to an active drug, the conditions are counter-balanced so that some rats receive the drug first and other rats receive the placebo first. This eliminates bias that could occur if the order in which drugs were given were to alter the results. In imaging studies, this can be more challenging. When using radiotracers with short half-lives (carbon-11 has a 20.3 minute half-life), it is possible and sometimes preferable to do baseline and drug-challenge scans on the same day. This can reduce the variation between scans that may occur if scans are conducted far apart in time. It also increases the likelihood that the subject will be able to easily complete the study (e.g., it is usually easier for a subject to commit to one day at the PET center rather than having to take off multiple days from their job or school). However, this also makes it more difficult to randomize the order of scans.

Consider scans of amphetamine-induced dopamine release. Amphetamine's effect on dopamine (and thus 11C-raclopride binding) is profound and long-lasting. It is not possible to do the drug-challenge scan on the same day before the baseline scan, since the effect of amphetamine would persist for hours (possibly longer) and corrupt a subsequent "baseline" meas-

http://dx.doi.org/10.5772/57414

urement. On the other hand, if effects of a drug or other stimulus are short-lived, it is generally possible to counter-balance the scans.

## 2.3. Expectation and reward-prediction error

We can learn from the work of Shultz and colleagues that dopamine neurons not only are activated in the presence of most drugs of abuse but that they are activated even before delivery of a drug, in response to cues and other stimuli that are "conditioned" or a conditioned stimulus (CS) (Schultz et al., 1997). Additionally, the dopamine neurons are sensitive to changes and errors in reward, which can be called prediction error. Dopamine neurons in the nonhuman primate brain fired after presentation of a reward that was not paired with a CS. When the reward and CS were paired, the dopamine neurons fired in response to the presentation of the CS and not to the subsequent presentation of the reward (Figure 15). That is, the dopamine neurons activated to the CS itself, because it was *predictive* of a reward (Doyon et al., 2005; Doyon et al., 2006). When the CS is presented and then the reward does not occur (negative prediction error), there is the typical activation to the CS, but then a dip in dopamine neuron activation when the expected reward does not occur. This study highlights how sensitive the dopamine system is to cues and expectation of reward, and care needs to be taken to design PET studies that take this sensitivity into account.

## 2.4. Sex differences

Sex differences are evident in many psychiatric disorders, medical disorders, and also in the normal human brain (Cosgrove, Mazure, et al., 2007). There are sex differences in structure (e.g., total volume of the human brain and some subdivisions), in function (e.g., emotional processing as measured with fMRI), and in chemistry (as measured with PET). These differences are important to measure, as they may clarify the clinical literature. It might be helpful, for instance, to know if the higher prevalence of depression in women vs. men can be explained by greater serotonergic dysfunction in women. Unfortunately, sex differences can also cloud the interpretation of data - if they are not carefully recognized and controlled. In one of our own studies, we were at first convinced of differences in nicotinic Acetylcholine receptor (nAChR) availability between healthy men and women when looking at a standard imaging outcome measure, volume of distribution ($V_T$). On further examination, however, we also found significant differences in total parent of the radiotracer (total unmetabolized radiotracer in the blood) and in $f_P$ (the fraction of radiotracer free in the blood and not bound to plasma proteins). When these two factors were included in the analysis (by use of the normalized outcome, $V_T/f_P$), the apparent sex difference disappeared (Figure 16) (Cosgrove, Mitsis, et al., 2007).

## 2.5. Patient management

Care must be taken in managing any study with human subjects, especially patients who are not typical healthy controls but may be individuals suffering from psychiatric disorders. There is a balance that must be struck between designing a study to answer every possible experimental question and keeping the demands on the participants within reason. As described

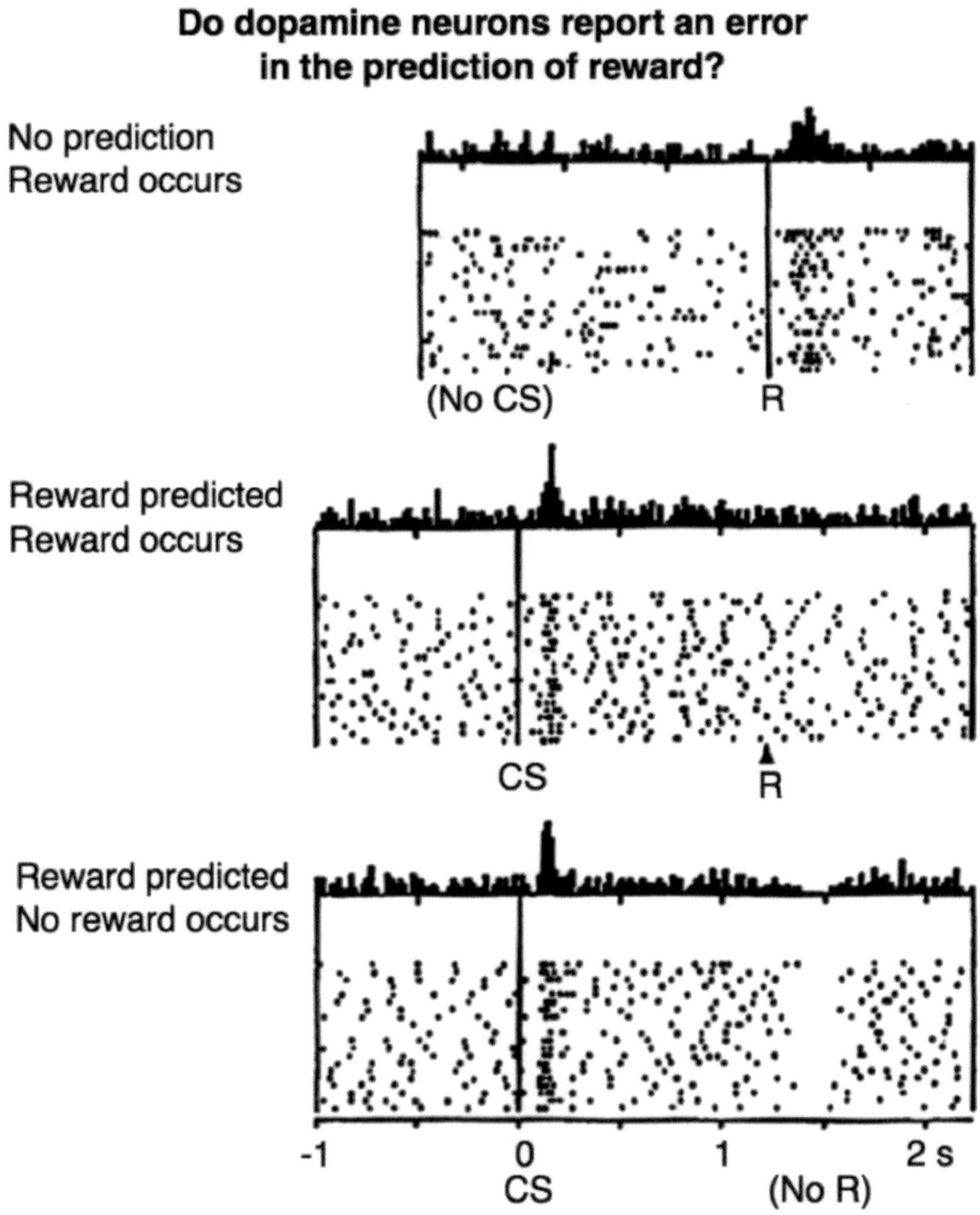


**Figure 15.** (Top) Prior to conditioning, reward without prediction causes a positive error in reward prediction, which increases DA neuron firing. (Middle) Following conditioning, the CS predicts the reward, leading to no prediction error. CS but not reward shows increase in DA neuron firing. (Bottom) After conditioning, CS but no reward causes a negative error in reward prediction. The CS causes increase in DA neuron firing, but the lack of reward causes a DECREASE in DA firing (Schultz et al., 1997).

http://dx.doi.org/10.5772/57414

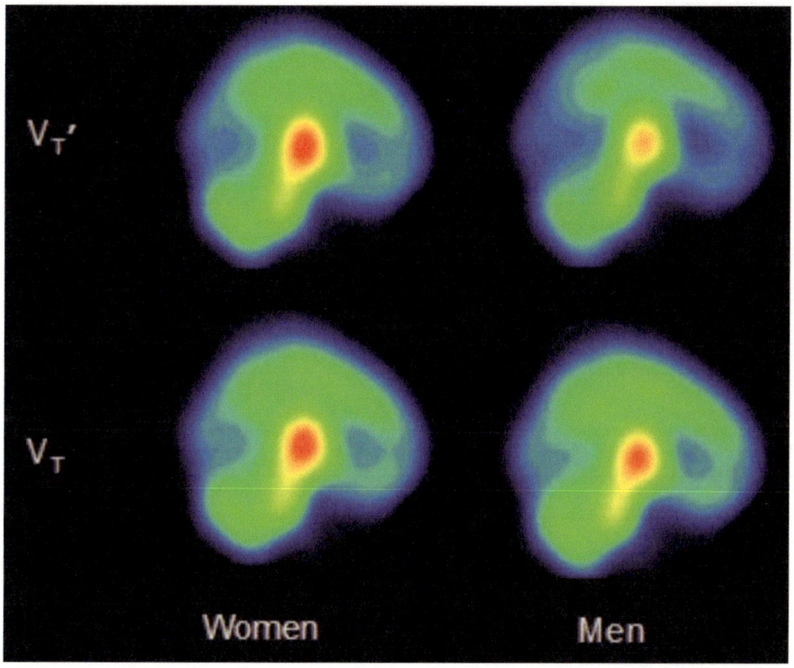


**Figure 16.** Mean parametric images illustrating $^{123}$1-5-IA-85380 activity in 10 men and 19 women in VT' (regional activity divided by total plasma parent between 6 and 8 h) and VT (regional activity divided by free plasma parent between 6 and 8 h). Across brain regions, the main VT' component was significantly greater in women than in men, but the main VT component did not significantly differ between the sexes. This research was originally published in *JNM*. 123I-5-IA-85380 SPECT Imaging of Nicotinic Acetylcholine Receptor Availability in Nonsmokers: Effects of Sex and Menstrual Phase. JNM. 2007;48:1637. © by the Society of Nuclear Medicine and Molecular Imaging, Inc.

below, in many smoking studies we asked our subjects to quit smoking. If this is for a short time, the subjects can manage. When it is for longer, we must implement strategies to help them quit. When we asked *schizophrenic* smokers to quit smoking, we took the additional step of having them stay in an inpatient facility for the week so they could be monitored.

There is also a huge effort that goes into subject recruitment and screening before individuals are invited to participate in studies. Subjects undergo batteries of psychological tests, thorough medical evaluations including a physical exam, complete blood tests, drug toxicology tests, electrocardiograms to ensure cardiac health, and structural MRs to rule out any obvious brain abnormalities. There is also a lengthy informed consent process that must be conducted with all potential subjects. SPECT and PET studies are complex and may involve a variety of risks including administration of radiotracers, placement of arterial lines, and drug administration. Each facet of the study demands discussion between investigator and subject of the potential risks. All of our studies are carefully evaluated and approved by a local radiation safety and a human subjects investigation committee (the latter is typically referred to as an Institutional Review Board or IRB).

| | Brody (2004) | Brody (2006) | Barrett (2004) | Scott (2007) |
|---|---|---|---|---|
| **Tracer** | [$^{11}$C]raclopride | [$^{11}$C]raclopride | [$^{11}$C]raclopride | [$^{11}$C]carfentanil & [$^{11}$C]raclopride |
| **Injection protocol** | Bolus + infusion | Bolus + infusion | Bolus | Bolus + infusion |
| **Tracer dose** | Slow bolus injection 5 mCi, followed by infusion 3mCi/hr | Slow bolus injection 185 MBq, followed by infusion 111 MBq/h | 10 mCi in 10 ml saline over 120 seconds | 10-15 mCi |
| **Scanner (resolution)** | ECAT 953 (5.6 mm FWHM) | GE Advance NXi | ECAT HR+ (42 mm FWHM) | Siemens HR+ (~5.5 x 5.0 mm FWHM) |
| **Design** | Inter-subject (1 scan) | Inter-subject (1 scan) | Intra-subject (2 scans) | Intra-subject (2 scans) |
| **Analysis** | Equilibrium | Equilibrium | SRTM | Logan Ref |
| **Phenomenon to test** | DA release in ventral striatum due to smoking | Gene variants of DA pathway & smoking | DA release due to smoking and hedonic response | $\mu$-opioid and DA D2 receptors and nicotine |
| **Subjects** | 20 nicotine dependent (5 female) | 45 tobacco-dependent smokers | 10 right-handed, non-medicated smokers (5 male) | 6 right-handed, healthy male smokers; 6 age- and sex- matched controls |
| **Subject characteristics** | ≥15 cigarettes/day | • 15-40 cigarettes per day<br>• No overlap with previous study group | Minimum of 2 DSM-IV criteria for nicotine dependence | 15-20 cig/day |
| **Time from last cigarette** | 2 hrs | 3 hrs | Minimum 12 hrs | ~12 hrs |
| **Protocol** | During the scan, subjects had a 10 min break OUTSIDE scanner; 10 smoked 1 cigarette; 10 controls | During the scan, subjects had a 10 min break OUTSIDE scanner; 35 smoked 1 cigarette; 10 controls | 2 scans, 1 control and 1 smoking; smoked in scanner prior to tracer delivery | Tracer infusion (randomized order), smoke 2 denicotinized cigarettes, 45 min, smoke 2 average nicotine cigarettes |
| **Timing** | 10 min break (smoking or not) 50 min post scan initiation | 1 hr scan, 10 min break in outdoor area (smoke/no smoke), 30 min scan | Cigarette 15 min pre [$^{11}$C]raclopride; aimed to smoke 1 cig / 12 min, max. 6 cigs | 90 min scans; smoked each cig for 5 min; smoke denicotinized cig at 2 & 12 min; smoke avg. nicotine cig at 40 & 50 min |
| **Self admin.** | Yes, outside scanner | Yes, outside scanner | Yes, in scanner | Yes, in scanner |
| **Cigarette type** | Usual brand | Either usual brand or standard study cigarette | Usual brand | Denicotinized & average nicotine |
| **Ventral striatum** | -4.3 ± 1.4% | | 3.12% | |
| **Putamen** | • Left -36.6%<br>• Right -29.7% | | • Anterior 2.9%<br>• Posterior -1.59% | |

http://dx.doi.org/10.5772/57414

| | Brody (2004) | Brody (2006) | Barrett (2004) | Scott (2007) |
|---|---|---|---|---|
| Caudate / N Acc | • Left -30.5%<br>• Right -25.9% | -8.4 ± 13.8% | -1.9% | |
| Basal ganglia | | | | 9.98% |
| Concerns | • Going outside for no-smoking group can still be a cue<br>• Not the first cigarette of the day, perhaps not a strong response.<br>• CT only done prior to break, not after return to scanner-possible attenuation issues<br>• Figure 2: 2 subjects driving the effect?<br>• Table 2: baselines are not the same in groups (smoking group higher in all regions, although not significant) | • Only one attenuation scan (following the return to the scanner) was applied to both the pre and post break scans<br>• Some subjects smoked favorite brand, some smoked study standard cigarette • Only 10 controls vs the 35 that smoked | • Not all subjects smoked the same number of cigarettes<br>• Some subjects reported aversive side effects which would alter hedonic ratings<br>• Large range of ΔBP in smoking group (ventral striatum: -57% to 70%) | • Denicotinized cigarettes possibly causing negative prediction error?<br>• Novel use of Logan graphical analysis to detect change in slope – not published elsewhere. |

**Table 3.** Smoking Studies

| | Salonen (1997) | Boileau (2003) | Urban (2010) | Yoder (2009) | Oberlin (2013) |
|---|---|---|---|---|---|
| Tracer | [$^{11}$C]raclopride | [$^{11}$C]raclopride | [$^{11}$C]raclopride | [$^{11}$C]raclopride | [$^{11}$C]raclopride |
| Injection protocol | Bolus | Bolus | Bolus + infusion | Bolus | Bolus |
| Tracer dose | 2.89 – 3.51 mCi | 10 mCi | ~ 7.8 mCi | 14.1 ± 0.99 mCi | 14.9 ± 0.10 mCi |
| Scanner (resolution) | ECAT 931 (6.1 X 6.7 mm) | ECAT HR+ (4.8 x 4.8 x 5.6 mm FWHM) | ECAT EXACT HR+ | EXACT HR+ (9 mm FWHM) | EXACT HR+ (9 mm FWHM effective res.) |
| Design | Intra-subject (2 scans) | Intra-subject (2 scans) | Intra-subject (2 scans) | Intra-subject (3 scans) | Intra-subject (2 scans) |
| Phenomenon to test | Acute alcohol effect on DA release in the striatum | Alcohol induced DA release | Sex differences in DA release post alcohol challenge | Alcohol & alcohol cues | Beer flavor induced DA release |
| Subjects | 7 healthy, right-handed men | 6 healthy male nonalcoholics | 21 healthy men and women | 8 healthy subjects (5 male, 3 female) | 49 healthy male drinkers |
| Subject characteristics | Non drug or alcohol dependent | Nonalcoholic moderate drinkers | Nonalcoholic, 10-15 drinks/wk | Non drug or alcohol dependent; 2 FH+; 5 surpassed hazardous drinking threshold | Non drug/alcohol dependent, except 4 meeting DSM-IV alcohol dependence; 12 FH+ |

| | Salonen (1997) | Boileau (2003) | Urban (2010) | Yoder (2009) | Oberlin (2013) |
|---|---|---|---|---|---|
| **Time from last drink** | ~12 hrs | 24 hours | Since night before | ~24 hours | ~48 hours |
| **Protocol** | • Drink BEFORE scan • 2 scans: 1) placebo, 2 hr break, 2) ethanol | Drink BEFORE scan, not told content of drink until this time | Scan order randomized | 3 scans: 1) neutral cues/no alcohol, 2) alcohol cues predict alcohol (but infusion delayed to post scan), 3) neutral cues with unexpected alcohol (infused during scan) | 2 scans, counterbalanced: 1) preferred beer flavor, 2) Gatorade® flavor |
| **Timing** | 3 separate drinks of placebo (75, 65, 55 min pre bolus), bolus, scan; 2 hr break; same schedule except using ethanol | Drink for 15 min, 30 min prior to bolus | Drink for 5-10 min, 5 min prior to bolus + infusion | Neutral or alcohol cues start 2 min after bolus, maintained 15 min | Beer or Gatorade flavor sprays (~15 ml) start 2 min after bolus, maintained 15 min |
| **Mode of alcohol administration** | Self | Self | Self | Investigator (IV infusion) | N/A |
| **Alcohol type** | Orange juice plus either tap water or ethanol | Orange juice with or without alcohol | Cranberry & soda with alcohol (~3 drinks worth) or trace alcohol | Ringer's lactate with or without alcohol | N/A |
| **Ventral striatum** | | 16.8 ± 16.3% | • Men: -12.1 ± 8% • Women: -6.2 ± 8% | • Cue condition w/ expected intoxication: -0.20 ± 0.1 • Unexpected alcohol condition: 0.12 ± 0.08 | • R ventral striatum: • FH+: 11.7 ± 4.1% (SE) • FH (ambig.): 3.8 ± 2.5% • FH-: 2.7 ± 2.7% |
| **N. acc.** | | 15.0 ± 15.9% | | | |
| **Putamen** | No significant difference: | 5.2 ± 17.5% Ventral 13.7 ± 17.5% | | | |
| **Caudate** | -0.10 ± 0.12 (P = 0.43) | 4.0 ± 16.4% | | | |
| **Concerns** | •Alcohol taken long time prior to scan. • Ethanol condition aversive to subjects? (1 subject too nauseous to have > 1 drink) | •Alcohol taken long time prior to scan. • Subjects drank large amount of alcohol – may have been aversive | • Biased to find greater ΔBP: control condition (smelling alcohol but not receiving any) may have caused negative prediction error | • No conditioning to cues (ala Shultz et al 997). Study assumes that cues are salient. | • Only FH+ subjects showed effect of beer flavor on DA • Lack of resting baseline makes definitive determination of effect direction difficult |

**Table 4.** Alcohol Studies

| | Weerts (2008) | Weerts (2011) |
|---|---|---|
| **Tracer** | [$^{11}$C]carfentanil & [$^{11}$C]methyl naltrindole | [$^{11}$C]carfentanil & [$^{11}$C]methyl naltrindole |
| **Injection protocol** | Bolus | Bolus |
| **Tracer dose** | [$^{11}$C]CAR (19.4 ± 2.1 mCi); [$^{11}$C]MeNTI (19.2 ± 3.2 mCi) | Avg. mCi: [$^{11}$C]CFN: 19.30 (AD), 19.99 (HC); [$^{11}$C]MeNTL: 18.87 (AD), 17.52 (HC) |
| **Scanner (resolution)** | GE (2 x 2 x 4.25 mm) | GE (5.5 x 6.1 mm FWHM) |
| **Design** | Inter-subject | Inter-subject |
| **Phenomenon to test** | Naltrexone occupancy of **δ**- and $\mu$- opioid receptors | **δ**- and $\mu$- opioid receptor availability at baseline |
| **Subjects** | 21 alcohol dependent & healthy control (15 male, 6 female) | 25 alcohol dependent & 30 healthy control |
| **Subject characteristics** | 60+ drinks/month, at least 5 drinks/occasion weekly | DSM-IV criteria for alcohol dependence; controls <8 drinks/wk women, <15 for men |
| **Time from last drink** | 15 days prior to naltrexone treatment | 5 days |
| **Protocol** | 15 days abstinence, followed by 4 days naltrexone | 2 PET scans in fixed order on the same day: [$^{11}$C]MeNTL followed by [$^{11}$C]CFN |
| **Timing** | 19 days inpatient, 50 mg p.o. 2x on day 15, then 1x daily for remainder of days; scan day | 5 days inpatient protocol; scans on day 5 |
| **Mode of alcohol administration** | N/A | N/A |
| **Alcohol type** | N/A | N/A |
| **Ventral striatum** | All ROIs:<br>[11C]CAR: 94.9 + 4.9% occupancy | • AD = 1.826 ± 0.068<br>• HC = 1.438 ± 0.061 |
| **Putamen** | [11C]MeNTI: 21.1 + 14.49% occupancy | • AD = 1.272 ± 0.044<br>• HC = 0.962 ± 0.040 |
| **Caudate** | | • AD = 1.395 ± 0.057<br>• HC = 1.113 ± 0.052 |

**Table 5.** Weerts Studies of Alcohol Dependence

# 3. Preclinical imaging of nicotinic acetylcholine receptors

## 3.1. Using nonhuman primate studies to aid in design of human studies

### *3.1.1. Wash-out of nicotine in the brain*

One key way that nonhuman primate (NHP) studies can help us to inform our clinical studies is to work out basics of experimental design before we inject radiotracers into humans. For imaging studies we conducted with the goal of measuring nicotine-induced "upregulation" of nAChRs in humans, preceding NHP studies played a critical role in experimental design. There is a wealth of literature showing that nicotine and tobacco smoking upregulate nAChRs throughout the brain (Abreu-Villaca et al., 2003; Breese et al., 1997; Kassiou et al., 2001; Marks et al., 1992). Nicotine studies with various doses and routes of administration to rats, mice, and monkeys - as well as postmortem human studies – have all demonstrated that nicotine and tobacco smoke result in significantly more nAChRs throughout the brain compared to saline (animals) or to not smoking (humans). We now know that nicotine itself is responsible for this upregulation. Nicotine acts in the cell to help the receptor subunits assemble and then acts to chaperone the receptors to the cell membrane (Srinivasan et al., 2010). Our goal was to measure this upregulation in living human tobacco smokers (Staley et al., 2006). But first, we needed to work out the proper experimental timing.

Nicotine and our radiotracer, $[^{123}I]$5-IA-85380, both bind to the same receptor in the brain – the nAChR containing the β2-subunit. When nicotine is present in the brain, it blocks the receptor and prevents the radiotracer from binding. Our preclinical experiment consisted of two monkeys drinking nicotine (diluted in water and sweetened with Tang to make it more appetizing) for 6 weeks. After 6 weeks, the monkeys were taken off nicotine. One monkey was scanned at 1 day into nicotine withdrawal, and the other was scanned at 2 days into nicotine withdrawal. Surprisingly, the data showed a *decrease* in radiotracer binding - suggesting that receptors may have been down-regulated! To probe further, we put the monkeys back on nicotine for two weeks and then scanned them both at 7 days of withdrawal. At that point, we saw the robust increase in radiotracer binding that was suggested by the preclinical literature. Taken together, the early data and the 7-day data suggested that nicotine remains in the brain during early withdrawal, and one must wait about 7 days for it to clear before measuring nicotine-induced upregulation. We also measured urine cotinine (the major metabolite of nicotine) levels in the monkeys over the 7 days of withdrawal. Cotinine progressively declined over the week, not completely clearing or reaching nonsmoker levels until 7 days of abstinence. The cotinine data nicely mirrored the brain closely. Once cotinine had cleared, we knew that we could proceed to measure nicotine-induced upregulation of nAChRs in the brain. In our human studies, discussed below, we routinely use low cotinine levels as an indicator that nicotine has cleared and that smokers can be scanned for nAChR.

### *3.1.2. Simplifying the analysis of nAChR availability*

As described in the Introduction, a reference region simplifies the estimation of receptor availability. β2-nAChRs are widely distributed throughout the whole brain with highest density in the thalamus, moderate binding in the cerebellum, striatum and brainstem, and low binding throughout the cortex. There is no region in the brain completely devoid of β2-nAChRs, so there is no appropriate reference region. For many of the studies imaging β2-nAChRs with SPECT or PET described herein, a bolus plus constant infusion paradigm was used to achieve equilibrium between the brain and the blood (see Section 1.2.10.1). The outcome measure was volume of distribution, $V_T$, which can be calculated as concentration of radioactivity in brain divided by concentration of radioactivity in blood, provided an equilibrium has been achieved between tissue and blood concentrations of tracer. $V_T$ is related to

http://dx.doi.org/10.5772/57414

binding potential (BP) and can be used as a measure of receptor availability. Because the bolus plus constant infusion paradigm in these studies reliably achieves equilibrium, the analysis is simplified, and there is no need for kinetic modeling. We refer to our outcome measure as receptor "availability", because we are not measuring all receptors. We cannot measure those receptors which, on average, are occupied by the endogenous neurotransmitter, acetylcholine, or by an exogenous ligand such as nicotine (hence the unexpected results at day 1 of withdrawal) (Staley et al., 2006).

### *3.1.3. Human nAChR scans in tobacco smokers*

Based on the preclinical monkey studies, our group imaged β2-nAChRs in human tobacco smokers at 7-9 days of smoking abstinence ('withdrawal'). In these studies, the subjects were required to quit smoking and not use any medications or nicotine replacement strategies such as the patch, because all forms of nicotine would bind the β2-nAChR and block the radiotracer from binding. In order to help the subjects quit smoking, we used contingency management (Staley et al., 2006). Put simply, subjects met with a member of the research group one to two times per day and gave evidence that they had not smoked. 'Evidence' is established by carbon monoxide breath readings less than 11 parts per million (the level of a nonsmoker) and urine cotinine levels that are at the level of a nonsmoker or decreased from the day before. *Contingent* upon successful tests, subjects are paid small sums of money, and they can typically earn up to $230 for abstaining for up to 9 days. In other words, we used *positive* reinforcement to help the subjects maintain abstinence for the duration of the study. In our first paper, we demonstrated that tobacco smokers at 7-9 days of abstinence have significantly higher β2-nAChR availability in the cortex, striatum, and cerebellum compared to a group of age- and sex-matched nonsmokers (Figure 17). This work confirmed that it is possible to measure the upregulation phenomenon in human smokers, *in vivo* (Staley et al., 2006).

There is also evidence from preclinical and postmortem studies that the β2-nAchRs do not stay upregulated but return to control levels. A postmortem study indicated that smokers who had quit smoking at least two months prior to their death had β2-nAChR levels similar to controls (Breese et al., 1997). However, smokers in the study had quit anywhere from 2 months to 30 years prior to their death, so the study did not shed light on the acute time course of receptor changes, e.g., during acute withdrawal in the first few months of abstinence. In our next study, we imaged β2-nAChR changes over the first few months of abstinence in tobacco smokers (Cosgrove et al., 2009). As shown in Figure 17, at one day of abstinence, nicotine is still present in the brain blocking the receptor, and there is no difference in β2-nAChR availability compared to the group of nonsmokers. At one week of abstinence, we again demonstrate there is higher β2-nAchR availability in smokers compared to nonsmokers. Then even at 2 and even 4 weeks of abstinence, receptor availability remains high and does not return to nonsmoker control levels until 6-12 weeks of abstinence. This study demonstrates that upregulation of β2-nAChRs is persistent, and these brain changes during acute abstinence are consistent with the clinical course of smoking cessation in which craving, relapse, and withdrawal symptoms occur over the first few months of abstinence, and relapse may occur months or years after the last cigarette. It is possible that nicotine replacement strategies are effective in some people,

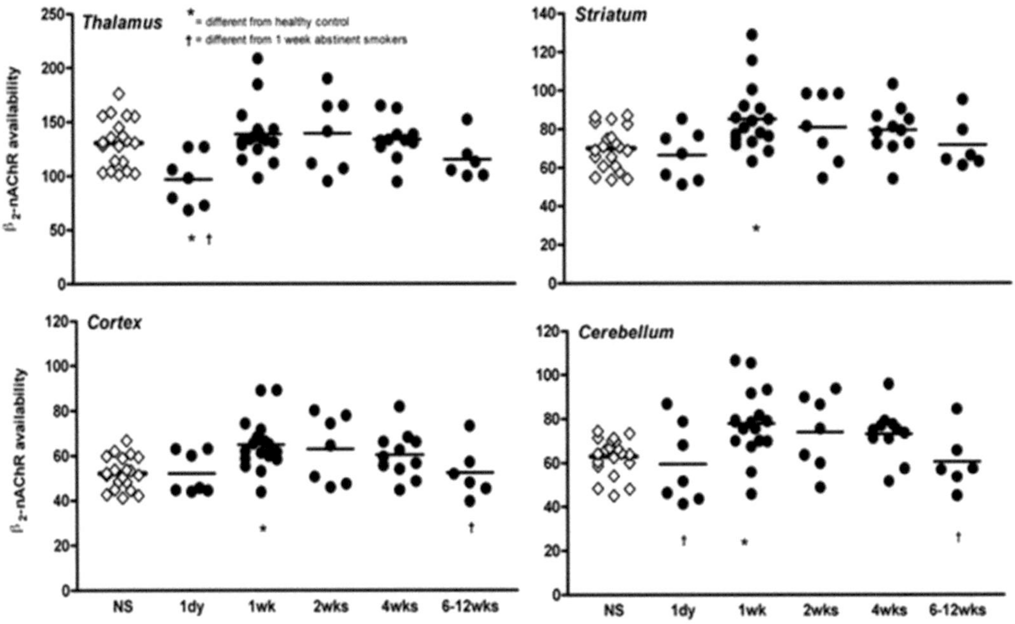


**Figure 17.** $\beta_2$-nAChR availability ($V_T/f_P$) is shown in individual nonsmokers (open diamonds) and tobacco smokers (filled circles) at 1 day, 1 week, 2 weeks, 4 weeks, and 6-12 weeks of abstinence in the thalamus, striatum (average of caudate and putamen), cortex (average of cortical regions including parietal, frontal, anterior cingulate, temporoinsular, and occipital cortex), and cerebellum. The line in each scatter plot represents the mean value of those subjects. * indicates significant difference from control nonsmokers after Bonferroni's correction using two-sample t-tests. † indicates significant difference from 1 week abstinent smokers after Bonferroni's correction using planned post-hoc between-group comparisons subsequent to the analysis of repeated measures mixed-effects regression models including the overall effect of abstinent smoker group.

because they continue to activate the pool of upregulated receptors and help "wean" the receptors off of nicotine as the dose of nicotine is decreased over time.

There is a large literature demonstrating sex differences in tobacco smoking behaviors. In general, men tend to smoke for the nicotine reinforcement, or nicotine *per se* in the cigarette, whereas women tend to smoke more for the sensory cues associated with smoking, as well as affect and stress regulation (Perkins, 2009; Perkins et al., 1999; Perkins et al., 2008). There are also two preclinical studies showing that male rats and mice exposed to nicotine exhibited greater nAChR upregulation than female rats and mice exposed to nicotine (Koylu et al., 1997; Mochizuki et al., 1998). We wanted to determine if there were sex differences in β2-nAChR availability between men and women smokers compared to nonsmokers. Consistent with the preclinical literature, we found that male smokers had significantly higher β2-nAChRs compared to male nonsmokers (between 9 and 17%) but that women smokers had similar β2-nAChR availability compared to women nonsmokers (between 1 and 3 %) (Cosgrove et al., 2012). This was a striking finding given all the studies demonstrating that nicotine and tobacco smoking upregulate β2-nAChRs throughout the brain. Considering known behavioral sex differences in tobacco smoking, these findings make sense and provide

http://dx.doi.org/10.5772/57414

a biological mechanism that may underlie some of the behaviors. Specifically, men smoke for the nicotine in cigarettes, they are more responsive to nicotine replacement therapy as a cessation strategy, and men's brains are responsive to nicotine, exhibiting upregulation of β2-nAChRs. Women smoke for affect regulation and for reasons other than the nicotine, they do not respond as well to nicotine replacement strategies, and their brains do not respond to nicotine by increasing β2-nAChRs. The bottom line is that novel treatment strategies targeting other receptor systems need to be evaluated to more effectively help women quit smoking. All the current strategies act at the β2-nAChR, and, of course, all nicotine replacement strategies act at that site. Varenicline (Chantix) is a partial agonist at the β2-nAChR, and even bupropion (Zyban) is a nicotinic antagonist.

In addition to receptor changes, imaging studies have informed our knowledge about what happens in the brain after someone smokes a cigarette. For example, after one puff of a cigarette, approximately 50% of all β2-nAChRs in the brain are occupied by nicotine. After smoking one or two cigarettes, the receptors are saturated, so 100% of β2-nAchRs are occupied by nicotine (Brody, Mandelkern, London, et al., 2006). We know that nicotine doesn't clear the brain right away, so if all the receptors are occupied by nicotine, why do people keep smoking throughout the day? This brings up some important points about tobacco smoking. People smoke for many different reasons, and nicotine reinforcement is only one component. The reinforcement or pleasure derived from nicotine, like many other drugs of abuse, is necessary in driving the initial phases of drug seeking behavior. But as the addiction progresses, many people continue to smoke in order to avoid withdrawal symptoms and due to the many conditioned cues that have become ingrained, which are a part of the repetitive nature of tobacco smoking. Additionally, there are 4000 chemical compounds that are produced when a cigarette burns; all of these compounds are in tobacco smoke and are inhaled. Thus, while nicotine is the primary addictive component of tobacco smoke, there are additional compounds such as MAO-A and MAO-B inhibitors that likely play a role.

Other imaging studies have demonstrated that even smoking a denicotinized cigarette, which supposedly has very low nicotine content, still occupies up to 20% of β2-nAChRs in the brain (Brody et al., 2008). This is similar to the level of occupancy produced by second hand smoke. Dr. Arthur Brody and colleagues at UCLA performed an elegant study examining the effect of second hand smoke on β2-nAChRs by having subjects sit in a car (the window was down a few inches) with a person smoking, and they reported up to 20% of β2-nAChRs were occupied by nicotine in the individual who was just sitting in the car, not smoking (Brody et al., 2012). Interestingly, a recent law in California prohibits smoking in the car with children under the age of 18.

#### *3.1.4. Use of microdialysis measurements*

Before PET made possible indirect measurement of dopamine release, *in vivo*, the only way to measure dopamine levels in a living brain was via microdialysis. Microdialysis is used primarily in rodents. During a surgery, a probe is placed through the skull into the region of interest, e.g., the nucleus accumbens. After recovery, dopamine levels can be sampled in the awake, behaving animal typically in response to a drug or a stimulus. Di Chiara and Imperato performed the seminal study showing that drugs abused by humans release DA in the nucleus accumbens of the rat brain using this technique (Di Chiara et al., 1988). Amphetamine (1.0 mg/kg, SC) raised DA levels over 1000% from baseline, whereas ethanol (1.0 g/kg, IP) and nicotine (0.6 mg/kg, SC) raised DA levels to 200% over baseline levels. This illustrates how powerful DA release can be when it is directly stimulated as with amphetamine, which is both a direct DA releaser and DA reuptake inhibitor. Put into context, a similar dose of amphetamine given to a monkey or a human in a PET experiment, which is an indirect measure of change in DA, would result in a 15-30% change in BP as measured with [$^{11}$C]raclopride or another D2/3 ligand.

## 4. Imaging dopamine release in response to nicotine, tobacco smoking, and alcohol in humans

As we have recounted, one natural strategy for using PET and SPECT to study smoking has been to image nAChR directly with a nicotinic ligand. Such studies have led to greater understanding of nicotine's persistence in the brain, sex differences in nAChR levels, and the role of nicotine in up-regulation of those levels. There is a second way that molecular imaging techniques can shed light on the neurochemistry of smoking (and drinking). As suggested by microdialysis studies, the mesolimibic DA system is important as the common pathway through which all drugs of abuse – and other rewarding inputs - are processed. With PET and a dopaminergic ligand that competes with DA for binding to a receptor, one could, in theory, image the effects of reward processing in the brain in response to an addictive substance or behavior. In practice, such studies have proved quite challenging and the reader must take care to consider the strengths and weaknesses of each attempt. One challenge is that neither alcohol nor nicotine causes large elevations of DA levels above baseline – probably only a doubling or tripling of baseline. And, the effects of both drugs are short-lived. A third challenge is that self-administration of the substances by a volunteer (smoking a cigarette, drinking a beer) is not easily performed within the confines of the PET scanner.

### 4.1. Nicotine and tobacco smoking

Most of the PET studies of the dopaminergic response to cigarette smoking and/or nicotine are summarized in Table 2. Barrett et al. did one of the earliest studies of smoking with PET; the first study with smokers actually smoking in the scanner (Barrett et al., 2004). The tracer was [11C]raclopride, a D2 antagonist that has been found to be sensitive to changes in endogenous DA (Dewey et al., 1993; Seeman et al., 1989). Barrett et al. used the paired-bolus design described in Figure 10 (left). But instead of administering the stimulus (i.e., smoking a cigarette) prior to the tracer, subjects were asked to smoke repeatedly (six times!) while in the scanner for the one-hour smoking scan. No task was performed during the baseline scan. The authors did not find any significant change in raclopride binding potential from baseline in any areas of the striatum when they looked at the results of all 10 smokers together. The study was, however, characterized by very large variation in ΔBP across smokers (range in ventral striatum: [-57%, 70%]). When the subjects who experienced "mood elevating effects in response

http://dx.doi.org/10.5772/57414

to [ ] smoking" (n=5) were broken out from the complete cohort, the authors found a 21% decrease in BP from baseline (i.e., increase in DA) in the caudate.

There were some notable innovations in the Barrett et al. study as well as some reasons for caution in interpretation. On the plus side, the smokers smoked in the scanner - thus any DA release detected could be attributed to the entire smoking behavior – something not possible with animals but highly relevant for medications development. The smokers were asked to smoke their own brand - another way of assuring that behavior in the scanner approximated subjects' smoking behavior. The authors recognized that, strictly speaking, the comparison of a baseline BP to one measured under a drug condition requires that a new level of DA be *constant* and maintained throughout the latter scan (we will return to this later). Because smoking probably causes only brief elevation of DA (Di Chiara et al., 1988), the investigators required repeated cigarettes – starting 15 minutes prior to tracer - in an attempt to achieve a constant elevated DA during the drug scan. Subjects were also asked to rate the "hedonic value" of their experience and their craving every 15 minutes during the smoking session. The investigators probed their data in creative and innovative ways. Across subjects (i.e., one data point per subject), they looked for correlations at every voxel in the striatum between change in BP from baseline and craving. $R^2$ values were then converted to t-scores, which were thresholded at $p < 0.05$. They found a relationship between craving and $\Delta$BP in dorsal and posterior areas of striatum.

On the downside, the extreme variability in BP values suggests the possibility of motion artifact and/or resolution limitations that would preferentially mar the measurement of activity in very small regions, such as the ventral striatum. Subject motion during smoking is unavoidable and could easily explain the wild variability between subjects. The protocol of six cigarettes in an hour is overly demanding and was very likely aversive to some of the subjects. Four subjects were unable to complete the prescribed regimen of cigarettes. Needless to say, imaging of aversive stimuli was not the intended aim of the study and would have constituted a confound. In our own experience, smokers move their heads when they smoke, and they are none too happy to be asked to smoke a second cigarette *even 25 minutes after* a first.

Scott et al. took an entirely different approach to both the experimental paradigm and the analysis (Scott et al., 2007). Their experiment contained only one scan per subject, and yet it involved a bolus of tracer rather than the more standard single-scan design with a bolus plus constant infusion. Two denicotinized cigarettes were smoked in succession early in the scan at 2 and 12 minutes post injection, and two regular nicotine-containing cigarettes were smoked at minutes 40 and 50 post-tracer injection. By virtue of this design, the investigators are asking a slightly different question than in other studies, namely, what role does the nicotine in cigarettes play in DA release? The cohort was extremely small (n=6 right-handed male smokers). There was also a nonsmoker group scanned at baseline and compared to smokers under denicotinized cigarettes. The value of this comparison is questionable at best. For smokers, there was no statistically significant decrease in raclopride binding from denicotinized to nicotine-containing cigarettes in any subregion of the striatum across the six smokers. In many of the regions, the reported standard deviations of the BP estimates were quite high, and the authors would have been well served simply to scan more subjects. As in the case of

Barrett et al., the investigators looked for and found a correlation between change in BP and a behavioral (or demographic) measure (Barrett et al., 2004). In the case of Scott, the significant relationship discovered was between greater decrease in BP (so presumed greater increase in DA) from denicotinized to nicotine-containing vs. degree of dependence on nicotine (as measured by the Fagerström score) (Scott et al., 2007). In contrast to Barrett, the Scott finding was in the ventral striatum. To their credit, Scott et al. corrected their statistical tests for multiple comparisons.

As with the Barrett paper, the Scott paper involved smoking in the scanner, so motion artifacts must be considered a real possibility. Although the paper mentions motion-correction, the state of the art in 2007 would have allowed correction of misalignment between reconstructed frames acquired over minutes. Nothing could have been done about motion of the subject that happened within the duration of a single time-frame (we note that with the advent of list-mode data, high frequency motion monitoring, and interative image reconstruction algorithms, within-frame motion correction is now possible). The investigators were able to carry out a bolus design rather than a bolus plus constant infusion because of their innovative analysis technique. They employed the Logan plot, mentioned above, to linearize the time-activity curves. Their claim was that they could find two separate slopes (two measures of the ratio of Vt in the striatum to Vt in the reference region) within the plot. The first slope would reflect binding of tracer in the early phase of the scan (corresponding to the denicotinized cigarettes), and the second slope would reflect the later phase (nicotine-containing). In our hands, this technique is extremely sensitive to the choice of data-range for each slope (Sullivan et al., 2013), and we have not seen any papers in the literature subsequent to Scott either using or evaluating said technique.

Two other studies should be mentioned. Like Scott et al., they were both focused on measuring the nicotine (as opposed to cigarette) effect on DA release in humans. Montgomery et al. administered nicotine to subjects via nasal spray (Montgomery et al., 2007); Takahashi et al. had subjects chew nicotine gum (Takahashi et al., 2008). Neither group found any significant change in BP with nicotine in any individual striatal region. Takahashi showed a significant decline in [11C]raclopride binding with nicotine administration in the striatum overall. The former seems like the best design; the latter would seem to be susceptible to motion from chewing - despite express instructions to subjects to chew with their lower jaw only. Following up on Scott et al. and Barrett et al., both newer studies looked for correlations between ΔBP and behavior. Montgomery found a correlation between "happiness" and ΔBP in associative striatum. In apparent agreement with Scott et al., Takahashi found voxels in the "ventral putamen" that showed a significant correlation between raclopride ΔBP and Fagerström score.

Finally, the most oft-cited smoking studies were performed by Brody et al. This is the same group at UCLA that did the study of second-hand smoke's ability to occupy nAChR, described above. Brody and colleagues employed yet a different experimental paradigm. Smokers were scanned with an [11C]raclopride bolus plus constant infusion for 90 minutes (Brody et al., 2004). From 50 to 60 minutes, the subjects went outside for a "smoke break". All the while, they were being infused with [11C]raclopride. Ten smokers smoked a cigarette while outside; ten did not. All returned and were repositioned in the scanner and scanned for a further 30

http://dx.doi.org/10.5772/57414

minutes. The data were analyzed with an equilibrium analysis (see Figure 10) comparing BP at baseline (period just preceding smoke break) with BP after smoking (period just following smoke break). The major finding was a large (but variable) amount of DA release in ventral caudate, ventral putamen, which was statistically greater in the smokers who smoked than in those who did not. In a follow up study, the same group used the same protocol two years later, and while they replicated the direction of the findings, the effect size was quite a bit smaller (Brody, Mandelkern, Olmstead, et al., 2006). In both studies, they found that the greater the reduction of craving for a cigarette from pre- to post-break, the greater the reduction in raclopride binding potential in the ventral caudate-nucleus accumbens region. The 2006 paper introduces genetic variation and its possible role in smoking. Subjects were typed for mutations in the genes that encode for dopamine receptors, dopamine transporter or catechol-O-methyltransferase (an enzyme that breaks down catecholamines) proteins. Their results suggest that differences in amount of DA released (change in tracer binding) could be related to mutation status, and this in turn helps to explain some of the inherent variability in the BP numbers in both studies.

There are some real strengths to the UCLA design. There is also some reason for concern. First, there is no smoking in the scanner, so there is no reason to worry about smoking-related head motion. On the other hand, repositioning the smokers without taking a new transmission scan could lead to reconstruction artifacts in the post-smoke-break images (transmission and emission data not aligned). In the investigators' defense, they also scanned a control group of smokers who take their break but do not smoke. There is no reason to expect that emission-transmission misalignment would be more likely in the smokers than in the controls, so it is probably not the driver of their results. The second – and more subtle – reason for caution in interpreting the Brody et al. data requires that we first compare their findings in 2004 with those in 2006.

In the equilibrium analysis, investigators must choose a data window at the end of the pre-break data to use for a baseline measurement. In both cases, the last 10 minutes of data – from 40-50 minutes – was used. In the 2004 paper, they used 10 minutes of data post-break; in 2006, they used 30 minutes. The investigators correctly asserted in their second paper that a key assumption of their analysis is that DA must remain elevated throughout the 30 minutes post-break (this is why Barrett et al. asked subjects to smoke multiple cigarettes) (Brody, Mandelkern, Olmstead, et al., 2006). Unfortunately, this assumption must be incorrect. If it were true, then both studies should have found exactly the same change in BP. But in 2006, they found less of an effect: only 8.4% change as compared to ~30% change in 2004. The explanations offered by the authors were not persuasive: motion-induced DA release in controls, repositioning error. None of these were any more likely to have occurred in the smoking group as opposed to the control. Rather, the discrepancy between 2006 and 2004 is entirely consistent with a change in the analysis procedure that, in essence, washed out the effect by averaging over a period that contains smoking induced DA release and a subsequent period in which DA levels are returning (have returned) to baseline. In other words, they used too wide a data window in their second paper. To be sure, we recently did a simulation study of smoking-induced DA release as measured by raclopride-PET and its dependence on the selection of the data window (Sullivan et al., 2013). While the simulations confirmed what we suspected, they raise an even more troubling concern about all previous attempts to image smoking effects on DA. That is, how can we compare across studies if people use even slightly different analysis techniques? How can we compare across groups if the time-period of response of dopamine to any drug stimulus is short and different between groups? And more generally, how can we apply standard models that assume "that DA concentration will remain elevated" to PET data when the assumption is not true? We address this important technical question in the final section of the chapter following our discussion of drinking studies.

### 4.2. Imaging dopamine release in response to alcohol

If smoking is difficult for subjects lying in the scanner, it is nevertheless possible. Drinking while lying in the scanner is not. Researchers have taken two approaches to this problem. The most obvious study design for measuring alcohol-induced DA release is for the subject to drink an alcoholic beverage shortly before being scanned and compare raclopride BP in this condition to either baseline or placebo. This is the approach that was employed by the three studies to look at drinking-induced DA release, per se. Salonen et al., Boileau et al., and Urban et al. each used two-scan designs (Boileau et al., 2003; Salonen, 1997; Urban et al., 2010). In each case, the conditions were either juice or alcohol plus juice. The conditions were randomized in the latter two studies. The Boileau and Salonen studies each consisted of 6 subjects; Urban scanned 11 men and 10 women. The subjects were social drinkers. The dose of alcohol was approximately 1 ml/kg in Boileau and Urban but about 1.3 ml/kg in Salonen. The blood alcohol levels in each study were consistent and generally reflected the respective doses (measurements were not taken at the same times, so direct comparisons are difficult). In any case, Urban claims that the dose in her study was equivalent to 3 standard drinks. Where the paradigms begin to diverge is the relative timing of alcohol and tracer. The alcohol was taken either 60 minutes, 30 minutes or 5 minutes prior to tracer injection in Salonen, Boileau and Urban, respectively. A second difference was that in the Urban study, the rim of the juice glass for the juice-only condition was coated with alcohol to minimize any difference in the subjects' expectation between conditions. A final noteworthy difference is that the Urban study used paired bolus plus infusion scans, whereas the other studies both used the more standard paired-bolus design.

The Salonen and Urban studies were essentially negative. No statistically significant decrease in [11C]raclopride binding was found in any region of the striatum in the alcohol condition compared to juice. Boileau reported decreases of 14-15% in raclopride BP in regions that they termed Nucleus Accumbens and Ventral Putamen. Despite finding no statistically significant drop in BP in any individual region, Urban reported a sex difference in decrease in BP in all regions taken together (see paper for further explanation). What is clear from these studies is that imaging effects of oral alcohol on DA in the striatum is not easy and that we may be at the limits of detectability for raclopride-PET. Perhaps if we scrutinize elements of each design, we may find something worth tweaking. In all studies, the amount of alcohol was quite large. Some subjects – even social drinkers – may have found it aversive. Each study reported at least one subject who dropped out. As with the smoking studies, the idea is to image drug-taking,

http://dx.doi.org/10.5772/57414

not aversion. In the Salonen study, the alcohol was taken a lengthy time before the tracer (from 75 – 55 min before). Although the authors were careful to document considerably elevated blood alcohol at both the beginning and end of the (1 hour) scanning period, one should not confuse elevated alcohol level with elevated DA. In fact, it is likely that DA responds early to drinking – possibly to the cues or the rapid rise in brain alcohol and then returns to baseline more quickly than alcohol level itself. In fact, it appears that Oberlin et al. have demonstrated that DA responds to the cues for alcohol rather than the alcohol itself (Oberlin et al., 2013). Consider nicotine. Nicotine remains in the brain for days, but the discrepancy (discussed above) between the 2004 and 2006 Brody papers (and microdialysis data) certainly suggests that nicotine-induced DA elevation is rather brief (Brody, Mandelkern, Olmstead, et al., 2006; Brody et al., 2004). All three alcohol-drinking designs suffer from lack of a baseline condition. Juice alone is used as a placebo, but if the taste of juice is rewarding then perhaps DA was released in this condition. There is always a difficulty interpreting any study that contains only placebo and drug. The difference could be due to changes during drug or changes during placebo. Consider the Urban design (Urban et al., 2010). In order to control expectation across conditions, the juice-only glass was rimmed with alcohol. But what if the smell of alcohol actually set up an expectation of alcohol? In that case, the juice condition was scanned while the subject experienced disappointment over not receiving the reward. This is called "reward prediction error" and in monkeys, it has been shown to be the cause of decreased dopaminergic firing rates as discussed previously (Schultz et al., 1997). Is there any evidence that reward prediction error leads to alteration of dopamine levels in humans? We must consider one last raclopride-PET paper to answer that question.

Yoder et al. took a different experimental approach to the study of alcohol-induced DA release (Yoder et al., 2009). Wary of the variability in alcohol absorption among people, they chose to administer the alcohol intravenously. The technique, called the "alcohol clamp", was developed by O'Connor et al. and is based on pharmacokinetic modeling of a variable-rate infusion of alcohol to maintain a constant blood alcohol level in each subject based on their height, weight, and gender (O'Connor et al., 1998). Second, expectation was controlled through visual and olfactory cues, which preceded – and predicted - the delivery of alcohol or saline, IV. There were three conditions scanned in three separate sessions – each scanned with a bolus of [11C]raclopride. The conditions were as follows: #1: neutral cues signaling IV saline, #2: alcohol cues signifying alcohol, and #3: neutral cues coupled with unexpected alcohol. This design was constructed to decouple expectation from consumption of alcohol. The alcohol in condition #2 was delivered *after* the data acquisition was complete, so the condition can be thought of "expectation of alcohol but no alcohol consumption" whereas condition #3 – thanks to a little trickery – can be thought of as "alcohol consumption with no expectation of alcohol". Subjects' answers to questionnaires during the scan confirmed that expectations were controlled as intended. The results were quite provocative: in left ventral striatum, BP of "alcohol consumption without expectation" went down relative to condition #1. That is, this comparison signifies increase in DA. But, in the contralateral ventral striatum, BP of "expectation of alcohol without alcohol consumption" was *higher* than condition #1. The authors explained this combination of results as follows. Expectation of reward without reward is equivalent to negative reward prediction error. Reward without expectation of reward is positive prediction error. The caveat in this interpretation is that the subjects (heavy drinkers) must be considered to have been "conditioned" by their drinking history to respond with appropriate expectation to the cues. Accepting the author's interpretation, this paper highlights the importance of controlling expectation in the study of drugs of abuse. To return to the Urban design (Urban et al., 2010), if the initial smell of alcohol on the rim of the juice-only glass was a cue for imminent alcohol reward, then we might expect DA to decrease during this scan. When compared to a second condition (i.e., alcohol drink), any apparent increase in DA with alcohol could, in fact, be the result of decrease in the juice-only condition.

Finally, in this section we should point out that there are many other important lines of investigation of alcohol abuse using PET other than examining DA release. Some have looked at receptor number (Martinez et al., 2005; Volkow et al., 1996), and others have looked at change in BP due to drugs for treatment of alcohol. We highlight two studies, briefly. Both studies are by Weerts et al. (Weerts et al., 2008; Weerts et al., 2011). Both studies looked at the Mu opioid receptor (MOR) and the Delta opioid receptor (DOR) thanks to the use of two selective tracers, [11C]carfentail and [11C]methyl-naltrindol. Collectively, the two studies looked at baseline level of MOR and DOR, as well as occupancy of the receptors due to four days of treatment with naltrexone, a non-selective opioid receptor antagonist that is prescribed for alcohol abuse. Baseline receptors in alcoholics were compared to healthy controls, and occupancy of naltrexone was measured in alcoholics only. The main findings were that clinical doses of naltrexone occupied 95% of MOR but only 75% of DOR. Second, MOR and DOR levels in high binding regions of the brain were higher in alcoholics than in controls (MOR was significant; DOR was not). The first finding suggests that any variability on efficacy of naltrexone is probably not mediated by binding to MOR, since all alcoholics were uniformly blocked. The second finding suggests that years of drinking may lead to upregulation of MOR and DOR, which is more like nAChR (Cosgrove et al., 2009) and less like D2 (Martinez et al., 2005).

## 5. Limitations of conventional modeling methods — Need for new ones

As previously stated, the "conventional" kinetic models used in all of the work discussed to this point treat BP as a surrogate for number of receptors (because $BP = B_{max}/K_D$ where $B_{max}$ is available, unoccupied receptors and $K_D$ is the affinity of the tracer for the receptor.) Depending on the circumstance, investigators treat ΔBP as change in available receptors due to altered number of receptors or altered level of endogenous transmitter occupying sites. Whether the analysis method is a full fitting of dynamic data or fitting of linearized data via the Logan plot or measurement of equilibrium levels, the underlying kinetic model is the same. In all cases, however, a fundamental assumption of the model(s) is that BP is not changing over the course of the study, because BP is a constant. Mathematically, we say that the kinetic model is time-invariant in parameters. The inadequacies of all three common methods of analysis in the face of transient DA release have been thoroughly studied in the recent paper by Sullivan et al (Sullivan et al., 2013). The reader is directed to that paper for more details. Any violation of the time-invariant parameters assumption could lead to misinterpretation of data. Many if not all of the investigators whose work is profiled herein appreciate this limitation of the kinetic models. As such, they asked subjects to smoke cigarettes every 15 minutes repeatedly (Barrett et al., 2004), or they were careful to assay blood alcohol level at start and end of scan and show that it was the same (Salonen, 1997). Nevertheless, no one can assure that DA remains constant throughout the PET scan. In fact, in the case of drinking or smoking, it almost certainly does not. Recall that if smoking-induced DA levels were constant in the Brody experiments, there would have been no discrepancy between the analyses of the 2004 and 2006 data sets (Brody, Mandelkern, Olmstead, et al., 2006; Brody et al., 2004). If alcohol drinking-induced DA levels were constant, there would be no discrepancy between the Boileau finding of change in BP and the Salonen negative result even though one gave alcohol 30 minutes before the scan, and the other gave it an hour before (Boileau et al., 2003; Salonen, 1997). What's more, if the timing of DA release is different across groups then – as Yoder et al. showed – the mere difference in timing could result in differences in BP and thus be interpreted as differences in magnitude of DA release (Yoder et al., 2004).

We have been working over the last ten years to develop kinetic models of tracer uptake and binding in the presence of transient neurotransmitter release (Constantinescu et al., 2007; Constantinescu et al., 2008; E. Morris et al., 1995; E. D. Morris et al., 2010; E. D. Morris et al., 2013; E. D. Morris et al., 2005; M. D. Normandin et al., 2008; M. D. Normandin et al., 2012; Sullivan et al., 2013). The earlier versions of the model were based on the idea that dopamine (or any other transmitter that competes with tracer) can exist in the free or bound states in addition to the various states of the tracer (refer back to Figures 4 and 11). New species in the model required new "boxes" which, in turn, meant more differential equations (E. Morris et al., 1995; E. D. Morris et al., 2005). The model described the data well (E. Morris et al., 1995; E. D. Morris et al., 2008) but was cumbersome to use. Subsequent work by Constantinescu and by Normandin et al. developed linearized versions of the model that could be solved quickly (and hence at each voxel) while retaining time-varying terms to describe brief changes in neurotransmitter level (M. Normandin et al., 2009). Validation of these models was carried out either (a) by configuring experiments in which a predictable pattern of DA change could be provoked in human subjects (Constantinescu et al., 2008; E. D. Morris et al., 2010), or (b) a comparison could be made between model predictions and microdialysis measurements made in the (rat) subjects at the same time as PET (E. D. Morris et al., 2008; M. D. Normandin et al., 2008; M. D. Normandin et al., 2012). Most recently, we have adapted the Normandin approach to the voxel level so that we can estimate time-courses of dopamine at each voxel in the striatum where "activation" is occurring due to drug stimulus. A critical step in such a process is some sort of statistical test to determine that change in DA really occurred at that location (voxel) in question. Finally, the outcome is a collection of curves in time at many voxels in the brain. The visualization technique that we have invented to display such 4-dimensional results is a "dopamine movie", wherein dopamine level is color-coded and the color in the activated voxels is displayed overlaid on MRI as a series of frames. The methods are described and demonstrated in a new publication in the Journal of Visualized Experiments (E. D. Morris et al., 2013). Validation and testing of these new dopamine movies is ongoing. We hope that they are a more sensitive probe of DA changes in the brain as a consequence of smoking and drinking behavior and that the increased sensitivity of the method will allow us to tease out patterns of response that are either "addictive" or "non-addictive".

## Author details

Evan D. Morris, Molly V. Lucas and Kelly P. Cosgrove

*Address all correspondence to: evan.morris@yale.edu

Yale PET Center, Yale University, USA

## References

[1] Abreu-Villaca, Y., F. J. Seidler, D. Qiao, C. A. Tate, M. M. Cousins, I. Thillai, & T. A. Slotkin. (2003). Short-term adolescent nicotine exposure has immediate and persistent effects on cholinergic systems: critical periods, patterns of exposure, dose thresholds. *Neuropsychopharmacology, 28*(11), 1935-1949.

[2] Alessio, A. M., S. Kohlmyer, K. Branch, G. Chen, J. Caldwell, & P. Kinahan. (2007). Cine CT for attenuation correction in cardiac PET/CT. *J Nucl Med, 48*(5), 794-801.

[3] Barrett, S. P., I. Boileau, J. Okker, R. O. Pihl, & A. Dagher. (2004). The hedonic response to cigarette smoking is proportional to dopamine release in the human striatum as measured by positron emission tomography and [11C]raclopride. *Synapse, 54*(2), 65-71.

[4] Biju, G., & R. de la Fuente-Fernandez. (2009). Dopaminergic function and progression of Parkinson's disease: PET findings. *Parkinsonism Relat Disord, 15 Suppl 4,* S38-40.

[5] Boileau, I., J. M. Assaad, R. O. Pihl, C. Benkelfat, M. Leyton, M. Diksic, R. E. Tremblay, & A. Dagher. (2003). Alcohol promotes dopamine release in the human nucleus accumbens. *Synapse, 49*(4), 226-231.

[6] Breese, C., M. Marks, J. Logel, C. Adams, B. Sullivan, A. Collins, & S. Leonard. (1997). Effect of smoking history on [$^3$H]nicotine binding in human postmortem brain. *J Pharmacol Exp Ther, 282,* 7-13.

[7] Brody, A. L., M. A. Mandelkern, M. R. Costello, A. L. Abrams, D. Scheibal, J. Farahi, E. D. London, R. E. Olmstead, J. E. Rose, & A. G. Mukhin. (2008). Brain nicotinic acetylcholine receptor occupancy: effect of smoking a denicotinized cigarette. *Int J Neuropsychopharmacol,* 1-12.

[8] Brody, A. L., M. A. Mandelkern, E. D. London, A. Khan, D. Kozman, M. R. Costello, E. E. Vellios, M. M. Archie, R. Bascom, & A. G. Mukhin. (2012). Effect of secondhand smoke on occupancy of nicotinic acetylcholine receptors in brain. *Arch Gen Psychiatry, 68*(9), 953-960.

[9] Brody, A. L., M. A. Mandelkern, E. D. London, R. E. Olmstead, J. Farahi, D. Scheibal, J. Jou, V. Allen, E. Tiongson, S. I. Chefer, A. O. Koren, & A. G. Mukhin. (2006). Ciga-

rette smoking saturates brain alpha 4 beta 2 nicotinic acetylcholine receptors. *Arch Gen Psychiatry, 63*(8), 907-915.

[10] Brody, A. L., M. A. Mandelkern, R. E. Olmstead, D. Scheibal, E. Hahn, S. Shiraga, E. Zamora-Paja, J. Farahi, S. Saxena, E. D. London, & J. T. McCracken. (2006). Gene variants of brain dopamine pathways and smoking-induced dopamine release in the ventral caudate/nucleus accumbens. *Arch Gen Psychiatry, 63*(7), 808-816.

[11] Brody, A. L., R. E. Olmstead, E. D. London, J. Farahi, J. H. Meyer, P. Grossman, G. S. Lee, J. Huang, E. L. Hahn, & M. A. Mandelkern. (2004). Smoking-induced ventral striatum dopamine release. *Am J Psychiatry, 161*(7), 1211-1218.

[12] Brooks, D. J., E. P. Salmon, C. J. Mathias, N. Quinn, K. L. Leenders, R. Bannister, C. D. Marsden, & R. S. Frackowiak. (1990). The relationship between locomotor disability, autonomic dysfunction, and the integrity of the striatal dopaminergic system in patients with multiple system atrophy, pure autonomic failure, and Parkinson's disease, studied with PET. *Brain, 113 ( Pt 5)*, 1539-1552.

[13] Carson, R. E., M. A. Channing, R. G. Blasberg, B. B. Dunn, R. M. Cohen, K. C. Rice, & P. Herscovitch. (1993). Comparison of bolus and infusion methods for receptor quantitation: application to [18F]cyclofoxy and positron emission tomography. *J Cereb Blood Flow Metab, 13*(1), 24-42.

[14] Constantinescu, C. C., C. Bouman, & E. D. Morris. (2007). Nonparametric extraction of transient changes in neurotransmitter concentration from dynamic PET data. *IEEE Trans Med Imaging, 26*(3), 359-373.

[15] Constantinescu, C. C., K. K. Yoder, D. A. Kareken, C. A. Bouman, S. J. O'Connor, M. D. Normandin, & E. D. Morris. (2008). Estimation from PET data of transient changes in dopamine concentration induced by alcohol: support for a non-parametric signal estimation method. *Phys Med Biol, 53*(5), 1353-1367.

[16] Cosgrove, K. P., J. Batis, F. Bois, P. K. Maciejewski, I. Esterlis, T. Kloczynski, S. Stiklus, S. Krishnan-Sarin, S. O'Malley, E. Perry, G. Tamagnan, J. P. Seibyl, & J. K. Staley. (2009). beta2-Nicotinic acetylcholine receptor availability during acute and prolonged abstinence from tobacco smoking. *Arch Gen Psychiatry, 66*(6), 666-676.

[17] Cosgrove, K. P., I. Esterlis, S. A. McKee, F. Bois, J. P. Seibyl, C. M. Mazure, S. Krishnan-Sarin, J. K. Staley, M. R. Picciotto, & S. S. O'Malley. (2012). Sex differences in availability of beta2*-nicotinic acetylcholine receptors in recently abstinent tobacco smokers. *Arch Gen Psychiatry, 69*(4), 418-427.

[18] Cosgrove, K. P., C. M. Mazure, & J. K. Staley. (2007). Evolving knowledge of sex differences in brain structure, function, and chemistry. *Biol Psychiatry, 62*(8), 847-855.

[19] Cosgrove, K. P., E. M. Mitsis, F. Bois, E. Frohlich, G. D. Tamagnan, E. Krantzler, E. Perry, P. K. Maciejewski, C. N. Epperson, S. Allen, S. O'Malley, C. M. Mazure, J. P. Seibyl, C. H. van Dyck, & J. K. Staley. (2007). 123I-5-IA-85380 SPECT imaging of nico-

tinic acetylcholine receptor availability in nonsmokers: effects of sex and menstrual phase. *J Nucl Med, 48*(10), 1633-1640.

[20] Cunningham, V. J., S. P. Hume, G. R. Price, R. G. Ahier, J. E. Cremer, & A. K. Jones. (1991). Compartmental analysis of diprenorphine binding to opiate receptors in the rat in vivo and its comparison with equilibrium data in vitro. *J Cereb Blood Flow Metab, 11*(1), 1-9.

[21] Dewey, S. L., G. S. Smith, J. Logan, J. D. Brodie, J. S. Fowler, & A. P. Wolf. (1993). Striatal binding of the PET ligand 11C-raclopride is altered by drugs that modify synaptic dopamine levels. *Synapse, 13*(4), 350-356.

[22] Di Chiara, G., & A. Imperato. (1988). Drugs abused by humans preferentially increase synaptic dopamine concentrations in the mesolimbic system of freely moving rats. *Proc Natl Acad Sci U S A, 85*(14), 5274-5278.

[23] Doyon, W. M., S. K. Anders, V. S. Ramachandra, C. L. Czachowski, & R. A. Gonzales. (2005). Effect of operant self-administration of 10% ethanol plus 10% sucrose on dopamine and ethanol concentrations in the nucleus accumbens. *J Neurochem, 93*(6), 1469-1481.

[24] Doyon, W. M., E. C. Howard, T. S. Shippenberg, & R. A. Gonzales. (2006). Kappa-opioid receptor modulation of accumbal dopamine concentration during operant ethanol self-administration. *Neuropharmacology, 51*(3), 487-496.

[25] Farde, L., L. Eriksson, G. Blomquist, & C. Halldin. (1989). Kinetic analysis of central [11C]raclopride binding to D2-dopamine receptors studied by PET--a comparison to the equilibrium analysis. *J Cereb Blood Flow Metab, 9*(5), 696-708.

[26] Farde, L., H. Hall, E. Ehrin, & G. Sedvall. (1986). Quantitative Analysis of D2 Dopamine Receptor Binding in the Living Human Brain by PET. *Science, 231*(4735), 258-261.

[27] Gunn, R. N., A. A. Lammertsma, S. P. Hume, & V. J. Cunningham. (1997). Parametric imaging of ligand-receptor binding in PET using a simplified reference region model. *Neuroimage, 6*(4), 279-287.

[28] Ichise, M., J. S. Liow, J. Q. Lu, A. Takano, K. Model, H. Toyama, T. Suhara, K. Suzuki, R. B. Innis, & R. E. Carson. (2003). Linearized reference tissue parametric imaging methods: application to [11C]DASB positron emission tomography studies of the serotonin transporter in human brain. *J Cereb Blood Flow Metab, 23*(9), 1096-1112.

[29] Innis, R. B., V. J. Cunningham, J. Delforge, M. Fujita, A. Gjedde, R. N. Gunn, J. Holden, S. Houle, S. C. Huang, M. Ichise, H. Iida, H. Ito, Y. Kimura, R. A. Koeppe, G. M. Knudsen, J. Knuuti, A. A. Lammertsma, M. Laruelle, J. Logan, R. P. Maguire, M. A. Mintun, E. D. Morris, R. Parsey, J. C. Price, M. Slifstein, V. Sossi, T. Suhara, J. R. Votaw, D. F. Wong, & R. E. Carson. (2007). Consensus nomenclature for in vivo imaging of reversibly binding radioligands. *J Cereb Blood Flow Metab, 27*(9), 1533-1539.

http://dx.doi.org/10.5772/57414

[30] Kassiou, M., S. Eberl, S. Meikle, A. Birrell, C. Constable, M. Fulham, D. Wong, & J. Musachio. (2001). In vivo imaging of nicotinic receptor upregulation following chronic (-)-nicotine treatment in baboon using SPECT. *Nuc Med Biol, 28*, 165-175.

[31] Koylu, E., S. Demirgoren, E. London, & S. Pogun. (1997). Sex difference in up-regulation of nicotinic acetylcholine receptors in rat brain. *Life Sci, 61*, PL 185-PL190.

[32] Lammertsma, A., & S. Hume. (1996). Simplified referene tissue model for PET receptor studies. *Neuroimage, 4*, 153-158.

[33] Lammertsma, A. A., C. J. Bench, S. P. Hume, S. Osman, K. Gunn, D. J. Brooks, & R. S. Frackowiak. (1996). Comparison of methods for analysis of clinical [11C]raclopride studies. *Journal of cerebral blood flow and metabolism : official journal of the International Society of Cerebral Blood Flow and Metabolism, 16*(1), 42-52.

[34] Liu, C., L. A. Pierce, 2nd, A. M. Alessio, & P. E. Kinahan. (2009). The impact of respiratory motion on tumor quantification and delineation in static PET/CT imaging. *Phys Med Biol, 54*(24), 7345-7362.

[35] Logan, J., J. S. Fowler, N. D. Volkow, G. J. Wang, Y. S. Ding, & D. L. Alexoff. (1996). Distribution volume ratios without blood sampling from graphical analysis of PET data. *J Cereb Blood Flow Metab, 16*(5), 834-840.

[36] Logan, J., J. S. Fowler, N. D. Volkow, A. P. Wolf, S. L. Dewey, D. J. Schlyer, R. R. MacGregor, R. Hitzemann, B. Bendriem, S. J. Gatley, & et al. (1990). Graphical analysis of reversible radioligand binding from time-activity measurements applied to [N-11C-methyl]-(-)-cocaine PET studies in human subjects. *J Cereb Blood Flow Metab, 10*(5), 740-747.

[37] Marks, M. J., J. R. Pauly, S. D. Gross, E. S. Deneris, I. Hermans-Borgmeyer, S. F. Heinemann, & A. C. Collins. (1992). Nicotine binding and nicotinic receptor subunit RNA after chronic nicotine treatment. *J Neurosci, 12*(7), 2765-2784.

[38] Martinez, D., R. Gil, M. Slifstein, D. R. Hwang, Y. Huang, A. Perez, L. Kegeles, P. Talbot, S. Evans, J. Krystal, M. Laruelle, & A. Abi-Dargham. (2005). Alcohol dependence is associated with blunted dopamine transmission in the ventral striatum. *Biol Psychiatry, 58*(10), 779-786.

[39] Martinez, D., M. Slifstein, A. Broft, O. Mawlawi, D. R. Hwang, Y. Huang, T. Cooper, L. Kegeles, E. Zarahn, A. Abi-Dargham, S. N. Haber, & M. Laruelle. (2003). Imaging human mesolimbic dopamine transmission with positron emission tomography. Part II: amphetamine-induced dopamine release in the functional subdivisions of the striatum. *J Cereb Blood Flow Metab, 23*(3), 285-300.

[40] Mathis, C. A., B. J. Bacskai, S. T. Kajdasz, M. E. McLellan, M. P. Frosch, B. T. Hyman, D. P. Holt, Y. Wang, G. F. Huang, M. L. Debnath, & W. E. Klunk. (2002). A lipophilic thioflavin-T derivative for positron emission tomography (PET) imaging of amyloid in brain. *Bioorg Med Chem Lett, 12*(3), 295-298.

[41] Mintun, M., M. Raichle, M. Kilbourn, G. Wooten, & M. Welch. (1984). A quantitative model for the in vivo assessment of drug binding sites with positron emission tomography. *Ann Neurol, 15*, 217-227.

[42] Mochizuki, T., V. Villemagne, U. Scheffel, R. Dannals, P. Finley, Y. Zhan, H. Wagner, & J. Musachio. (1998). Nicotine induced up-regulation of nicotinic receptors in CD-1 mice demonstrated with an in vivo radiotracer: gender differences. *Synapse, 30*, 116-118.

[43] Montgomery, A. J., A. R. Lingford-Hughes, A. Egerton, D. J. Nutt, & P. M. Grasby. (2007). The effect of nicotine on striatal dopamine release in man: A [11C]raclopride PET study. *Synapse, 61*(8), 637-645.

[44] Morris, E., R. Fisher, N. Alpert, S. Rauch, & A. Fischman. (1995). In vivo imaging of neuromodulation using positron emission tomography: optimal ligand characteristics and task length for detection of activation. . *Human Brain Mapping*, 35-55.

[45] Morris, E. D., S. I. Chefer, M. A. Lane, R. F. Muzic, Jr., D. F. Wong, R. F. Dannals, J. A. Matochik, A. A. Bonab, V. L. Villemagne, S. J. Grant, D. K. Ingram, G. S. Roth, & E. D. London. (1999). Loss of D2 receptor binding with age in rhesus monkeys: importance of correction for differences in striatal size. *J Cereb Blood Flow Metab, 19*(2), 218-229.

[46] Morris, E. D., C. C. Constantinescu, J. M. Sullivan, M. D. Normandin, & L. A. Christopher. (2010). Noninvasive visualization of human dopamine dynamics from PET images. *Neuroimage, 51*(1), 135-144.

[47] Morris, E. D., S. J. Kim, J. M. Sullivan, S. Wang, M. D. Normandin, C. C. Constantinescu, & K. P. Cosgrove. (2013). Creating Dynamic Images of Short-lived Dopamine Fluctuations with lp-ntPET: Dopamine Movies of Cigarette Smoking. *J Vis Exp*(78).

[48] Morris, E. D., M. D. Normandin, & W. K. Schiffer. (2008). Initial comparison of ntPET with microdialysis measurements of methamphetamine-induced dopamine release in rats: support for estimation of dopamine curves from PET data. *Mol Imaging Biol, 10*(2), 67-73.

[49] Morris, E. D., K. K. Yoder, C. Wang, M. D. Normandin, Q. H. Zheng, B. Mock, R. F. Muzic, Jr., & J. C. Froehlich. (2005). ntPET: a new application of PET imaging for characterizing the kinetics of endogenous neurotransmitter release. *Mol Imaging, 4*(4), 473-489.

[50] Normandin, M., R. Badgaiyan, W. Schiffer, & E. Morris. (2009). A linear simplification of the parametric ntPET model for estimation of neurotransmitter response kinetics. *J Nucl Med, May*(Suppl).

[51] Normandin, M. D., & E. D. Morris. (2008). Estimating neurotransmitter kinetics with ntPET: a simulation study of temporal precision and effects of biased data. *Neuroimage, 39*(3), 1162-1179.

[52] Normandin, M. D., W. K. Schiffer, & E. D. Morris. (2012). A linear model for estimation of neurotransmitter response profiles from dynamic PET data. *Neuroimage, 59*(3), 2689-2699.

[53] O'Connor, S., S. Morzorati, J. Christian, & T. K. Li. (1998). Clamping breath alcohol concentration reduces experimental variance: application to the study of acute tolerance to alcohol and alcohol elimination rate. *Alcohol Clin Exp Res, 22*(1), 202-210.

[54] Oberlin, B. G., M. Dzemidzic, S. M. Tran, C. M. Soeurt, D. S. Albrecht, K. K. Yoder, & D. A. Kareken. (2013). Beer flavor provokes striatal dopamine release in male drinkers: mediation by family history of alcoholism. *Neuropsychopharmacology, 38*(9), 1617-1624.

[55] Patlak, C. S., & R. G. Blasberg. (1985). Graphical evaluation of blood-to-brain transfer constants from multiple-time uptake data. Generalizations. *J Cereb Blood Flow Metab, 5*(4), 584-590.

[56] Patlak, C. S., R. G. Blasberg, & J. D. Fenstermacher. (1983). Graphical evaluation of blood-to-brain transfer constants from multiple-time uptake data. *J Cereb Blood Flow Metab, 3*(1), 1-7.

[57] Pellerin, L., & P. J. Magistretti. (1994). Glutamate uptake into astrocytes stimulates aerobic glycolysis: a mechanism coupling neuronal activity to glucose utilization. *Proc Natl Acad Sci U S A, 91*(22), 10625-10629.

[58] Perkins, K. A. (2009). Sex differences in nicotine reinforcement and reward: influences on the persistence of tobacco smoking. *Nebr Symp Motiv, 55*, 143-169.

[59] Perkins, K. A., E. Donny, & A. R. Caggiula. (1999). Sex differences in nicotine effects and self-administration: review of human and animal evidence. *Nicotine Tob Res, 1*(4), 301-315.

[60] Perkins, K. A., & J. Scott. (2008). Sex differences in long-term smoking cessation rates due to nicotine patch. *Nicotine Tob Res, 10*(7), 1245-1250.

[61] Salonen, I., Hietala, J., Laihinen, A., Lehikoinen, P., Leino, L., Nagren, K., Ruotsalainene, U., Oikonen, V., Tuokkola, T., Nanto, V. (1997). A PET Study on the Acute Effect of Ethanol on Striatal D2 Dopamine Receptors with [11C]Raclopride in Healthy Males. *Human Psychopharmacology, 12*, 145-152.

[62] Schultz, W., P. Dayan, & P. R. Montague. (1997). A neural substrate of prediction and reward. *Science, 275*(5306), 1593-1599.

[63] Scott, D. J., E. F. Domino, M. M. Heitzeg, R. A. Koeppe, L. Ni, S. Guthrie, & J. K. Zubieta. (2007). Smoking modulation of mu-opioid and dopamine D2 receptor-mediated neurotransmission in humans. *Neuropsychopharmacology, 32*(2), 450-457.

[64] Seeman, P., H.-C. Guan, & H. Niznik. (1989). Endogenous dopamine lowers the dopamine $D_2$ receptor density as measured with [$^3$H]raclopride: implications for positron emission tomography of the human brain. *Synapse, 3*, 96-97.

[65] Slifstein, M., & M. Laruelle. (2000). Effects of statistical noise on graphic analysis of PET neuroreceptor studies. *J Nucl Med, 41*(12), 2083-2088.

[66] Srinivasan, R., R. Pantoja, F. J. Moss, E. D. Mackey, C. D. Son, J. Miwa, & H. A. Lester. (2010). Nicotine up-regulates alpha4beta2 nicotinic receptors and ER exit sites via stoichiometry-dependent chaperoning. *J Gen Physiol, 137*(1), 59-79.

[67] Staley, J. K., S. Krishnan-Sarin, K. P. Cosgrove, E. Krantzler, E. Frohlich, E. Perry, J. A. Dubin, K. Estok, E. Brenner, R. M. Baldwin, G. D. Tamagnan, J. P. Seibyl, P. Jatlow, M. R. Picciotto, E. D. London, S. O'Malley, & C. H. van Dyck. (2006). Human tobacco smokers in early abstinence have higher levels of beta2* nicotinic acetylcholine receptors than nonsmokers. *J Neurosci, 26*(34), 8707-8714.

[68] Sullivan, J. M., S. J. Kim, K. P. Cosgrove, & E. D. Morris. (2013). Limitations of SRTM, Logan graphical method, and equilibrium analysis for measuring transient dopamine release with [(11)C]raclopride PET. *Am J Nucl Med Mol Imaging, 3*(3), 247-260.

[69] Takahashi, H., Y. Fujimura, M. Hayashi, H. Takano, M. Kato, Y. Okubo, I. Kanno, H. Ito, & T. Suhara. (2008). Enhanced dopamine release by nicotine in cigarette smokers: a double-blind, randomized, placebo-controlled pilot study. *Int J Neuropsychopharmacol, 11*(3), 413-417.

[70] Urban, N. B., L. S. Kegeles, M. Slifstein, X. Xu, D. Martinez, E. Sakr, F. Castillo, T. Moadel, S. S. O'Malley, J. H. Krystal, & A. Abi-Dargham. (2010). Sex differences in striatal dopamine release in young adults after oral alcohol challenge: a positron emission tomography imaging study with [(1)(1)C]raclopride. *Biol Psychiatry, 68*(8), 689-696.

[71] Volkow, N. D., G. J. Wang, J. S. Fowler, J. Logan, S. J. Gatley, R. Hitzemann, A. D. Chen, S. L. Dewey, & N. Pappas. (1997). Decreased striatal dopaminergic responsiveness in detoxified cocaine-dependent subjects. *Nature, 386*(6627), 830-833.

[72] Volkow, N. D., G. J. Wang, J. S. Fowler, J. Logan, R. Hitzemann, Y. S. Ding, N. Pappas, C. Shea, & K. Piscani. (1996). Decreases in dopamine receptors but not in dopamine transporters in alcoholics. *Alcohol Clin Exp Res, 20*(9), 1594-1598.

[73] Wagner, H. N., Burns, H.D., Dannals, R.F., Wong, D.F., Langstrom, B., Duelfer, T., Frost, J.J., Ravert, H.T., Rosenbloom, J.B., Lukas, S.E., Kramer, A.V., Kuhar, M.J. . (1983). Imaging Dopamine Receptors in the Humans Brain by Positron Tomography. *Science, 221*(4617), 1264-1266.

[74] Weerts, E. M., Y. K. Kim, G. S. Wand, R. F. Dannals, J. S. Lee, J. J. Frost, & M. E. McCaul. (2008). Differences in delta- and mu-opioid receptor blockade measured by

positron emission tomography in naltrexone-treated recently abstinent alcohol-dependent subjects. *Neuropsychopharmacology, 33*(3), 653-665.

[75] Weerts, E. M., G. S. Wand, H. Kuwabara, C. A. Munro, R. F. Dannals, J. Hilton, J. J. Frost, & M. E. McCaul. (2011). Positron emission tomography imaging of mu- and delta-opioid receptor binding in alcohol-dependent and healthy control subjects. *Alcohol Clin Exp Res, 35*(12), 2162-2173.

[76] Yoder, K. K., E. D. Morris, C. C. Constantinescu, T. E. Cheng, M. D. Normandin, S. J. O'Connor, & D. A. Kareken. (2009). When what you see isn't what you get: alcohol cues, alcohol administration, prediction error, and human striatal dopamine. *Alcohol Clin Exp Res, 33*(1), 139-149.

[77] Yoder, K. K., C. Wang, & E. D. Morris. (2004). Change in binding potential as a quantitative index of neurotransmitter release is highly sensitive to relative timing and kinetics of the tracer and the endogenous ligand. *J Nucl Med, 45*(5), 903-911.

[78] Zhou, Y., M. K. Chen, C. J. Endres, W. Ye, J. R. Brasic, M. Alexander, A. H. Crabb, T. R. Guilarte, & D. F. Wong. (2006). An extended simplified reference tissue model for the quantification of dynamic PET with amphetamine challenge. *Neuroimage, 33*(2), 550-563.

Chapter 6

# PET Imaging of the Serotoninergic 5-HT1A System

Amélie Lothe, Sandrine Bouvard and Philippe Ryvlin

Additional information is available at the end of the chapter

http://dx.doi.org/10.5772/57122

## 1. Introduction

Serotonin (5-hydroxytryptophan, 5-HT) is a modulating neurotransmitter of the central nervous system involved in a large spectrum of emotional and cognitive processes and physiological activities [1, 2], including sleep, locomotion, eating, memory, endocrine modulation, and sexual behaviour. The serotoninergic system is modulated in humans by both genetic and environmental factors. Furthermore, the central serotoninergic system is altered in multiple diseases such as depression [3, 4], migraine [5, 6], epilepsy [7-9], Alzheimer's disease [10, 11], eating disorders [12], anxiety [13], schizophrenia [14] and autism [15, 16]. Various radioligands are currently available for *in vivo* brain imaging of the serotoninergic system in humans, including antagonists for the 5-$HT_{1A}$, 5-$HT_{1B}$, 5-$HT_{2A}$, and 5-$HT_4$ receptors, and for the serotonin transporter (SERT) [17].

5-HT exerts its multiplicity of actions though seven classes of 5-HT receptors (17 subtypes identified to date), involving different signal transduction pathways [18, 19, 2]. The 5-$HT_{1A}$ receptors were the first to be cloned in humans and are probably the best-characterized subtype of 5-HT receptors [20]. These receptors are G protein coupled receptors (GPCRs); 5-HT binding to 5-$HT_{1A}$ receptors causes neuronal hyperpolarization through the G-protein-coupled opening of K+ channels [21, 22]. The 5-$HT_{1A}$ receptors are mostly expressed in neurons, either as heteroreceptors when located in target regions of 5-HT neurons with a particularly high concentration in limbic areas, such as cingulate cortex and hippocampus, or as autoreceptors on the soma and dendrites of 5-HT neurons in raphe nuclei, where they exert negative feedback on the serotoninergic neuron firing rate and 5-HT release [23, 24]. Thus, serotoninergic neurotransmission is strongly modulated by 5-$HT_{1A}$ receptors.

Several PET tracers have been developed for imaging 5-$HT_{1A}$ receptors [25]. The most commonly used radioligands are [$^{11}$C]WAY-100635 (N- [2-[4-(2-methoxyphenyl)-1-piperazin-

INTECH
open science | open minds

© 2013 Lothe et al.; licensee InTech. This is a paper distributed under the terms of the Creative Commons Attribution License (http://creativecommons.org/licenses/by/3.0), which permits unrestricted use, distribution, and reproduction in any medium, provided the original work is properly cited.

yl]ethyl]-N-(2-pyridinyl)cyclohexane carboxamide) and [$^{18}$F]MPPF (4-(2′-methoxyphenyl)-1-[2′-(N-2-pirydynyl)-p-fluorobenzamido]-ethyl-piperazine) (see figure 1).

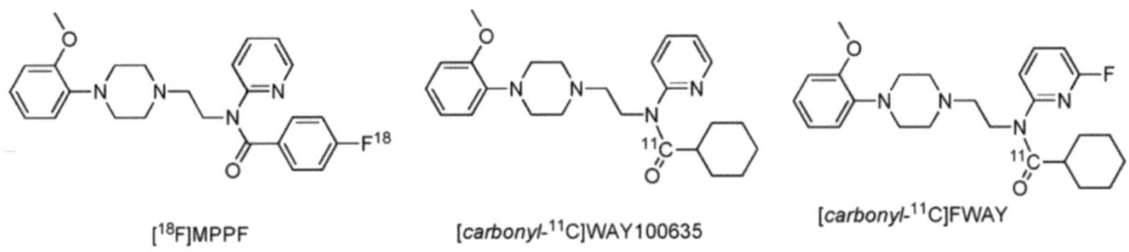


**Figure 1.** Chemical structure of antagonist PET tracers of 5-HT$_{1A}$ receptors

In this chapter, we will start by reviewing the different binding properties of [$^{18}$F]MPPF versus [$^{11}$C]WAY-100635. We will then discuss in more detail PET data obtained with [$^{18}$F]MPPF in comparison with those obtained with [$^{11}$C]WAY-100635 in various pathological conditions, including major depressive disorder, depressive comorbidity in temporal lobe epilepsy, and schizophrenia.

## 2. Binding properties of [$^{18}$F]MPPF versus [$^{11}$C]WAY-100635

[$^{18}$F]MPPF and [$^{11}$C]WAY-100635 are both selective and potent antagonists at 5-HT$_{1A}$ autoreceptors and heteroreceptors, but differ in their binding properties at 5-HT$_{1A}$ receptors.

Firstly, [$^{18}$F]MPPF is characterized by a lower affinity for 5-HT$_{1A}$ receptors (Ki=3.3 nM in rat hippocampal membrane homogenates) than [$^{11}$C]WAY-100635 (Ki=0.8 nM) [26] and [$^{18}$F]FCWAY (Ki=0.25 nM) [27].

The high affinity of [$^{11}$C]WAY-100635 for 5-HT$_{1A}$ receptors would make it relatively insensitive to changes in endogenous 5-HT concentration. Indeed, the binding of [$^{11}$C]WAY-100635 remained unchanged after injection of fenfluramine or after depletion of 5-HT by treatment with p-chlorophenylalanine (p-CPA) or with reserpine in rodents [28, 29]. In this regard, a decreased [$^{11}$C]WAY-100635 binding will be interpreted as reflecting a reduction in the density of 5-HT$_{1A}$ receptors.

Conversely, the affinity of [$^{18}$F]MPPF is closer to that of endogenous 5-HT for 5-HT$_{1A}$ receptors (Ki=4.2 nM in rat frontal cortex homogenates) [30]. Thus, [$^{18}$F]MPPF appears to be sensitive to the extra-cellular concentration of endogenous 5-HT [31, 32, 33]. Several studies using β-sensitive microprobes and microdialysis in the brain of rats demonstrated decreases in [$^{18}$F]MPPF binding after pharmacologically or electrical stimulation induced increases in the concentration of extracellular 5-HT [31, 32], while the binding of [$^{18}$F]MPPF is increased in the hippocampus following a reduction in the extracellular 5-HT concentration in rats treated with p-EPA, an inhibitor of tryptophan hydroxylase [33]. These findings were confirmed with simulated [$^{18}$F]MPPF PET data [34]. Moreover, an original PET study using [$^{18}$F]MPPF and alpha-[$^{11}$C]Methyl-L-Tryptophan (AMT), a precursor of 5-HT, reported a significant negative correlation between 5-HT synthesis and 5-HT$_{1A}$ binding potential (BP) bilaterally in hippocampus and anterior insula and in the left anterior cingulate gyrus in healthy subjects [35].

Accordingly, in contrast to [$^{11}$C]WAY-100635, a decreased [$^{18}$F]MPPF binding could either reflect lower 5-HT$_{1A}$ receptor density or a higher extracellular concentration of 5-HT that could be associated with various changes in the number of 5-HT$_{1A}$ receptors.

Secondly, [$^{18}$F]MPPF binds to externalized 5-HT$_{1A}$ receptors only, while [$^{11}$C]WAY-100635 also binds to internalized receptors [36]. As a result of this property, [$^{18}$F]MPPF may allow indirect assessment of the internalization of 5-HT$_{1A}$ autoreceptors [37].

Using β-sensitive microprobes in rats, a significant decrease of [$^{18}$F]MPPF binding was observed in the dorsal raphe nucleus (autoreceptors), but not in the hippocampus (heteroreceptors), after acute treatment with 8-OH-DPAT, a 5-HT$_{1A}$ receptor agonist, or with fluoxetine, a selective serotonin reuptake inhibitor (SSRI) [37, 38]. This reduction is associated with the internalization of 5-HT$_{1A}$ autoreceptors of dorsal raphe nucleus observed in parallel using quantitative electron microscopic immunocytochemistry [38]. Similarly, a [$^{18}$F]MPPF PET study conducted in cats reported a decreased BP in the dorsal raphe nucleus after acute fluoxetine administration [39]. Finally, an interesting [$^{18}$F]MPPF PET study has examined this property by investigating healthy subjects five hours after the randomized, double-blind administration of a single oral dose of fluoxetine [40]. As expected, [$^{18}$F]MPPF binding in raphe nuclei is decreased in response to fluoxetine in each healthy subject [40].

Thirdly, the 5-HT$_{1A}$ binding of both ligand was found to be differentially influenced by several factors, including genetic factors, age and gender.

Several genetic factors, including the triallelic 5-HT transporter gene-linked polymorphic region (5-HTTLPR) and 5-HT$_{1A}$ promoter polymorphism, have a significant impact on [$^{18}$F]MPPF and [$^{11}$C]WAY-100635 binding [41-47].

Two [$^{11}$C]WAY-100635 PET studies showed a significant impact of the 5-HTTLPR polymorphism on the 5-HT$_{1A}$ receptor binding, but in different directions [41-42]. One of the two studies reported lower [$^{11}$C]WAY-100635 BP in various limbic and neocortical brain regions in healthy subjects (predominantly men) with S/S or S/L genotypes compared to those with L/L genotype [41], whereas the other series found greater BP in the cingulate gyri in healthy women with S/S and S/L genotypes compared to those with L/L genotype [42]. Similarly, we observed a greater [$^{18}$F]MPPF non displaceable $BP_{ND}$ ($BP_{ND} = f_{ND}.B_{avail}/K_D$ where $f_{ND}$ is the fraction of radioligands free and non specifically bound, $B_{avail}$ is the total number of available receptors for binding and $1/K_D$ is the affinity of the radioligand) [48] in homozygote women carriers of the S allele of 5-HTTLPR compared with carriers of at least one $L_A$ allele over large brain regions including temporal and parietal lobes as well as the insula, cingulate gyri and left orbitofrontal cortex [43]. In contrast, a recent PET study failed to show a significant effect of the 5-HTTLPR polymorphism on the [$^{11}$C]WAY-100635 BP in a large population of 54 healthy volunteers, but that included men predominantly [47].

The association of C(-1019)G 5-$HT_{1A}$ promoter polymorphism and 5-$HT_{1A}$ receptor binding has also been evaluated in humans in three [$^{11}$C]WAY-100635 PET studies and one [$^{18}$F]MPPF study [41, 44-46]. One of these [$^{11}$C]WAY-100635 studies reported no association between C(-1019)G 5-$HT_{1A}$ promoter polymorphism and 5-$HT_{1A}$ receptor BP in a homogenous group of healthy subjects [41]. We also failed to detect a significant relationship between C(-1019)G 5-$HT_{1A}$ promoter polymorphism and [$^{18}$F]MPPF binding in healthy subjects. However our data suggest that women homozygote for the G allele have greater [$^{18}$F]MPPF $BP_{ND}$ compared to other individuals primarily over the frontal and temporal neocortex. The other two [$^{11}$C]WAY-100635 PET studies, performed in a mixed population of depressed and healthy individuals, demonstrated greater BP in limbic regions and the raphe nuclei, in carriers with at least one G allele compared to the C/C genotype [45, 46].

5-$HT_{1A}$ receptor binding measured by either [$^{18}$F]MPPF and [$^{11}$C]WAY-100635 significantly declines with age [49-52]. However, this effect was especially observed on [$^{18}$F]MPPF binding in women [50] and, conversely, on [$^{11}$C]WAY-100635 binding in men [52]. Note that one [$^{11}$C]WAY-100635 PET study failed to show any significant correlation between age and 5-$HT_{1A}$ receptor binding [53].

With regard to the gender factor, greater [$^{18}$F]MPPF $BP_{ND}$ values independent of age were demonstrated in women compared to men, in limbic and paralimbic regions, predominantly in the right hemisphere [50]. Furthermore, after controlling for age and 5-HTTLPR polymorphism, a higher [$^{18}$F]MPPF $BP_{ND}$ to 5-$HT_{1A}$ receptors was also observed in women than in men over a very restricted set of brain regions, including the left temporal pole and parahippocampal gyrus [43]. Thus, we might speculate that the larger gender difference could partly reflect unbalanced 5-HTTLPR polymorphism between men and women.

A few PET studies have also examined the effects of gender on [$^{11}$C]WAY-100635 binding to 5-$HT_{1A}$ receptors, reporting contradictory findings. Two previous studies found no effect of gender on [$^{11}$C]WAY-100635 binding [51, 54], whereas other series reported higher binding in women compared to men [47, 53, 55].

Overall, [$^{18}$F]MPPF and [$^{11}$C]WAY-100635 are likely to yield different and complementary PET findings in different pathological conditions.

## 3. Major depressive disorder

Depression is a common mental disorder, affecting about 121 million people worldwide. By the year 2020, depression is projected to become the second most important cause of disease burden, as measured by Disability-Adjusted Life Years (DALYs) (World Health Organization). The average lifetime prevalence of Major Depressive Disorder (MDD) is 14.6% in high-income countries [56], with the typically reported rates of 5% to 12% for men and 10% to 26% for women.

According to the Diagnostic Statistical Manual of Mental Disorders [57], Fourth edition, Text revision (DSM-IV-R), a Major Depressive Episode is characterized by a depressed mood and/

or a markedly diminished interest or pleasure in all or almost all activities most of the day during the same 2-week period. In addition, three or more of the following symptoms must be present: gain or loss of weight, insomnia or hypersomnia, psychomotor agitation or retardation, fatigue, feelings of worthlessness or guilt, diminished ability to concentrate, and recurrent thoughts of death or suicidal ideation.

MDD is associated with diminished role functioning, poor health-related quality of life, medical comorbidity, such as cardiovascular disease [58], and increased risk of mortality [59].

Since roughly the 1970s, 5-HT has been involved in the pathophysiology of MDD [60, 61]. Numerous studies reported a reduction of 5-HT plasma concentrations and 5-HT metabolite levels in the cerebro-spinal fluid of patients with MDD [62, 63]. In addition, pharmacological agents that reduce brain 5-HT levels (e.g. reserpine) can induce depressive symptoms in healthy subjects as well as in recovered depressed patients [4, 64-66]. More recently, PET studies using alpha-[$^{11}$C]Methyl-L-Tryptophan (AMT) showed a reduction of this tracer uptake in the anterior cingulate gyrus and left mesial temporal cortex in MDD patients, supporting the possibility of reduced extracellular 5-HT concentration in depression [67, 68].

The involvement of 5-$HT_{1A}$ receptors in depression is well recognized; however the nature of their modifications is still controversial (see for review [69, 70]). A large number of PET studies have investigated 5-$HT_{1A}$ receptors in patients with MDD using [$^{11}$C]WAY-100635 [3, 69, 71-81].

Most previous [$^{11}$C]WAY-100635 PET studies showed a reduction of 5-$HT_{1A}$ receptor $BP_{ND}$ in various limbic and neocortical brain regions, as well as in the raphe nuclei, of untreated, treated, remitted MDD patients as well as in drug-naïve primary-care patients with MDD [3, 71, 73, 74-76, 79]. Interestingly, a [$^{18}$F]MPPF PET study performed in a monkey model of depression also reported a reduced BP in limbic regions and raphe nuclei [82]. It is in agreement with the majority of post-mortem data demonstrating decreased 5-$HT_{1A}$ receptor density in depressed suicide victims in different brain regions including the raphe nuclei, the hippocampus, and the frontal cortex [83-89]. The reduction of 5-$HT_{1A}$ receptor binding could be partly the consequence of a possible hypersecretion of endogenous corticosteroids (see for review [69, 90]).

However, other PET studies using [$^{11}$C]WAY-100635 reported an increased ratio of specifically bound ligand over free ligand ($BP_F$) in the same regions in MDD patients never or not recently exposed to antidepressants, compared with controls [77-79]. Similarly, an increased 5-$HT_{1A}$ $BP_F$ has been shown in patients with MDD during sustained remission and not having taken antidepressant medications for at least six months, compared with healthy controls [81]. These authors suggest that higher 5-$HT_{1A}$ autoreceptor binding in the raphe nuclei could lead to greater inhibition of 5-HT neuron firing rate and decreased 5-HT release in the target regions of 5-HT neurons, possibly leading to compensatory up-regulation of 5-$HT_{1A}$ receptors in the same regions [78].

These discordant PET findings might partly reflect differences in the modeling methods used to calculate BP ($BP_{ND}$ versus $BP_F$) [48], the choice of the reference region (e.g. inclusion of cerebellar vermis and gray matter in the reference region or use of white matter) [91], MDD severity, treatment status, and genetic polymorphism status (e.g. for the C-1019G 5-$HT_{1A}$

receptor and 5-HTTLPR polymorphisms) of the patients selected [79] (see for review [70]). Thus, regarding the choice of the reference region, scans from the same patient population, analysed with SRTM and a cerebellar reference region, could either demonstrate reduced 5-$HT_{1A}$ $BP_{ND}$ when using cerebellar gray matter, or increased or unchanged $BP_{ND}$ when using cerebellar white matter [79, 81]. Indeed, the grey matter of cerebellum contains limited but significant amount of 5-$HT_{1A}$ receptors, while its white matter does not and thus represents a more appropriate reference. Furthermore, as already mentioned, [$^{18}$F]MPPF and [$^{11}$C]WAY-100635 $BP_{ND}$ were reported to be influenced by the triallelic 5-HTTLPR polymorphism, which S allele is associated with depressive disorder [92, 93].

### 3.1. Effects of antidepressants

A small number of PET studies have examined the potential impact of chronic antidepressant medication on 5-$HT_{1A}$ receptor binding.

Three test-retest [$^{11}$C]WAY-100635 studies reported no change of $BP_{ND}$ after selective serotonin recapture inhibitor (SSRI) treatment in MDD patients [75, 94, 95]. Contrary to these findings, a reduction of [$^{11}$C]WAY-100635 $BP_F$ was found in MDD patients previously treated by antidepressants (most of the antidepressant exposure ended between 21 and 14 days prior to PET scans) when compared with medication naiøve MDD patients, but not when compared with healthy controls [77]. In line with this result, a decreased 5-$HT_{1A}$ $BP_{ND}$ was observed following at least 12 weeks of SSRI treatment in patients suffering from social phobia or panic disorder [96]. These data suggest that chronic antidepressant treatment could induce a down-regulation of 5-$HT_{1A}$ receptors.

In a recent test-retest [$^{18}$F]MPPF PET study, we explored the potential dynamic changes in [$^{18}$F]MPPF $BP_{ND}$ in six patients with untreated MDD, before, and after five and 30 days of SSRI treatment [97]. No change of [$^{18}$F]MPPF $BP_{ND}$ after SSRI medication was observed within the raphe nuclei and a significant increase of [$^{18}$F]MPPF $BP_{ND}$ from baseline to 30 days of SSRI treatment was reported primarily in the medial orbital region and the anterior cingulate gyrus. These findings are in contradiction with the three previous test-retest [$^{11}$C]WAY-100635 studies which have addressed this issue [75, 94, 95].

After 30 days of SSRI treatment, no more significant modification of [$^{18}$F]MPPF $BP_{ND}$ was found in MDD patients compared with healthy subjects in the medial orbital region and the anterior cingulate gyrus. Thus effective SSRI treatment is associated with a trend toward normalisation of the serotoninergic function. In agreement with these human PET imaging data, no change in the in vivo [$^{18}$F]MPPF binding was found in the dorsal raphe nucleus, frontal cortex and hippocampus of rats undergoing chronic SSRI treatment, as measured with β-microprobes or with the small animal PET scanner YAP-(S)PET system [98, 99].

Overall these preliminary [$^{18}$F]MPPF data suggest the existence of SSRI-mediated serotoninergic adaptative mechanisms in patients with MDD. However, due to the small sample size, it is necessary to confirm these findings in a larger population.

Apart from the discrepancy of the used radioligands, several points of difference between our [$^{18}$F]MPPF study and the three previous [$^{11}$C]WAY-100635 studies should be noted [75, 94,

95]. Firstly, one of these [$^{11}$C]WAY-100635 studies did not evaluate specifically the medial orbital region and the anterior cingulate gyrus [94]. Moreover, the treatment response, the treatment duration, the polymorphism status for serotoninergic genes as well as the cortisol plasma levels [69] of the patients selected could partly explain these discrepancies. For instance, in one of the [$^{11}$C]WAY-100635 studies, only half of the patients studied were responders [75], whereas in our [$^{18}$F]MPPF study all patients were responders.

## 4. Depressive comorbidity in temporal lobe epilepsy

Epilepsy is a common chronic neurological disorder characterized by recurrent unprovoked seizures, due to an abnormal, excessive, and synchronous neuronal discharges, affecting about 50 million people worldwide. Depressive disorders are the most frequent psychiatric comorbidity in epilepsy but often remain under-recognized and untreated [100-103]. The lifetime prevalence of major depression ranged from 11 and 60% in patients with recurrent seizures [103] and increased in patients with temporal lobe epilepsy (TLE), particularly in those with left TLE and possibly hippocampal sclerosis (for review see [101, 104-108]). The rate of suicide in patients with epilepsy is about two to five times that of the general population, and this rate rises to six to seven times in the case of TLE [109, 110]. In addition, comorbid depression is a strong predictor of poor quality of life in patients with epilepsy [111]. This higher incidence of depressive disorders in patients with epilepsy, in particular in those with TLE, may reflect the existence of common pathogenic mechanisms between mood disorders and epilepsy [112]. In this paragraph, we are referring to the presence of depressive symptoms in interictal period. Indeed, depressive symptoms may also occur transiently during ictal or post-ictal [103].

A large body of evidence from preclinical studies indicates an anticonvulsant and antiepileptic effect of 5-HT mediated by 5-HT$_{1A}$ receptors [113]. The activation of 5-HT$_{1A}$ receptors retards the development of the kindling process in rats [114] and in cats [115, 116] and inhibits epileptiform activity in various cellular models of epilepsy [117, 118]. In addition, agents that raise endogenous 5-HT levels (e.g. SSRI) have an anticonvulsant effect, mediated by 5-HT$_{1A}$ receptors [119], in genetically epilepsy-prone rats [120], in partial seizures generated by low-frequency electrical stimulation in rats [121], as well as in kindled rats [116]. Finally, given their multiple cellular localizations, the 5-HT$_{1A}$ receptors may mediate inhibition of excitatory neurons, but also of inhibitory neurons, leading to opposite effects on the neural network [122]. Accordingly, a possible mechanism of neuronal hyperexcitability in epilepsy could be an excitatory/inhibitory shift mediated by changes in serotoninergic transmission.

Abnormalities of the 5-HT$_{1A}$ receptors were reported in TLE using various radioligands, including [$^{11}$C]WAY-100635, [$^{18}$F]FCWAY and [$^{18}$F]MPPF. All showed a BP reduction that predominated over the epileptogenic temporo-limbic structures [123-130] (see figure 2).

This reduction of 5-HT$_{1A}$ binding on the side of the epileptogenic zone support the hypothesis of a decrease in 5-HT$_{1A}$ receptors density in TLE. In line with these imaging studies, a decrease of binding of the agonist [$^{3}$H]8-OH-DPAT (8-hydroxy-2-(di-n-propylamino) tetralin) to 5-HT$_{1A}$ receptors was reported in the hippocampus of genetically epilepsy-prone rats [131].

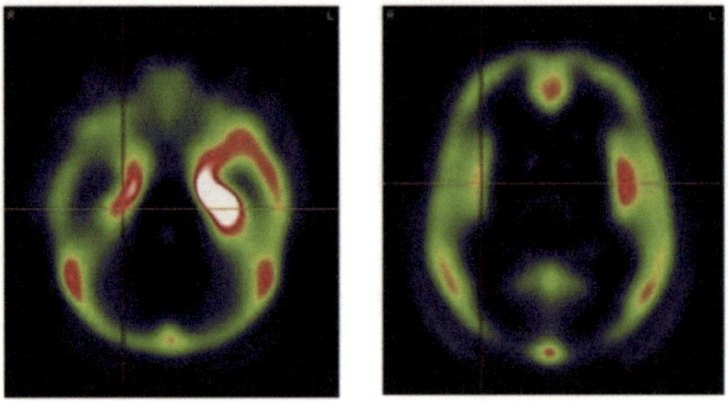

**Figure 2.** Typical pattern of [$^{18}$F]MPPF $BP_{ND}$ in patients with TLE.

Nevertheless, it should be stressed that the P-glycoprotein (PGP) expression could compromise this interpretation of PET findings. PGP is an ATP-driven transmembrane efflux pump, which is located at the blood-brain barrier and transports a wide variety of substrates from the brain to blood and cerebrospinal fluid. [$^{18}$F]MPPF being a substrate for PGP, its brain uptake is modulated. An overexpression of PGP is reported in epileptic foci, probably leading to drug resistance in epilepsy [132]. Thus, the reduction of [$^{18}$F]MPPF $BP_{ND}$ observed in patients with TLE could reflect a combination between decreased number of 5-$HT_{1A}$ receptors and a more active PGP pump.

In epilepsy and depression, PET studies of the serotoninergic system focused on 5-$HT_{1A}$ receptors in patients with TLE. Previous PET investigations of 5-$HT_{1A}$ receptors using [$^{11}$C]WAY-100635 and [$^{18}$F]FC-WAY observed greater BP reduction in the more depressed patients with TLE, suggesting decreased expression of 5-$HT_{1A}$ receptors [126, 127, 133, 134]. This abnormality was primarily reported ipsilateral to the epileptogenic temporal lobe, and more specifically over the anterior cingulate gyrus [126] and the hippocampus [127, 133]. Recently this finding was confirmed in a larger sample of TLE patients, reporting a significant inverse relation between Beck depression inventory (BDI) scores and [$^{18}$F]FC-WAY 5$HT_{1A}$ receptor plasma free-fraction corrected volume of distribution (V/f1) in the hippocampus ipsilateral to the patient's epileptic focus [134]. In 37 TLE patients with or without hippocampal sclerosis, Hasler et al. [135] also showed lower [$^{18}$F]FCWAY binding in patients with a history of MDD compared with those without such a history, in hippocampus, temporal neocortex, anterior insula, anterior cingulate and raphe nuclei. However, a recent [$^{11}$C]WAY-100635 PET study performed in a small population of 13 TLE patients with or without hippocampal sclerosis failed to report any correlation between binding potential and depression [130].

In contrast with these findings, we observed greater $BP_{ND}$ of [$^{18}$F]MPPF in the more depressed TLE patients with hippocampal sclerosis and no previous antidepressant exposure, particularly within the insula contralateral to seizure onset as well as in the raphe nuclei [8]. Interestingly, a different set of brain regions was associated with each of the main dimensions explored by the BDI-2, with the insula and raphe abnormalities being associated with symptoms of psychomotor anhedonia and negative cognition, whereas somatic symptoms correlated with [$^{18}$F]MPPF $BP_{ND}$ in the anterior cingulate gyrus and hippocampus ipsilateral to seizure onset. Considering the sensitivity of [$^{18}$F]MPPF to the extra-cellular concentration of endogenous 5-HT, the greater [$^{18}$F]MPPF $BP_{ND}$ observed in the more depressed patients suggests a combination of an underlying depletion in the extra-celllular concentration of 5-HT and a decreased density in 5-$HT_{1A}$ receptors.

As previously mentioned, discordance between PET studies of 5-$HT_{1A}$ receptors in patients with epilepsy and depression might also reflect a difference in the modeling methods used to calculate BP [79], the choice of the reference region, as well as the studied patient samples. Indeed, in our [$^{18}$F]MPPF PET study, we have selected a more homogeneous group of patients than those of previous [$^{11}$C]WAY-100635 studies; all patients were naïve to previous antidepressant exposure and showed MRI signs of hippocampal sclerosis. Conversely, the proportion of patients with hippocampal sclerosis varied in other series [126, 127, 133, 134]. The pathophysiology of epilepsy-related depression might differ between TLE patients with and without hippocampal sclerosis [136, 137]. Furthermore, the brain distribution of 5-$HT_{1A}$ receptors would be influenced by previous antidepressant treatment [77]. Finally, it should be noted that antiepileptic drugs, such as carbamazepine [138], could modify the intracerebral concentration of 5-HT. Thus, differences in the proportion of patients with and without depressive symptoms receiving carbamazepine could also play a role in the discordances observed between [$^{18}$F]MPPF and [$^{11}$C]WAY-100635 PET findings.

## 5. Schizophrenia

Schizophrenia is a severely disabling and complex psychiatric disorder with a lifetime prevalence of approximately 1% in the general population [139]. The diagnosis of schizophrenia encompasses the presence of positive (delusions, hallucinations, thought disorder) and negative (emotional blunting, paucity of speech, loss of motivation, self neglect, and social withdrawal) symptoms, and cognitive deficits (deficits in attention, executive function, and memory). According to DSM-IV-TR, two or more positive symptoms have occurred for at least one month, unless hallucinations or delusions are especially bizarre, in which case one alone suffices for diagnosis. The onset of symptoms typically occurs during adolescence and young adulthood, with men having an earlier age of onset than women. Medical and psychiatric comorbidities, such as substance abuse, anxiety and depressive disorders, are frequent in patients with schizophrenia [140]. Furthermore patients with schizophrenia have higher rates of mortality in comparison to the general population [141].

Schizophrenia has a multifactorial etiology, involving a combination of genetic and environmental risk factors. Several neurotransmitters systems (dopamine, glutamate, acetylcholine, GABA, serotonin) are altered in schizophrenia. Until recently, the predominant focus of research in the pathophysiology of schizophrenia was the dopaminergic neurotransmission. The current dopamine hypothesis postulates that dopaminergic systems in schizophrenia might be characterized by a cortical/subcortical imbalance. Subcortical mesolimbic dopaminergic projections might be hyperactive (underlying positive symptoms), while mesocortical dopaminergic projections to the prefrontal cortex might be hypoactive (underlying negative symptoms and cognitive impairments) [142]. However, despite over 100 years of research, the precise pathophysiologic mechanisms of schizophrenia still remain unclear.

Over the years, there is increasing evidence that the serotonergic 5-$HT_{1A}$ system is involved in the pathophysiology of schizophrenia and its treatment [143]. Abnormalities of 5-$HT_{1A}$ receptors were reported in patients suffering from schizophrenia or schizoaffective disorder. Firstly, most post-mortem studies observed an increased 5-$HT_{1A}$ receptor density (between 17% and 79%) in different brain regions of patients with schizophrenia, including the dorsolateral prefrontal cortex [144-148]. It should be noted that the majority of patients included in post-mortem studies had generally lengthy histories of psychiatric illness and of antipsychotic chronic treatment and/or other medications that could have an impact on the 5-$HT_{1A}$ receptor distribution.

Only few [$^{11}$C]WAY-100635 PET studies were performed in patients with schizophrenia or schizoaffective disorder and have reported inconsistent results. The first [$^{11}$C]WAY-100635 PET study showed an increased $BP_{ND}$ in the left medial temporal cortex in patients with schizophrenia who were untreated and never previously exposed to antipsychotic drug (APD) compared to healthy subjects [149]. However, other PET series demonstrated a decreased [$^{11}$C]WAY-100635 BP in the amygdala in drug-free and drug-naïve patients with schizophrenia or schizophreniform disorder (predominantly drug-naïve) [150] or failed to show BP alterations in various populations of APD-treated, untreated or never exposed to APDs patients with schizophrenia or schizoaffective disorder [151, 152]. There are several possible explanations for these discrepancies including differences in the brain regional distribution of PET changes, in the modeling methods used to calculate BP, in the selected patient samples as well as in their antipsychotic treatment.

Antipsychotic medications are used to treat schizophrenia. Since mid-1950's, numerous APDs with different pharmacological profiles were developed. In agreement with the dopamine hypothesis of schizophrenia, the first generation antipsychotics, such as haloperidol, are dopamine $D_2$ antagonists and are effective for reducing positive symptoms of schizophrenia. However, they are ineffective against negative symptoms and have high propensity for induction of extrapyramidal symptoms. The second generation antipsychotics, such as clozapine, olanzapine or risperidone, present enhanced efficacy in treating positive and negative symptoms and lower rates of extrapyramidal side effects [153]. The latter are potent 5-$HT_{2A/2C}$ receptor antagonists and relatively weak dopamine $D_2$ antagonists.

To date, the development of new APDs focuses on agonist properties at 5-$HT_{1A}$ receptors, pharmacologic profile involved in the treatment of negative symptoms and cognitive deficits of schizophrenia and in the reduction of extrapyramidal side effects [154]. Indeed, preclinical studies reported that 5-$HT_{1A}$ agonists reduced $D_2$-antagonist-induced catalepsy and increased the outflow of dopamine in the striatum [155] and in the medial prefrontal cortex [156, 157]. Aripiprazole is the first APDs with a unique pharmacologic profile combining a partial agonist activity at dopamine $D_2$ receptors, an antagonism at 5-$HT_2$ receptors and a partial agonism at 5-$HT_{1A}$ receptors [158]. In rats, aripiprazole modulates the in-vivo 5-HT and dopamine release in the medial prefrontal cortex through the activation of 5-$HT_{1A}$ receptors [159]. Furthermore, aripiprazole does not induce extrapyramidal symptoms in patients with schizophrenia or schizoaffective disorder [160].

The effects of different APDs on 5-$HT_{1A}$ receptors have been evaluated using PET and [$^{11}$C]WAY-100635 or [$^{18}$F]MPPF as radioligand, but these series reported conflicting results [151, 161-163]. Two [$^{11}$C]WAY-100635 PET studies showed contradictory findings in treated schizophrenic patients, reporting either no difference between patients taking clozapine or second generation antipsychotics and age-matched controls [151] or a reduction in $BP_{ND}$ obtained after treatment with aripiprazole in comparison to age-matched controls [163]. In addition a recent test-retest study failed to observe a significant effect of chronic treatment of ziprasidone on the 5-$HT_{1A}$ binding in six schizophrenic patients [162].

To investigate the impact of various APDs on the serotoninergic system, we performed a [$^{18}$F]MPPF PET study in 19 schizophrenic patients treated with either aripiprazole or second generation antipsychotics [161]. We reported a reduced [$^{18}$F]MPPF $BP_{ND}$ mainly in the frontal and orbitofrontal cortex, in treated schizophrenic patients compared to age- and gender-matched healthy subjects. These findings may reflect either the pathophysiology of schizophrenia or medication effects. Furthermore, the schizophrenic patients treated with aripiprazole showed a reduction of global [$^{18}$F]MPPF $BP_{ND}$ in comparison to healthy subjects and schizophrenic patients with second generation antipsychotic treatment. In addition, in comparison to matched controls, the reduction of regional [$^{18}$F]MPPF $BP_{ND}$ was more marked in the schizophrenic patients treated with aripiprazole in comparison to those receiving second generation antipsychotic treatment. These abnormalities were localized in larger clusters encompassing the right and left frontal and orbitofrontal cortex, precunei and cingulate regions, the left temporal region as well as the raphe nuclei. These findings could be due to either occupancy by aripiprazole at 5-$HT_{1A}$ receptors or a decreased 5-$HT_{1A}$ receptor density. These findings may possibly reflect the partial agonist of aripiprazole activity at 5-$HT_{1A}$ receptors. However, no modifications of 5-$HT_{1A}$ receptor density and mRNA expression were found in limbic regions in rats after 12 weeks of aripiprazole treatment [164]. In our opinion, our [$^{18}$F]MPPF PET data most likely reflect the partial agonist activity of aripiprazole at 5-$HT_{1A}$ receptors. Importantly, in contrast with previous [$^{11}$C]WAY-100635 PET studies, we take into account cortical atrophy as a confounding factor, by excluding the affected clusters in the right temporal gyrus and insula from our [$^{18}$F]MPPF PET analyses. These contradictory 5-$HT_{1A}$ receptors PET findings could be attributable to differences in the used radioligands, the choice of the reference region, in sample populations, including duration of illness, as well as the in vivo agonist properties at the 5-$HT_{1A}$ receptors of studied APDs.

## 6. Conclusion

Discordance between [$^{18}$F]MPPF and [$^{11}$C]WAY-100635 PET studies of 5-$HT_{1A}$ receptors might reflect their differential sensitivity to extracellular concentration of endogenous 5-HT and to the internalization of 5-$HT_{1A}$ autoreceptors, but also differences in the data modeling strategies used to calculate BP, including the choice of the reference region (inclusion of cerebellar vermis and gray matter in the reference region)[79], and the population studied. We should also bear in mind that the genetic background for each subject and the gene-by-environment interaction can have a significant influence in different directions on [$^{18}$F]MPPF and [$^{11}$C]WAY-100635 PET findings, which is difficult to control for in the small samples of patients and healthy subjects included in PET studies [41-46].

In future PET studies of 5-$HT_{1A}$ receptors, a more detailed clinical description of studied patients would improve the understanding of discrepancies between studies. Furthermore, particular attention should be paid to the constitution of a group of healthy subjects matched for confounding factors, such as age and sex. For instance, a PET study reported a lower cortical trapping of the alpha-[$^{11}$C]Methyl-L-Tryptophan (AMT) in women compared to men [165].

Future studies should aim at disentangling these issues by using a traditional multi-injection [$^{18}$F]MPPF protocol that enables a precise quantification of binding parameters (B'MAX; Kd) and the estimation of extracellular 5-HT concentration [166] or by coupling [$^{18}$F]MPPF and [$^{11}$C]WAY-100635 PET studies in the same individuals taking advantage of their different affinities for 5-$HT_{1A}$ receptors. Another future challenge will be to image endogenous 5HT release in humans [167].

## Acknowledgements

We thank Didier Le Bars for [$^{18}$F]MPPF radiosynthesis and the medical team of the CERMEP – Imagerie du vivant. We are indebted to Nicolas Costes and Jérôme Redouté.

The Article Processing Charge was funded by the Translational and Integrative Group in Epilepsy Research (TIGER) (CRNL).

## Author details

Amélie Lothe[1*], Sandrine Bouvard[1] and Philippe Ryvlin[1,2]

*Address all correspondence to: amelie.lothe@cermep.fr

1 INSERM U1028, CNRS UMR5292, and University Claude Bernard Lyon 1, Lyon Neuroscience Research Center, Translational and Integrative Group in Epilepsy Research (TIGER), Lyon, France

2 Department of Functional Neurology and Epileptology and Institute for Children and Adolescents with Epilepsy (IDEE), Hospices Civils de Lyon, Lyon, France

## References

[1] Lucki I. The spectrum of behaviors influenced by serotonin. Biol. Psychiatry 1998;44:151-16

[2] Barnes NM, Sharp T. A review of central 5-HT receptors and their function. Neuropharmacology 1999;38(8):1083-1152.

[3] Drevets WC, Thase ME, Moses-Kolko EL, Price J, Frank E, Kupfer DJ, et al. Serotonin-1A receptor imaging in recurrent depression: replication and literature review. Nucl. Med. Biol. 2007;34(7):865-877.

[4] Maes M, Meltzer H. The serotonin hypothesis of major depression. In: Bloom, FE, Kupfer, DJ (Eds.), Psychopharmacology. The Fourth Generation of Progress. Raven Press Ltd, New York, NY 1995:933-944.

[5] Demarquay G, Lothe A, Royet JP, Costes N, Mick G, Mauguière F, et al. Brainstem changes in 5-HT1A receptor availability during migraine attack. Cephalalgia 2011;31(1):84-94.

[6] Lothe A, Merlet I, Demarquay G, Costes N, Ryvlin P, Mauguière F. Interictal brain 5-HT(1A) receptors binding in migraine without aura: a (18)F-MPPF-PET study. Cephalalgia 2008;28(12):1282-1291.

[7] Didelot A, Ryvlin P, Lothe A, Merlet I, Hammers A, Mauguiere F. PET imaging of brain 5-$HT_{1A}$ receptors in the preoperative evaluation of temporal lobe epilepsy. Brain 2008;131(Pt 10):2751-2764.

[8] Lothe A, Didelot A, Hammers A, Costes N, Saoud M, Gilliam F, et al. Comorbidity between temporal lobe epilepsy and depression: a [$^{18}$F]MPPF PET study. Brain 2008b; 131(Pt 10):2765-2782.

[9] Merlet I, Ryvlin P, Costes N, Dufournel D, Isnard J, Faillenot I, et al. Statistical parametric mapping of 5-$HT_{1A}$ receptor binding in temporal lobe epilepsy with hippocampal ictal onset on intracranial EEG. Neuroimage 2004;22(2):886-896.

[10] Truchot L, Costes N, Zimmer L, Laurent B, Le Bars D, Thomas-Antérion C, et al. A distinct [$^{18}$F]MPPF PET profile in amnestic mild cognitive impairment compared to mild Alzheimer's disease. Neuroimage 2008;40(3):1251-1256.

[11] Buhot MC, Martin S, Segu L. Role of serotonin in memory impairment. Ann. Med. 2000;32(3):210-221.

[12] Hainer V, Kabrnova K, Aldhoon B, Kunesova M, Wagenknecht M. Serotonin and norepinephrine reuptake inhibition and eating behavior. Ann. N. Y. Acad. Sci. 2006;1083:252-269.

[13] Gross C, Zhuang X, Stark K, Ramboz S, Oosting R, Kirby L, et al. Serotonin 1A receptor acts during development to establish normal anxiety-like behaviour in the adult. Nature 2002;416(6879):396-400.

[14] Iqbal N, van Praag HM. The role of serotonin in schizophrenia. Eur Neuropsychopharmacol. 1995;5 Suppl:11-23.

[15] Burgess NK, Sweeten TL, McMahon WM, Fujinami RS. Hyperserotoninemia and altered immunity in autism. J. Autism. Dev. Disord. 2006;36(5):697-704.

[16] Chugani DC. Serotonin in autism and pediatric epilepsies. Ment. Retard. Dev. Disabil. Res. Rev. 2004;10(2):112-116.

[17] Paterson LM, Kornum BR, Nutt DJ, Pike VW, Knudsen GM. 5-HT radioligands for human brain imaging with PET and SPECT. Med Res Rev. 2011;Jun 14.doi: 10.1002/med.20245.

[18] Hannon J, Hoyer D. Molecular biology of 5-HT receptors. Behav Brain Res. 2008;195(1):198-213.

[19] Bockaert J, Claeysen S, Bécamel C, Dumuis A, Marin P. Neuronal 5-HT metabotropic receptors: fine-tuning of their structure, signaling, and roles in synaptic modulation. Cell Tissue Res. 2006;326(2):553-72.

[20] Fargin A, Raymond JR, Lohse MJ, Kobilka BK, Caron MG, Lefkowitz RJ. The genomic clone G-21 which resembles a betaadrenergic receptor sequence encodes the 5-HT1A receptor. Nature 1988;335, 358-360.

[21] Beck SG, Choi KC. 5-Hydroxytryptamine hyperpolarizes CA3 hippocampal pyramidal cells through an increase in potassium conductance. Neurosci Lett. 1991; 133: 93–6.

[22] Okuhara DY, Beck SG. 5-HT1A receptor linked to inward-rectifying potassium current in hippocampal CA3 pyramidal cells. J Neurophysiol. 1994; 71: 2161–7.

[23] Richer M, Hen R, Blier P. Modification of serotonin neuron properties in mice lacking 5-HT1A receptors. Eur. J. Pharmacol. 2002;435(2-3):195-203

[24] Weissmann-Nanopoulos D, Mach E, Magre S, Demassay Y, Pujol JF. Evidence for the localization of 5HT1-A binding sites on serotonin containing neurons in the raphe dorsalis and raphe centralis nuclei of the rat brain. Neurochem. Int. 1985;7:1061-1072.

[25] Kumar JS, Mann JJ. PET tracers for 5-HT(1A) receptors and uses thereof. Drug Discov Today 2007;Sep 12(17-18):748-56.

[26] Zhuang ZP, Kung MP, Chumpradit S, Mu M, Kung HF. Derivatives of 4-(2′- methoxyphenyl)-1-[2′-(N-2″-pyridinyl-p-iodobenzamido)ethyl]pipera zine (p-MPPI) as 5-HT1A ligands. J. Med. Chem. 1994;37(26):4572-4575.

[27] Lang L, Jagoda E, Schmall B, Vuong BK, Adams HR, Nelson DL, et al. Development of fluorine-18-labeled 5-HT1A antagonists. J Med Chem. 1999 May 6;42(9):1576-86.

[28] Rice OV, Gatley SJ, Shen J, Huemmer CL, Rogoz R, DeJesus OT et al., 2001. Effects of endogenous neurotransmitters on the in vivo binding of dopamine and 5-HT radiotracers in mice. Neuropsychopharmacology;25(5):679-89.

[29] Maeda J, Suhara T, Ogawa M, Okauchi T, Kawabe K, Zhang MR et al. In vivo binding properties of [carbonyl-11C]WAY-100635:effect of endogenous serotonin. Synapse 2001;40(2):122-9.

[30] Van Wijngaarden I, Tulp MT, Soudijn W. The concept of selectivity in 5-HT receptor research. Eur. J. Pharmacol. 1990;188(6): 301-312.

[31] Rbah L, Leviel V, Zimmer L. Displacement of the PET ligand $^{18}$F-MPPF by the electrically evoked serotonin release in the rat hippocampus. Synapse 2003;49(4):239-245.

[32] Zimmer L, Mauger G, Le Bars D, Bonmarchand G, Luxen A, Pujol JF. Effect of endogenous serotonin on the binding of the 5-$HT_{1A}$ PET ligand $^{18}$F-MPPF in the rat hippocampus: kinetic beta measurements combined with microdialysis. J. Neurochem. 2002; 80(2):278-286.

[33] Zimmer L, Rbah L, Giacomelli F, Le Bars D, Renaud B. A reduced extracellular serotonin level increases the 5-HT1A PET ligand 18FMPPF binding in the rat hippocampus. Journal of Nuclear Medicine 2003;44 (9):1495-501.

[34] Millet P, Moulin M, Bartoli A, Del Guerra A, Ginovart N, Lemoucheux L, et al. In vivo quantification of 5-HT1A-[18F]MPPF interactions in rats using the YAP-(S)PET scanner and a beta-microprobe. Neuroimage. 2008 Jul 1;41(3):823-34.

[35] Frey BN, Rosa-Neto P, Lubarsky S, Diksic M. Correlation between serotonin synthesis and 5-HT1A receptor binding in the living human brain: a combined alpha-[11C]MT and [18F]MPPF positron emission tomography study. Neuroimage 2008;42(2):850-7.

[36] Gozlan H, Thibault S, Laporte AM, Lima L, Hamon M. The selective 5-$HT_{1A}$ antagonist radioligand [$^3$H]WAY 100635 labels both G-protein coupled and free 5-$HT_{1A}$ receptors in rat brain membranes. Eur J Pharmacol. 1995;288:173-186.

[37] Zimmer L, Riad M, Rbah L, Belkacem-Kahlouli A, Le Bars D, Renaud B, et al. Toward brain imaging of serotonin 5-HT1A autoreceptor internalization. Neuroimage 2004;22(3):1421-1426.

[38] Riad M, Zimmer L, Rbah L, Watkins KC, Hamon M, Descarries L. Acute treatment with the antidepressant fluoxetine internalizes 5-HT1A autoreceptors and reduces the in vivo binding of the PET radioligand [18F]MPPF in the nucleus raphe dorsalis of rat. J Neurosci 2004;24(23):5420-6.

[39] Aznavour N, Rbah L, Riad M, Reilhac A, Costes N, Descarries L et al. A PET imaging study of 5-HT(1A) receptors in cat brain after acute and chronic fluoxetine treatment. Neuroimage 2006;33(3):834-42.

[40] Sibon I, Benkelfat C, Gravel P, Aznavour N, Costes N, Mzengeza S et al. Decreased [18F]MPPF binding potential in the dorsal raphe nucleus after a single oral dose of fluoxetine: a positron-emission tomography study in healthy volunteers. Biol Psychiatry 2008;63(12):1135-40.

[41] David SP, Murthy NV, Rabiner EA, Munafó MR, Johnstone EC, Jacob R et al. A functional genetic variation of the serotonin (5-HT) transporter affects 5-HT1A receptor binding in humans. J Neurosci. 2005;25(10):2586-90.

[42] Lee M, Bailer UF, Frank GK, Henry SE, Meltzer CC, Price JC et al. Relationship of a 5-HT transporter functional polymorphism to 5-HT1A receptor binding in healthy women. Mol Psychiatry 2005;10(8):715-6.

[43] Lothe A, Boni C, Costes N, Gorwood P, Bouvard S, Le Bars D et al. Association between triallelic polymorphism of the serotonin transporter and [18F]MPPF binding potential at 5-HT1A receptors in healthy subjects. Neuroimage 2009;47(2):482-492.

[44] Lothe A, Boni C, Costes N, Bouvard S, Gorwood P, Lavenne F, et al. 5-$HT_{1A}$ gene promoter polymorphism and [$^{18}$F]MPPF binding potential in healthy subjects: a PET study. Behav Brain Funct. 2010;Jul 7;6:37.

[45] Parsey RV, Oquendo MA, Ogden RT, Olvet DM, Simpson N, Huang YY et al. Altered serotonin 1A binding in major depression: a [carbonyl-C-11]WAY100635 positron emission tomography study. Biol Psychiatry 2006;59(2):106-13.

[46] Sullivan GM, Ogden RT, Oquendo MA, Kumar JS, Simpson N, Huang YY, et al. Positron emission tomography quantification of serotonin-1A receptor binding in medication-free bipolar depression. Biol Psychiatry 2009;66:223-30.

[47] Borg J, Henningsson S, Saijo T, Inoue M, Bah J, Westberg L, et al. Serotonin transporter genotype is associated with cognitive performance but not regional 5-HT1A receptor binding in humans. Int. J. Neuropsychopharmacol. 2009;1–10.

[48] Innis RB, Cunningham VJ, Delforge J, Fujita M, Gjedde A, Gunn RN, et al. Consensus nomenclature for in vivo imaging of reversibly binding radioligands. J. Cereb. Blood Flow Metab. 2007;27(9):1533-1539.

[49] Møller M, Jakobsen S, Gjedde A. Parametric and regional maps of free serotonin 5HT1A receptor sites in human brain as function of age in healthy humans. Neuropsychopharmacology 2007;32:1707-14.

[50] Costes N, Merlet I, Ostrowsky K, Faillenot I, Lavenne F, Zimmer L, et al. A 18F-MPPF PET normative database of 5-HT1A receptor binding in men and women over aging. J Nucl Med 2005;46:1980-9.

[51] Tauscher J, Verhoeff NP, Christensen BK, Hussey D, Meyer JH, Kecojevic A, et al. Serotonin 5-HT1A receptor binding potential declines with age as measured by [11C]WAY-100635 and PET. Neuropsychopharmacology 2001;24:522-30.

[52] Cidis Meltzer C, Drevets WC, Price JC, Mathis CA, Lopresti B, Greer PJ, et al. Gender-specific aging effects on the serotonin 1A receptor. Brain Res 2001;895:9-17.

[53] Parsey RV, Oquendo MA, Simpson NR, Ogden RT, Van Heertum R, Arango V et al. Effects of sex, age, and aggressive traits in man on brain serotonin 5-HT1A receptor binding potential measured by PET using [C-11]WAY-100635. Brain Res. 2002;954(2): 173-82.

[54] Stein P, Savli M, Wadsak W, Mitterhauser M, Fink M, Spindelegger C, et al. The serotonin-1A receptor distribution in healthy men and women measured by PET and [carbonyl-11C]WAY-100635. Eur. J. Nucl. Med. Mol. Imaging 2008;35, 2159–2168.

[55] Jovanovic H, Lundberg J, Karlsson P, Cerin A, Saijo T, Varrone A, et al. Sex differences in the serotonin 1A receptor and serotonin transporter binding in the human brain measured by PET. NeuroImage 2008;39(3), 1408–1419.

[56] Bromet E, Andrade LH, Hwang I, Sampson NA, Alonso J, de Girolamo G, et al. Cross-national epidemiology of DSM-IV major depressive episode. BMC Med. 2011 Jul 26;9:90.

[57] American Psychiatric Association. Diagnostic Statistical Manual of Mental Disorders, Forth edition, Wasghiton, American psy press, 2000

[58] Fenton WS, Stover ES. Mood disorders: cardiovascular and diabetes comorbidity. Curr Opin Psychiatry. 2006 Jul;19(4):421-7.

[59] Ustün TB, Ayuso-Mateos JL, Chatterji S, Mathers C, Murray CJ. Global burden of depressive disorders in the year 2000. Br J Psychiatry. 2004 May;184:386-92.

[60] Dhaenen H. Imaging the serotonergic system in depression. Eur Arch Psychiatry Clin Neurosci. 2001;251 (Suppl 2): II76–80.

[61] Jans LA, Riedel WJ, Markus CR, Blokland A. Serotonergic vulnerability and depression: assumptions, experimental evidence and implications. Mol Psychiatry 2007 Jun; 12(6):522-43.

[62] Asberg M, Thoren P, Traskman L, Bertilsson L, Ringberger V. 'Serotonin depression'–a biochemical subgroup within the affective disorders? Science 1976; 191: 478–80.

[63] Meltzer HY. Role of serotonin in depression. Ann N Y Acad Sci. 1990; 600:486–99.

[64] Delgado PL, Charney DS, Price LH, Aghajanian GK, Landis H, Heninger GR. Serotonin function and the mechanism of antidepressant action. Reversal of antidepressant-induced remission by rapid depletion of plasma tryptophan. Arch Gen Psychiatry. 1990 May;47(5):411-8.

[65] Smith KA, Fairburn CG, Cowen PJ. Relapse of depression after rapid depletion of tryptophan. Lancet 1997 Mar 29;349(9056):915-9.

[66] Young SN, Smith SE, Pihl RO, Ervin FR. Tryptophan depletion causes a rapid lowering of mood in normal males. Psychopharmacology 1985;87(2):173-7.

[67] Berney A, Nishikawa M, Benkelfat C, Debonnel G, Gobbi G, Diksic M. An index of 5-HT synthesis changes during early antidepressant treatment: alpha-[11C]methyl-L-tryptophan PET study. Neurochem Int. 2008;52(4-5):701-8.

[68] Rosa-Neto P, Diksic M, Okazawa H, Leyton M, Ghadirian N, Mzengeza S et al. Measurement of brain regional alpha-[11C]methyl-L-tryptophan trapping as a measure of serotonin synthesis in medication-free patients with major depression. Arch Gen Psychiatry 2004; 61(6):556-63.

[69] Savitz JB, Drevets WC. Neuroreceptor imaging in depression. Neurobiol Dis. 2012 Jun 9. [Epub ahead of print]

[70] Shrestha S, Hirvonen J, Hines CS, Henter ID, Svenningsson P, Pike VW, et al. Serotonin-1A receptors in major depression quantified using PET: controversies, confounds, and recommendations. Neuroimage 2012 Feb 15;59(4):3243-51.

[71] Saijo T, Takano A, Suhara T, Arakawa R, Okumura M, Ichimiya T, et al. Effect of electroconvulsive therapy on 5-HT1A receptor binding in patients with depression: a PET study with [11C]WAY 100635. Int J Neuropsychopharmacol. 2010 Jul;13(6): 785-91.

[72] Mickey BJ, Ducci F, Hodgkinson CA, Langenecker SA, Goldman D, Zubieta JK. Monoamine oxidase A genotype predicts human serotonin 1A receptor availability in vivo. J Neurosci. 2008; 28:11354-9.

[73] Drevets WC, Frank E, Price JC, Kupfer DJ, Holt D, Greer PJ, et al. PET imaging of serotonin 1A receptor binding in depression. Biol Psychiatry 1999;46:1375-1387.

[74] Drevets WC, Frank E, Price JC, Kupfer DJ, Greer PJ, Mathis C. Serotonin type-1A receptor imaging in depression. Nucl Med Biol. 2000;27:499-507.

[75] Sargent PA, Kjaer KH, Bench CJ, Rabiner EA, Messa C, Meyer J, et al. Brain serotonin 1A receptor binding measured by positron emission tomography with [$^{11}$C]WAY-100635: effects of depression and antidepressant treatment. Arch Gen Psychiatry 2000;57:174-180.

[76] Bhagwagar Z, Rabiner EA, Sargent PA, Grasby PM, Cowen PJ. Persistent reduction in brain serotonin 1A receptor binding in recovered depressed men measured by positron emission tomography with [$^{11}$C]WAY-100635. Mol Psychiatry 2004;9:386-392.

[77] Parsey RV, Oquendo MA, Ogden RT, Olvet DM, Simpson N, Huang YY, et al. Altered serotonin 1A binding in major depression: a [carbonyl-C-11]WAY100635 positron emission tomography study. Biol Psychiatry 2006a;59:106-113.

[78] Parsey RV, Olvet DM, Oquendo MA, Huang YY, Ogden RT, Mann JJ. Higher 5-HT1A receptor binding potential during a major depressive episode predicts poor treatment response: preliminary data from a naturalistic study. Neuropsychopharmacology 2006b;31:1745-9.

[79] Parsey RV, Ogden RT, Miller JM, Tin A, Hesselgrave N, Goldstein E, et al. Higher serotonin 1A binding in a second major depression cohort: modeling and reference region considerations. Biol Psychiatry 2010;68:170-178.

[80] Hirvonen J, Karlsson H, Kajander J, Lepola A, Markkula J, Rasi-Hakala H et al. Decreased brain serotonin 5-HT1A receptor availability in medication-naive patients with major depressive disorder: an in-vivo imaging study using PET and [carbonyl-11C]WAY-100635. Int J Neuropsychopharmacol. 2008;11(4):465-76.

[81] Miller JM, Brennan KG, Ogden TR, Oquendo MA, Sullivan GM, Mann JJ, et al. Elevated serotonin 1A binding in remitted major depressive disorder: evidence for a trait biological abnormality. Neuropsychopharmacology 2009;34:2275-2284.

[82] Shively CA, Friedman DP, Gage HD, Bounds MC, Brown-Proctor C, Blair JB, et al. Behavioral depression and positron emission tomography-determined serotonin 1A receptor binding potential in cynomolgus monkeys. Archives of General Psychiatry 2006;63, 396-403.

[83] Bowen DM, Najlerahim A, Procter AW, Francis PT, Murphy E. Circumscribed changes of the cerebral cortex in neuropsychiatric disorders of later life. Proc. Natl. Acad. Sci. USA 1989;86:9504-8.

[84] Cheetham SC, Crompton MR, Katona CL, Horton RW. Brain 5-HT1 binding sites in depressed suicides. Psychopharmacology (Berl). 1990;102(4):544-8.

[85] Francis PT, Pangalos MN, Stephens PH, Bartlett JR, Bridges PK, Malizia AL, et al. Antemortem measurements of neurotransmission: possible implications for pharmacotherapy of Alzheimer's disease and depression. J Neurol Neurosurg Psychiatry. 1993 Jan;56(1):80-4.

[86] Arango V, Underwood MD, Boldrini M, Tamir H, Kassir SA et al. Serotonin 1A receptors, serotonin transporter binding and serotonin transporter mRNA expression in the brainstem of depressed suicide victims. Neuropsychopharmacology 2001;25(6):892-903.

[87] Lopez-Figueroa AL, Norton CS, Lopez-Figueroa MO, Armellini-Dodel D, Burke S, Akil H et al. Serotonin 5-HT1A, 5-HT1B, and 5-HT2A receptor mRNA expression in subjects with major depression, bipolar disorder, and schizophrenia. Biol. Psychiatry 2004;55(3):225-33.

[88] Boldrini M, Underwood MD, Mann JJ, Arango V. Serotonin-1A autoreceptor binding in the dorsal raphe nucleus of depressed suicides. J Psychiatr Res. 2008; 42:433-42.

[89] Anisman H, Du L, Palkovits M, Faludi G, Kovacs GG, Szontagh-Kishazi P, et al. Serotonin receptor subtype and p11 mRNA expression in stress-relevant brain regions of suicide and control subjects. J Psychiatry Neurosci. 2008 Mar;33(2):131-41.

[90] Lopez JF, Chalmers DT, Little KY, Watson SJ. Regulation of serotonin1A, glucocorticoid, and mineralocorticoid receptor in rat and human hippocampus: implications for the neurobiology of depression. Biol. Psychiatry 1998;43(8):547-73.

[91] Hirvonen J, Kajander J, Allonen T, Oikonen V, Någren K, Hietala J. Measurement of serotonin 5-HT1A receptor binding using positron emission tomography and [carbonyl-(11)C]WAY-100635-considerations on the validity of cerebellum as a reference region. J Cereb Blood Flow Metab. 2007;27(1):185-95.

[92] Kendler KS, Kuhn JW, Vittum J, Prescott CA, Riley B. The interaction of stressful life events and a serotonin transporter polymorphism in the prediction of episodes of major depression: a replication. Arch Gen Psychiatry 2005 May;62(5):529-35.

[93] Caspi A, Sugden K, Moffitt TE, Taylor A, Craig IW, Harrington H, et al. Influence of life stress on depression: moderation by a polymorphism in the 5-HTT gene. Science 2003;301(5631):386–389.

[94] Moses-Kolko EL, Price JC, Thase ME, Meltzer CC, Kupfer DJ, Mathis CA, et al. Measurement of 5-$HT_{1A}$ receptor binding in depressed adults before and after antidepressant drug treatment using positron emission tomography and [$^{11}$C]WAY-100635. Synapse 2007;61:523-530.

[95] Karlsson H, Hirvonen J, Kajander J, Markkula J, Rasi-Hakala H, Salminen JK, et al. Research letter: Psychotherapy increases brain serotonin 5-HT1A receptors in patients with major depressive disorder. Psychological Medicine 2010;40(3):523-528.

[96] Spindelegger C, Lanzenberger R, Wadsak W, Mien LK, Stein P, Mitterhauser M, et al. Influence of escitalopram treatment on 5-HT 1A receptor binding in limbic regions in patients with anxiety disorders. Mol Psychiatry 2009 Nov;14(11):1040-50.

[97] Lothe A, Saoud M, Bouvard S, Redouté J, Lerond J, Ryvlin P. 5-$HT_{1A}$ receptor binding in patients with major depressive disorder before and after antidepressant treatment : A pilot [$^{18}$F]MPPF positron emission tomography study. Psychiatry Research : Neuroimaging 2012;Jul 30;203(1):103-4

[98] Riad M, Rbah L, Verdurand M, Aznavour N, Zimmer L, Descarries L. Unchanged density of 5-HT(1A) autoreceptors on the plasma membrane of nucleus raphe dorsalis neurons in rats chronically treated with fluoxetine. Neuroscience 2008;151(3): 692-700.

[99] Moulin-Sallanon M, Charnay Y, Ginovart N, Perret P, Lanfumey L, Hamon M, et al. Acute and chronic effects of citalopram on 5-HT1A receptor-labeling by [18F]MPPF and -coupling to receptors-G proteins. Synapse. 2009 Feb;63(2):106-16.

[100] Téllez-Zenteno JF, Dhar R, Hernandez-Ronquillo L, Wiebe S. Long-term outcomes in epilepsy surgery: antiepileptic drugs, mortality, cognitive and psychosocial aspects. Brain 2007;130(Pt 2):334-45.

[101] Jones JE, Hermann BP, Barry JJ, Gilliam F, Kanner AM, Meador KJ. Clinical assessment of axis I psychiatric morbidity in chronic epilepsy: a multicenter investigation. J Neuropsychiatry Clin Neurosci Spring 2005;17:172-9.

[102] Jones JE, Bell B, Fine J, Rutecki P, Seidenberg M, Hermann B. A controlled prospective investigation of psychiatric comorbidity in temporal lobe epilepsy. Epilepsia 2007;48(12):2357-60.

[103] Kanner AM. Depression in epilepsy: prevalence, clinical semiology, pathogenic mechanisms, and treatment. Biol Psychiatry 2003;54:388-98.

[104] Hermann B, Seidenberg M, Jones J. The neurobehavioural comorbidities of epilepsy: can a natural history be developed? Lancet Neurol. 2008;7(2):151-60.

[105] Gilliam FG, Santos J, Vahle V, Carter J, Brown K, Hecimovic H. Depression in epilepsy: ignoring clinical expression of neuronal network dysfunction? Epilepsia. 2004;45 Suppl 2:28-33.

[106] Quiske A, Helmstaedter C, Lux S, Elger CE. Depression in patients with temporal lobe epilepsy is related to mesial temporal sclerosis. Epilepsy Res. 2000;39:121-5.

[107] Victoroff JI, Benson F, Grafton ST, Engel J Jr, Mazziotta JC. Depression in complex partial seizures. electroencephalography and cerebral metabolic correlates. Arch Neurol. 1994; 51: 155–63.

[108] Altshuler LL, Devinsky O, Post RM, Theodore W. Depression, anxiety, and temporal lobe epilepsy. Laterality of focus and symptoms. Arch Neurol. 1990; 47: 284–8.

[109] Bell GS, Sander JW. Suicide and epilepsy. Curr Opin Neurol. 2009 Apr;22(2):174-8.

[110] Christensen J, Vestergaard M, Mortensen PB, Sidenius P, Agerbo E. Epilepsy and risk of suicide: a population-based case-control study. Lancet Neurol. 2007 Aug;6(8): 693-8.

[111] Kanner AM. Depression and epilepsy: a review of multiple facets of their close relation. Neurol Clin. 2009 Nov;27(4):865-80.

[112] Kanner AM. Mood disorder and epilepsy: a neurobiologic perspective of their relationship. Dialogues Clin Neurosci. 2008;10(1):39-45.

[113] Bagdy G, Kecskemeti V, Riba P, Jakus R. Serotonin and epilepsy. J Neurochem. 2007;100(4):857-73.

[114] Wada Y, Shiraishi J, Nakamura M, Koshino Y. Role of serotonin receptor subtypes in the development of amygdaloid kindling in rats. Brain Res. 1997;747:338-42.

[115] Wada Y, Nakamura M, Hasegawa H, Yamaguchi N. Role of serotonin receptor subtype in seizures kindled from the feline hippocampus. Neurosci Lett. 1992;141:21-4.

[116] Wada Y, Nakamura M, Hasegawa H, Yamaguchi N. Intra-hippocampal injection of 8-hydroxy-2-(di-n-propylamino)tetralin (8-OH-DPAT) inhibits partial and generalized seizures induced by kindling stimulation in cats. Neurosci Lett. 1993;159:179-182.

[117] Salgado-Commissariat D, Alkadhi KA. Serotonin inhibits epileptiform discharge by activation of 5-HT1A receptors in CA1 pyramidal neurons. Neuropharmacology 1997; 36: 1705-12.

[118] Tokarski K, Zahorodna A, Bobula B, Hess G. Comparison of the effects of 5-HT1A and 5-HT4 receptor activation on field potentials and epileptiform activity in rat hippocampus. Exp Brain Res. 2002 Dec;147(4):505-10.

[119] Lu KT, Gean PW. Endogenous serotonin inhibits epileptiform activity in rat hippocampal CA1 neurons via 5-hydroxytryptamine1A receptor activation. Neuroscience 1998;86:729-37.

[120] Yan QS, Jobe PC, Dailey JW. Further evidence of anticonvulsant role for 5-hydroxytryptamine in genetically epilepsy-prone rats. Br J Pharmacol. 1995; 115:1314-8.

[121] Watanabe K, Minabe Y, Ashby CR, Katsumori H. Effect of acute administration of various 5-HT receptor agonists on focal hippocampal seizures in freely moving rats. Eur J Pharmacol. 1998; 350:181-8.

[122] Levkovitz Y, Segal M. Serotonin 5-HT1A receptors modulate hippocampal reactivity to afferent stimulation. J Neurosci. 1997; 17:5591-8.

[123] Toczek MT, Carson RE, Lang L, Ma Y, Spanaki MV, Der MG, et al. PET imaging of 5-HT1A receptor binding in patients with temporal lobe epilepsy. Neurology 2003;60:749-56.

[124] Merlet I, Ryvlin P, Costes N, Dufournel D, Isnard J, Faillenot I, et al. Statistical parametric mapping of 5-HT1A receptor binding in temporal lobe epilepsy with hippocampal ictal onset on intracranial EEG. Neuroimage 2004a;22(2):886-96.

[125] Merlet I, Ostrowsky K, Costes N, Ryvlin P, Isnard J, Faillenot I et al. 5-HT1A receptor binding and intracerebral activity in temporal lobe epilepsy: an [18F]MPPF-PET study. Brain 2004b; 127(Pt 4):900-13.

[126] Savic I, Lindstrom P, Gulyas B, Halldin C, Andree B, Farde L. Limbic reductions of 5-HT1A receptor binding in human temporal lobe epilepsy. Neurology 2004;62:1343-51.

[127] Giovacchini G, Toczek MT, Bonwetsch R, Bagic A, Lang L, Fraser C et al. 5-HT 1A receptors are reduced in temporal lobe epilepsy after partial volume correction. J Nucl Med. 2005; 46:1128–35.

[128] Ito S, Suhara T, Ito H, Yasuno F, Ichimiya T, Takano A et al. Changes in central 5-HT(1A) receptor binding in mesial temporal epilepsy measured by positron emission tomography with [(11)C]WAY100635. Epilepsy Res. 2007;73:111-8.

[129] Didelot A, Ryvlin P, Lothe A, Merlet I, Hammers A, Mauguière F. PET imaging of brain 5-HT1A receptors in the preoperative evaluation of temporal lobe epilepsy. Brain 2008;131(Pt 10):2751-64.

[130] Assem-Hilger E, Lanzenberger R, Savli M, Wadsak W, Mitterhauser M, Mien LK, et al. Central serotonin 1A receptor binding in temporal lobe epilepsy: a [carbonyl-(11)C]WAY-100635 PET study. Epilepsy Behav. 2010 Nov;19(3):467-73.

[131] Statnick MA, Dailey JW, Jobe PC, Browning RA. Abnormalities in brain serotonin concentration, high-affinity uptake, and tryptophan hydroxylase activity in severe-seizure genetically epilepsy-prone rats. Epilepsia 1996;37: 311-21.

[132] Kwan P, Brodie MJ. Potential role of drug transporters in the pathogenesis of medically intractable epilepsy. Epilepsia 2005;46(2):224-35.

[133] Theodore WH, Hasler G, Giovacchini G, Kelley K, Reeves-Tyer P, Herscovitch P, et al. Reduced hippocampal 5HT1A PET receptor binding and depression in temporal lobe epilepsy. Epilepsia 2007;48:1526-1530.

[134] Theodore WH, Wiggs EA, Martinez AR, Dustin IH, Khan OI, Appel S, et al. Serotonin 1A receptors, depression, and memory in temporal lobe epilepsy. Epilepsia. 2012 Jan;53(1):129-33.

[135] Hasler G, Bonwetsch R, Giovacchini G, Toczek MT, Bagic A, Luckenbaugh DA, et al. 5-$HT_{1A}$ receptor binding in temporal lobe epilepsy patients with and without major depression. Biol Psychiatry 2007;62:1258-1264.

[136] Quiske A, Helmstaedter C, Lux S, Elger CE. Depression in patients with temporal lobe epilepsy is related to mesial temporal sclerosis. Epilepsy Res. 2000;39:121-5.

[137] Hecimovic H, Goldstein JD, Sheline YI, Gilliam FG. Mechanisms of depression in epilepsy from a clinical perspective. Epilepsy Behav 2003;4 (Suppl 3): S25–30.

[138] Ahmad S, Fowler LJ, Whitton PS. Lamotrigine, carbamazepine and phenytoin differentially alter extracellular levels of 5-hydroxytryptamine, dopamine and amino acids. Epilepsy Res. 2005;63(2-3):141-9.

[139] Perala J, Suvisaari J, Saarni S, Kuoppasalmi K, Isomesta E, Pirkola S, et al. Lifetime prevalence of psychotic and bipolar disorders in a general population. Arch Gen Psychiatry 2007;1 :19-28.

[140] Buckley PF, Miller BJ, Lehrer DS, Castle DJ. Psychiatric comorbidities and schizophrenia. Schizophr Bull. 2009 Mar;35(2):383-402.

[141] Saha S, Chant D, McGrath J. Meta-analyses of the incidence and prevalence of schizophrenia: conceptual and methodological issues. Int J Methods Psychiatr Res. 2008;17(1):55-61.

[142] Abi-Dargham A. Do we still believe in the dopamine hypothesis? New data bring new evidence. Int J Neuropsychopharmacol. 2004 Mar;7 Suppl 1:S1-5.

[143] Bantick RA, Deakin JF, Grasby PM. The 5-$HT_{1A}$ receptor in schizophrenia: a promising target for novel atypical neuroleptics? J Psychopharmacol 2001;15(1):37-46.

[144] Hashimoto T, Nishino N, Nakai H and Tanaka C. Increase in serotonin 5-HT1A receptors in prefrontal and temporal cortices of brains from patients with chronic schizophrenia. Life Sci 1991;48:355–363.

[145] Joyce JN, Shane A, Lexow N, Winokur A, Casanova MF and Kleinman JE. Serotonin uptake sites and serotonin receptors are altered in the limbic system of schizophrenics. Neuropsychopharmacology 1993;8: 315–336.

[146] Burnet PW, Eastwood SL, Harrison PJ. 5-HT1A and 5-HT2A receptor mRNAs and binding site densities are differentially altered in schizophrenia. Neuropsychopharmacology 1996; 15(5):442-55.

[147] Simpson MD, Lubman DI, Slater P and Deakin JF. Autoradiography with [3H]8-OH-DPAT reveals increases in 5-HT(1A) receptors in ventral prefrontal cortex in schizophrenia. Biol Psychiatry 1996;39: 919–928.

[148] Sumiyoshi T, Stockmeier CA, Overholser JC, Dilley GE and Meltzer HY. Serotonin1A receptors are increased in postmortem prefrontal cortex in schizophrenia. Brain Res 1996;708: 209–214.

[149] Tauscher J, Kapur S, Verhoeff NP, Hussey DF, Daskalakis ZJ, Tauscher-Wisniewski S, et al. Brain serotonin 5-HT(1A) receptor binding in schizophrenia measured by positron emission tomography and [11C]WAY-100635. Arch Gen Psychiatry 2002 Jun;59(6):514-20.

[150] Yasuno F, Suhara T, Ichimiya T, Takano A, Ando T, Okubo Y. Decreased 5-HT1A receptor binding in amygdala of schizophrenia. Biol Psychiatry 2004;55(5):439-44.

[151] Bantick RA, Montgomery AJ, Bench CJ, Choudhry T, Malek N, McKenna PJ et al. A positron emission tomography study of the 5-HT1A receptor in schizophrenia and during clozapine treatment. J Psychopharmacol 2004;18(3):346-354.

[152] Frankle WG, Lombardo I, Kegeles LS, Slifstein M, Martin JH, Huang Y, et al. Serotonin 1A receptor availability in patients with schizophrenia and schizo-affective disorder: a positron emission tomography imaging study with [11C]WAY 100635. Psychopharmacology (Berl). 2006 Dec;189(2):155-64.

[153] Davis JM, Chen N, Glick ID. A meta-analysis of the efficacy of second-generation antipsychotics. Arch Gen Psychiatry 2003;60:553–564

[154] Newman-Tancredi A, Kleven MS. Comparative pharmacology of antipsychotics possessing combined dopamine D2 and serotonin 5-HT1A receptor properties. Psychopharmacology (Berl). 2011 Aug;216(4):451-73.

[155] Ichikawa J, Meltzer HY. Valproate and carbamazepine increase prefrontal dopamine release by 5-HT1A receptor activation. Eur J Pharmacol 1999;380(1):R1-3.

[156] Arborelius L, Nomikos GG, Hacksell U, and Svensson TH. (R)-8-OH-DPAT preferentially increases dopamine release in rat medial prefrontal cortex. Acta Physiol Scand 1993;148(4):465-466.

[157] Rollema H, Lu Y, Schmidt AW, and Zorn SH. Clozapine increases dopamine release in prefrontal cortex by 5-HT1A receptor activation. Eur J Pharmacol 1997;338(2):R3-5.

[158] Jordan S, Koprivica V, Chen R, Tottori K, Kikuchi T, Altar CA. The antipsychotic aripiprazole is a potent, partial agonist at the human 5-HT1A receptor. Eur J Pharmacol 2002;441(3):137-140.

[159] Bortolozzi A, Díaz-Mataix L, Toth M, Celada P, Artigas F. In vivo actions of aripiprazole on serotonergic and dopaminergic systems in rodent brain. Psychopharmacology (Berl.). 2007;191(3):745-758.

[160] Kane JM, Carson WH, Saha AR, McQuade RD, Ingenito GG, Zimbroff DL, et al. Efficacy and safety of aripiprazole and haloperidol versus placebo in patients with schizophrenia and schizoaffective disorder. J Clin Psychiatry. 2002 Sep;63(9):763-71.

[161] Lerond J, Lothe A, Ryvlin P, d'Amato T, Bouvard S, Ciumas C, et al. Effects of aripiprazole, risperidone and olanzapine on $5\text{-HT}_{1A}$ receptors in patients with schizophrenia. J Clinic Psychopharmacol 2012 (in press).

[162] Frankle WG, Lombardo I, Kegeles LS, Slifstein M, Martin JH, Huang Y et al. Measurement of the serotonin 1A receptor availability in patients with schizophrenia during treatment with the antipsychotic medication ziprasidone. J Psychopharmacol. 2011; 25(6):734-743.

[163] Mamo D, Graff A, Mizrahi R, Shammi CM, Romeyer F, Kapur S. Differential effects of aripiprazole on D(2), 5-HT(2), and 5-HT(1A) receptor occupancy in patients with schizophrenia: a triple tracer PET study. Am J Psychiatry 2007;164(9):1411-1417.

[164] Han M, Huang XF, du Bois TM, Deng C. The effects of antipsychotic drugs administration on 5-HT1A receptor expression in the limbic system of the rat brain. Neuroscience 2009;164(4):1754-1763.

[165] Sakai Y, Nishikawa M, Leyton M, Benkelfat C, Young SN, Diksic M. Cortical trapping of alpha-[(11)C]methyl-l-tryptophan, an index of serotonin synthesis, is lower in females than males. Neuroimage. 2006 Nov 15;33(3):815-24.

[166] Costes N, Benkelfat C, Zimmer L, Dagher A, Le Bars D. Toward a quantification of extra-cellular brain endogenous serotonin concentration with [$^{18}$F]MPPF in PET and a multi-injection protocol. NeuroReceptor Mapping 08, Pittsburg. Neuroimage 2008;T149.

[167] Paterson LM, Tyacke RJ, Nutt DJ, Knudsen GM. Measuring endogenous 5-HT release by emission tomography: promises and pitfalls. J Cereb Blood Flow Metab. 2010;30(10):1682-706.

Chapter 7

# Pathological Gambling: PET Studies

Daniela Santoro and Stefano Pallanti

Additional information is available at the end of the chapter

http://dx.doi.org/10.5772/57125

## 1. Introduction

Pathological gambling(PG) affects 1–3% of the adult population, and has high comorbidity [1].

PG is a persistent or maladaptive gambling behavior characterized by excessive time consumed to gambling or thinking about gambling, needing togamble with increasing amounts of money, chasing one's losses, unsuccessful efforts to stop gambling and financial/social problems due to gambling. Hence, PG can also be considered as a behavioral addiction since the characteristics and diagnostic criteria share many common features with substance addictions [2].

PG can be classified as an impulse control disorder, that can be described as a "chain" of subjective states including arousal, craving and acting, accompanied by a feeling of elation and followed by disphoria, all of which are supposed related to an underpinning neurobiology [3].

It is widely suggested that gambling excitement is central to the disorder, and that it is associated with physiological measures of arousal, that are increased during the gambling [4].

It's become a common opinion among researchers that the use of imaging studies as Magnetic Resonance Imaging (MRI) and Positron Emission Tomography (PET) can be a way to learn more about pathophysiology of this disorder.

## 2. Brain areas involved

Functional imaging studies of the prefrontal and orbitofrontal cortex have implicated dysfunction of these structures both in the pathological gambling.

A recently published functional magnetic resonance imaging (fMRI) study reported that the healthy controls activated their ventromedial and subgenual prefrontal cortex during a 'loss-

INTECH
open science | open minds

© 2013 Santoro and Pallanti; licensee InTech. This is an open access article distributed under the terms of the Creative Commons Attribution License (http://creativecommons.org/licenses/by/3.0), which permits unrestricted use, distribution, and reproduction in any medium, provided the original work is properly cited.

chasing game' more then during decisions to quit. The authors suggested that PG patients may have a neural substrate involving these areas, as loss-chasing is one of the cardinal symptoms of the disorder [1]. Compared to controls, patients with PG had greater activation of the prefrontal cortex Brodmann Areas (BA) 9 and 44 while watching gambling-related images [5], lending evidence to the hypothesis that prefrontal cortex areas were also involved in craving aspects of pathological gambling.

Hollander et al. in a previous study [6], in an entirely different cohort of PG patients assessed with FDG-PET, found that monetary-rewarded blackjack was associated with a significantly higher relative metabolic rate in the primary visual cortex (BA 17), the cingulate gyrus (BA 24), the putamen, and prefrontal BA areas 47 and 10 compared to playing blackjack for points only.

An fMRI study of the Iowa Gambling Task (IGT) confirmed medial frontal/cingulated activation during decision-making and greater activation in gamblers than controls in ventral medial frontal areas [7]. This pattern suggests heightened limbic and sensory activation in gambling for monetary reward with increased emotional valence, and confirms the salience of monetary reward in PG.

Other MRI studies on healthy volunteers responding to monetary consequences reported an activation in prefrontal and premotor cortices. This has been interpreted as related to the integration of reward choice salience and preparatory behaviors for obtaining rewards. The basal ganglia and the caudate nucleus in particular are fundamental structures for liking behavior to rewarding and aversive outcome, and they are also involved in modulation decision-making and risk-taking behaviours. These structures have a key role in learning and reasoning processes, and this is reflected in basal ganglia dysfunction.

Some studies have proposed that the salience of monetary reward would be correlated to caudate and nucleus accumbens activation [3]

## 3. Investigations on neural circuits involved

Over the past 2 decades, National Institute of Mental Health (NIMH) has supported research to understand mental disorders as brain disorders. NIMH has therefore launched the Research Domain Criteria (RDoC) project.

RDoC is an experimental approach to the classification of mental disorders that incorporates multiple dimensions: behavior, thought patterns, neurobiological measures, and genetics. RDoC uses genetics, imaging, and cognitive science for understanding deficits in social behavior. The RDoC project has a primary focus on neural circuits. While genes cut across the current diagnostic labels, neuroimaging often helps us to sub-divide current groups. This is particularly interesting when we consider the PG and signs of behavioral alterations related.

The RDoC framework is a heuristic to facilitate the incorporation of behavioral neuroscience in the study of psychopathology. RDoC first aims to identify reliable and valid psychological and biological mechanisms and their disruptions, with an eventual goal of understanding how anomalies in these mechanisms drive psychiatric symptoms [8].

http://dx.doi.org/10.5772/57125

RDoC classification rests on three assumptions. First, the RDoC framework conceptualizes mental illnesses as brain disorders. In contrast to neurological disorders with identifiable lesions, mental disorders can be addressed as disorders of brain circuits. Second, RDoC classification assumes that the dysfunction in neural circuits can be identified with the tools of clinical neuroscience, including electrophysiology, functional neuroimaging, and new methods for quantifying connections in vivo. Third, the RDoC framework assumes that data from genetics and clinical neuroscience will yield biosignatures that will augment clinical symptoms and signs for clinical management.

Examples where clinically relevant models of circuitry-behavior relationships augur future clinical use include fear/extinction, reward, executive function, and impulse control. The practitioner of the future could supplement a clinical evaluation of mental disorders with data from functional or structural imaging, genomic sequencing, and laboratory-based evaluations of fear conditioning and extinction to determine prognosis and appropriate treatment, analogous to what is done routinely today in many other areas of medicine.

The RDoC focuses on neural circuitry, with levels of analysis progressing in one of two directions: upwards from measures of circuitry function to clinically relevant variation, or downwards to the genetic and molecular/cellular factors that ultimately influence such function. [9] Fear circuitry and executive functioning are examples of two functional domains where the relevant circuitry and behaviors seem relatively clear, and these have been selected as the initial areas to be developed; other examples might include reward circuitry and frontostriatal circuits. So, we could begin to create neurobiological circuit maps of behavioral and cognitive functioning and explicate the ways in which activity in these circuits becomes dysregulated in mental disorders.

Patient subjects with relevant presenting psychopathology might be grouped on the basis of a genetic polymorphism or a particular response to a neuroimaging task rather than a DSM/ICD diagnosis; in this manner, investigators can query relevant mechanisms as they cut across traditional categories. [10]

The rationale for the RDoC approach is to facilitate translation of modern molecular biology, neuroscience, and behavioral approaches toward explicating the pathophysiology of disorders. By targeting circuit functioning and relevant behaviors, one particular goal is that this process will direct the search for treatment targets in various domains. [11]

RDoC's integrative approach includes cognition along with social processes, arousal/regulatory systems, and negative and positive valence systems as the major domains, because these neurobehavioral systems have all evolved to serve the motivational and adaptive needs of the organism. With its focus on neural circuits informed by the growing evidence of the neurodevelopmental nature of many disorders and its capacity to capture the patterns of co-occurrence of behaviors and symptoms, the RDoC approach holds promise to advance our understanding of the nature of mental disorders. [12]

Based on RDoC approach, we could identify some neural circuits supposed involved in PG: Nucleos Accumbes (NA) - Orbital Frontal Cortex (OFC) relatively to craving; OFC - Caudates Nucleus (NC) respect to inhibition failure; Limbic system – OFC concerning to affective instability; Anterior Cingulate Cortex (ACC) – OFC about economic decision making. These networks represent hypotheses to be studied to understand the mechanisms underpinning the PG, a disorder regarding addiction and decision making.

In this respect, PET could become a key tool in this evolving diagnostic and therapeutic process.

## 4. The role of dopamine

Brain dopamine neurons code rewarding environmental stimuli by releasing endogenous dopamine (DA), a transmission signal that is important for reinforcement learning. Human reward-seeking gambling behavior, and especially PG, has been presumed to be modulated by brain DA [13].

Several neurotransmitters, and especially DA, have been implicated in the neurobiology of PG [4]. Its release is associated with change in subjective experience and reinforcement of behavior.

Linnet et al. [4] in their study proposed that DA release would be associated with increased excitement levels in PG compared with healthy controls. The study showed that PG with decreased binding potentials in the ventral striatum had significantly higher excitement levels than healthy controls. DA is a neurotransmitter associated with addictive behaviours through a heightened sensitivity to certain types of "reward" such as foods high in sugar or fat content and substances such as cocaine or metamphetamine.

Even if systemic pharmacological interventions such as cocaine and amphetamine lead to release of DA in the whole dorsal and ventral striatum, it appears that more specific types of stimulation leads to regionally restricted dopamine release. And this is supported by the segregation of cortical and and sub-cortical imputs to the striatum.

The relation between DA release and bahavioural reward suggests that the DA system is associated with maladaptative behavior in PG [14].

The salience of monetary reward was reported as correlated to caudate and nucleus accumbens activation. It has been supposed that a dopaminergic neuron activity in these regions may be involved in the acquisition of the associations between salient contextual stimuli and rewarding events [3].

The role of DA in PG is further supported by reports of associations between dopaminergic medications and impulse control disorders in patients with Parkinson's disease (PD) [15]. There are only a few reported functional imaging studies in pathological gamblers with contradicting support for the concept of reward deficiency.

In pathological gamblers, DA release correlated positively with gambling symptom severity. The gamblers who have the most severe symptoms release the most DA. Correlation analyses showed that the most severely addicted gamblers released more DA during high reward gambling than less addicted gamblers. A Positron Emission Tomography (PET) study investigating PD patients with and without PG, showed increased DA release during gambling in patients with PG [16]. Personality traits commonly associated with PD, such as impulsivity and antisociality, are also associated with increased, and not decreased, mesolimbic DA responses [17,18, 19].

Striatal DA is released during gambling irrespective of gambling outcome suggesting that the mere expectation/prediction of reward is sufficient to induce dopaminergic changes. Greater gambling symptom severity is associated with greater dopaminergic responses. The dopaminergic response to reward-predicting stimulus and the linkage between addiction severity and DA release in pathological gamblers may play roles in the development and the symptomatology of the maladaptive gambling behavior [20].

Individuals suffering from substance abuse and dependence have cognitive and behavioural decision-making impairments similar to PG, that could be associated with dopaminergic dysregulations. Recent researches suggest that the dopamine system and ventral striatum play a central role in PG as well as substance dependence. In healthy controls DA appears to be associated with, instead in PG dopamine might be also associated with monetary losses. This suggest a dopaminergic base of susceptibility to immediate reward seeking in PG [21].

In PG the DA system may be associated with dysfunctional learning (reward prediction error), that is associated with increased activation of midbrain DA neurons, which stimulate synaptic DA release in the striatum and through the brain.

Impulse control disorders such as PG are a serious and common adverse effect of DA replacement medication in PD. Patients with PG have increased impulsivity and abnormalities in striatal DA, in common with behavioural and substance addictions in the non-PD population. Symptomatic relief of motor symptoms in PD is achieved by increasing endogenous dopamine levels using levodopa, or by synthetic activation of DA receptors using DA agonists. DA agonists in particular may contribute to the development of impulse control disorders (ICDs) in about 13% of PD patients [22, 23]. PD patients with PG have dysfunctional activation of DA autoreceptors in the midbrain and low DA tone in the anterior cingulated cortex. Thus, altered striatal and cortical DA homeostasis may incur vulnerability for the development of PG in PD, linked with the impulsive personality trait. Natural variation in DA homeostasis in the midbrain and cortex can impact an individuals' propensity for impulsivity and, as such, modulate risk for ICDs in PD. DA agonists may exaggerate these dopaminergic influences over behaviour, turning a previous tendency to engage in rewarding activities into a pathological inability to abstain from them [24].

More recently, Linnet et al. [25] investigated the dopaminergic coding of reward and uncertainty in PG sufferers and healthy controls. They used PET with the tracer [(11)C]raclopride to measure DA release, and they used performance on the Iowa Gambling Task (IGT) to determine overall reward and uncertainty. The data supported an inverse relation between striatal DA release and IGT performance if the PG group, but not in the healthy control group. These findings are consistent with the hypothesis of dopaminergic sensitivity toward uncertainty, and show as dopaminergic sensitivity to uncertainty is pronounced in PG, but not among non-gambling healthy controls. So it's reasonable to assume that, in PG patients, decisions with maximum uncertainty and variance are associated with the highest dopaminergic activation. Morevover, dopaminergic coding of variance in IGT performance in PG was strongest in the combined striatum and in the ROI(Return On Investment) analysis, only the putamen reached significance level. This may suggest a strong role of the putamen in relation to uncertainty, which may exceed that of the ventral striatum by a factor of 2 to 3.

## 5. PET specific studies

Hollander et al. [26] therefore hypothesized that lithium effects would decrease relative metabolic rate in at least some portions of the cingulate and orbitofrontal systems. Since they have recently reported elevated relative white matter metabolic rates in frontal regions in patients with schizophrenia [20], and since the statistical parametric mapping analysis in fMRI gambling studies showed group difference clusters partially encompassing white matter underlying cortical areas [7], they assessed white matter metabolic rates underlying each BA on an exploratory basis. In another previous treatment study, lithium was effective in reducing both gambling behavior and affective instability [27].

Although mood stabilizers and serotonin reuptake inhibitors have shown some efficacy in the treatment of this condition, there is little known about how these pharmacological interventions work. In patients with PG, relative glucose metabolic rates (rGMR) in the orbitofrontal cortex and medial frontal cortex were significantly increased at baseline compared to normal controls. Lithium administration was associated with widespread effects in the prefrontal cortex and cingulate gyrus. Lithium increased rGMR further in the orbitofrontal cortex, heightening normal/patient differences, but it also increased the rGMR of the posterior cingulate and the dorsolateral frontal cortex normalizing the metabolic rate in these regions.

Cortical areas implicated in impulse control disorders show increased rGMR in PG at baseline. Lithium treatment, while alleviating the symptoms, further increases rGMR in these areas [18].

Buckholtz et al. [17, 18], using the PET ligand [18F] Fallypride, found that trait impulsivity was negatively associated with binding to DA D2/3 receptors in the midbrain. DA receptors in this region are dominated by autoreceptors [28], which function to limit striatal DA release following reward. This suggests that midbrain autoreceptors influence individuals' propensity for impulsivity, and opens the possibility that excessive striatal DA release following gambling rewards in PD patients with PG, shown in Steeves et al. [29], stems from reduced control overstriatal DA by midbrain autoreceptors.

Ray et al. [19] reported the results of their PET and [11C] FLB-457 study, a radiotracer with high affinity for DA D2/3 receptors, and therefore sensitivity to extrastriatal, showing midbrain and prefrontal cortex dopaminergic differences in PD patients with and without PG. They suggested that impaired DA homeostasis in the midbrain, resulting in increased striatal DA release during reward, may be responsible for increased impulsivity and therefore vulnerability for addiction in these patients.

Recently, Boileau et al. [30] used PET to test whether PG is associated with abnormalities in D2 and D3 receptor levels, as observed in substance use disorder (SUD). They used Two PET scans, one with the D3 receptor preferring agonist [11C]-(+)-propyl-hexahydro-naphthooxazin (PHNO) and the other with [11C]raclopride, to assess D2/3 DA receptor availability, and behavioural measures (self-report questionnaires and slot-machine game) to assess subjective effects and relationships to PET measures. The key findings of this study are two: first, in contrast to SUD, PG subjects'binding profile for both D2 and D3 receptor subtypes did not differ significantly from those of healthy controls, suggesting different neurobiological signatures between PG and SUD. Secondly, the study provides novel information regarding the D3 receptor in PG, showing a relationship between D3 levels across PG subjects and symptom severity and impulsiveness. So, D3 may be a viable marker for vulnerability across addictions and a potential target for intervention. The apparent ability of DA agonists in general, and D3-preferring agonists, in particular, to induce impulse control disorders in some patients, suggested an important role for this receptor in PG: its distribution on brain structures receiving afferent ventral striatal projections suggests that its activity can modify limbic output, and thus motivation for reward.

Savitz et al. [31] have tested the effect of a functional missense mutation in the dopamine 3 receptor (DRD3) gene (Ser9Gly, rs6280) on reward-associated DA release in the Striatum. They used two PET scans with [$^{11}$C]raclopride using the bolus plus constant infusion method. On one occasion subjects completed a sensorimotor task (control condition) and on another occasion subjects completed a gambling task (reward condition). Since PET- [11C]raclopride technique allows exploration of the effects of genetic variation on the amount of DA released under conditions associated with increased phasic release of DA, such as during receipt of unpredicted reward, during receipt of unpredictable monetary reward the glycine allele was associated with a greater reduction in D2/3 receptor binding in the middle caudate and the ventral striatum. Moreover they showed as the glycine allele yields D3 autoreceptors have a higher affinity for DA and display more robust intracellular signaling.

As discussed in Joutsa et al. [13], the binding of [$^{11}$C]raclopride is sensitive to changes in striatal DA concentration during receipt of non-pharmacological rewards such as a video game, large monetary wins versus large monetary losses and the monetary incentive delay task. Notably, in this study of pathological gamblers and healthy controls who completed 3 PET scans with [$^{11}$C]raclopride while gambling with a slot machine, the severity of addiction to gambling was positively associated with the degree of DA release in the basal ganglia during gambling.

Consistent with these results, highly impulsive individuals, who are thought to be vulnerable to developing addiction disorders, were shown to have diminished availability of striatal D2/3 autoreceptors, potentially predisposing them to a greater phasic DA response [18].

## 6. Conclusions

The PET imaging data are potentially important because genetically & not genetically-driven differences in DA receptor function may influence the changes in dopaminergic signaling that modulate emotional, motivational and stress responses.

Although large sample sizes are uncommon in PET studies because of cost and radiation exposure, PET has an advantage over MRI because it allows a particular molecular target to be assayed directly. Thus it is likely that true signals can be detected with relatively small sample sizes. Nevertheless, it would be interesting to examine large samples.

A number of studies have successfully applied multi-modal imaging in order to examine the relationship between serotonergic function or dopamine storage capacity and the hemodynamic response to affective stimuli in regions such as the amygdala. A gambling task could be implemented in a cohort of subjects who complete both [11C]raclopride PET and fMRI. So, it's therefore desirable that future multi-modal imaging studies can combine fMRI and PET data.

These studies would also be compatible with the new way of approaching to mental disorders proposed by NIMH.

## Author details

Daniela Santoro and Stefano Pallanti

Careggi University Hospital, Department of Psychiatry, Florence, Italy

## References

[1] Campbell-Meiklejohn DK, Woolrich MW, Passingham RE, Rogers RD: Knowing when to stop: the brain mechanisms of chasing losses. Biol Psychiatry 2008; 63: 293–300.

[2] Potenza, M.N., 2008. Review. The neurobiology of pathological gambling and drug addiction: an overview and new findings. Philos. Trans. R. Soc. Lond. B Biol. Sci. 363, 3181–3189.

[3] Pallanti S, Haznedar MM, Hollander E, LiClzi E, Bernardi S, Newmark R, Buchsbaum MS: Basal ganglia activity in Pathological Gambling: a fluorodexoxyglucose Positron Emission Tomography study. Neuropsychobiology,2010;62:132-138.

[4] Linnet J, Moller A, Peterson E, Gjedde A, Doudet D: Dopamine release in ventral striatum during lowa Gambling Task performance is associated with increase excitement levels in pathological gambling.Research Report 2010;106:383-390.

[5] Crockford DN, Goodyear B, Edwards J, Quickfall J, el-Guebaly N: Cue-induced brain activity in pathological gamblers. Biol Psychiatry 2005; 58: 787–795.

[6] Hollander E, Pallanti S, Baldini Rossi N, Sood E, Baker BR, Buchsbaum MS: Imaging monetary reward in pathological gamblers. World J Biol Psychiatry 2005; 6: 113–120.

[7] Tanabe J, Thompson L, Claus E, Dalwani M, Hutchison K, Banich MT: Prefrontal cortex activity is reduced in gambling and nongambling substance users during decision-making. Hum Brain Mapp 2007; 28: 1276–1286.

[8] Sanislow CA, Pine DS, Quinn KJ, Kozak MJ, Garvey MA, Heinssen RK, Wang PS, Cuthbert BN. Developing constructs for psychopathology research: research domain criteria. J Abnorm Psychol. 2010 Nov;119(4):631-9

[9] Insel T, Cuthbert B, Garvey M, Heinssen R, Pine DS, Quinn K, Sanislow C, Wang P. Research domain criteria (RDoC): toward a new classification framework for research on mental disorders. Am J Psychiatry. 2010 Jul;167(7):748-51.

[10] Cuthbert, BN & Insel, TR. Classification issues in women's mental health: Clinical utility and etiological mechanisms. Archives of Women's Mental Health, 2010. Epub ahead of print.

[11] Cuthbert BN, Insel TR. Toward new approaches to psychotic disorders: the NIMH Research Domain Criteria project. Schizophr Bull. 2010 Nov;36(6):1061-2. Epub 2010 Oct 7.

[12] Morris SE, Cuthbert BN. Research Domain Criteria: cognitive systems, neural circuits, and dimensions of behavior. Dialogues Clin Neurosci. 2012 Mar; 14(1):29-37.

[13] Joutsa J, Johansson J, Niemela S, Ollikainen A, Hirvonen MM, Piepponen P, Arponen E, Alho H, Voon V, Rinne JO, Hietala J, Kaasinen V. Mesolimbic dopamine release is linked to symptom severity in pathological gambling. NeuroImage 60(2012)

[14] Linnet J,MollerA, Peterson E, Gjedde A, Doudet D: Inverse association between dopaminergic neurotransmission and lowa Gambling Task performance in Pathological gamblers and healthy controls,2010; 52:28-34.

[15] Voon, V., Fernagut, P.O., Wickens, J., Baunez, C., Rodriguez, M., Pavon, N., Juncos, J.L., Obeso, J.A., Bezard, E., 2009. Chronic dopaminergic stimulation in Parkinson's disease: from dyskinesias to impulse control disorders. Lancet Neurol. 8, 1140–1149.

[16] Steeves, T.D., Miyasaki, J., Zurowski, M., Lang, A.E., Pellecchia, G., Van Eimeren, T., Rusjan, P., Houle, S., Strafella, A.P., 2009. Increased striatal dopamine release in Parkinsonian patients with pathological gambling: a [11C] raclopride PET study. Brain 132, 1376–1385.

[17] Buckholtz, J.W., Treadway, M.T., Cowan, R.L., Woodward, N.D., Benning, S.D., Li, R., Ansari, M.S., Baldwin, R.M., Schwartzman, A.N., Shelby, E.S., Smith, C.E., Cole, D., Kessler, R.M., Zald, D.H., 2010a. Mesolimbic dopamine reward system hypersensitivity in individuals with psychopathic traits. Nat. Neurosci. 13, 419–421.

[18] Buckholtz, J.W., Treadway, M.T., Cowan, R.L., Woodward, N.D., Li, R., Ansari, M.S., Baldwin, R.M., Schwartzman, A.N., Shelby, E.S., Smith, C.E., Kessler, R.M., Zald, D.H., 2010b. Dopaminergic network differences in human impulsivity. Science 329, 532.

[19] Forbes, E.E., Brown, S.M., Kimak, M., Ferrell, R.E., Manuck, S.B., Hariri, A.R., 2009. Genetic variation in components of dopamine neurotransmission impacts ventral striatal reactivity associated with impulsivity. Mol. Psychiatry 14, 60–70.

[20] Buchsbaum MS, Buchsbaum BR, Hazlett EA, Haznedar M, Newmark R, Tang C, Hof PR: Relative glucose metabolic rate higher in white matter in schizophrenia. Am J Psychiatry 2007; 164: 1072–1081.

[21] Linnet J,MollerA, Peterson E, Gjedde A, Doudet D: Dopamine release in ventral striatum of pathological gamblers losing money,2010;122:326-333.

[22] Voon, V., Hassan, K., Zurowski, M., et al., 2006. Prevalence of repetitive and reward-seeking behaviors in Parkinson disease. Neurology 67 (7), 1254–1257.

[23] Weintraub, D., Koester, J., Potenza, M.N., et al., 2010. Impulse control disorders in Parkinson disease: a cross-sectional study of 3090 patients. Arch. Neurol. 67 (5), 589–595.

[24] Ray NJ, Miyasaki JM, Zurowski M, Ko JH, Cho SS, Pellecchia G, Antonelli F, Houle S, Lang AE, Strafella AP. Extrastriatal dopaminergic abnormalities of DA homeostasis in Parkinson's patients with medication-induced pathological gambling: A [11C] FLB-457 and PET study. Neurobiology of Disease 48 (2012) 519–525

[25] Linnet J, Mouridsen K, Peterson E, Moller A, Doudet DS, Gjedde A: Striatal dopamine release codes uncertainty in pathological gambling. Psychiatry Research: Neuroimaging, 2012; 204: 55-60.

[26] Hollander E, Buchsbaum MS, Haznedar MM, Berenguer J, Berlin HA, Chaplin W, Goodman CR, LiCalzi EM, Newmark R, Pallanti S. FDG-PET Study in Pathological Gamblers (Lithium increases Orbotofrontal, Dorsolateral and Cingulate Metabolism). Neuropsychobiology 2008;58:37-47

[27] Hollander E, Pallanti S, Allen A, Sood E, Baldini Rossi N: Does sustained-release lithium reduce impulsive gambling and affective instability versus placebo in pathological gamblers with bipolar spectrum disorders? Am J Psychiatry 2005; 162: 137–145.

[28] Khan, Z.U., Mrzljak, L., Gutierrez, A., de la Calle, A., Godman-Rakic, P.S., 1998. Prominence of the dopamine D2 short isoform in dopaminergic pathways. Proc. Natl. Acad. Sci. U. S. A. 95 (13), 7731–7736.

[29] Steeves, T.D.L., Miyasaki, J., Zurowski, M., et al., 2009. Increased striatal dopamine releasein Parkinsonian patients with pathological gambling: a [11C] raclopride PET study. Brain 132 (Pt 5), 1376–1385.

[30] Boileau I, Payer D, Chugani B, Lobo D, Behzadi A, RusjanPM, Houle S, Wilson AA, Warsh J, Kish SJ, Zack M: The D2/3 dopamine receptor in pathological gambling: a positron emission tomography study with [11C]-(+)-propyl-hexahydro-naphtho-oxazin and [11C]raclopride. Addiction. 2012 Nov 20. doi: 10.1111/add.12066.

[31] Savitz J, Hodgkinson CA, Martin-Soelch C, Shen PH, Szczepanik J, Nugent A, Herscovitch P, Grace AA, Goldman D, Drevets WC: The Functional DRD3 Ser9Gly Polymorphism (rs6280) Is Pleiotropic, Affecting Reward as Well as Movement. PLoS One. 2013; 8(1): e54108.

Section 3

# PET Imaging in Clinical Oncology

# Chapter 8

# PET – Assessment of Oncologic Treatment Response

Inga S. Grills and Victor S. Mangona

Additional information is available at the end of the chapter

http://dx.doi.org/10.5772/57127

## 1. Introduction

Positron Emission Tomography (PET), particularly with 18-Fluorodeoxyglucose (FDG), continues to define and expand its role in oncologic management. Beyond tumor size, as definable by computed tomography (CT), PET provides a measure of metabolic activity in tumors and is integral in initial workup for multiple disease sites including head/neck squamous cell carcinoma, non-small cell lung cancer (NSCLC), lymphoma, and many others. For head and neck cancers, FDG PET imaging facilitates early detection of persistent and recurrent head/neck squamous cell carcinoma after chemoradiotherapy, increasing deferral of surgical neck dissection to the salvage setting in many cases. In the setting of non-small-cell lung cancer, PET is further considered standard of care for radiotherapy treatment planning. Post-treatment PET has further shown to facilitate assessment of treatment response, with metabolic response seen on PET pre-dating CT-based radiographic response. Though routine post-therapy PET after definitive non-surgical management is standard management for head/neck squamous cell carcinomas, evidence to support this routine use for other subsites is lacking and thus currently not recommended for various organ sites including lung. This chapter herein discusses various PET imaging techniques and assessment variables that have been used to investigate assessment of response to oncologic treatment. In particular, assessment of response with early and late post-radiotherapy PET imaging for head and neck, NSCLC, rectal cancer, esophageal cancer, and lymphoma are discussed. Recent research involving on-treatment PET imaging as well as future work are further presented.

INTECH
open science | open minds

© 2013 Grills and Mangona; licensee InTech. This is a paper distributed under the terms of the Creative Commons Attribution License (http://creativecommons.org/licenses/by/3.0), which permits unrestricted use, distribution, and reproduction in any medium, provided the original work is properly cited.

## 2. PET technique

### 2.1. $^{18}$F-FDG

PET is a medical imaging technique employing the unique parameters of decay of positron-emitting isotopes. Today, PET is routinely used in conjunction with computed tomography (CT) in a combined medical imaging device, PET-CT, allowing anatomic image correlation with the functional imaging obtained by PET.

A number of PET radiotacers have been used in oncology, though $^{18}$F-Flourodeoxyglucose (FDG) is FDA-approved and most commonly employed. Other agents including $^{18}$F-FMISO ($^{18}$F-Fluoromisonidazole), $^{18}$FLT ($^{18}$F-Fluorothymidine), 16b-$^{18}$F-Fluoro-5a-Dihydrotestosterone ($^{18}$F-FDHT), $^{60}$Cu-ATSM (Copper-diacetyl-bis(N4-methylthiosemicarbazone)), $^{18}$F-FES (16a-$^{18}$F-fluoro-17b-estradiol), $^{11}$C-MET (11C-methionine), show significant potential to monitor the response to therapy before, during, or after therapeutic intervention[1].

$^{18}$F-FDG chemically is 2-deoxy-2-$^{18}$F-fluoro-D-glucose, a glucose analog. On $^{18}$FDG, the positron-emitting radioactive isotope fluorine-18 is substituted at the 2' position of the glucose molecule preventing glycolysis, which requires a hydroxyl group at the 2′ position. It has significantly increased uptake in tissues with increased metabolic activity, in particular, most malignancies [2]. With increased demand for gluose, tumors tend to have increased expression of glucose transport proteins at the cellular membrane as well as increased hexokinase [3]. With its relatively short half-life of 110 minutes, in tissues with rapid uptake, the $^{18}$F decay occurs primarily when trapped intracellularly, helping visualize these areas on PET. Malignancies with moderate to high $^{18}$F-FDG uptake include most lung cancers, colorectal cancers, esophageal cancers, gastric cancers, head and neck cancers, cervical cancers, ovarian cancers, breast cancers, lymphomas, and melanoma [4]. Hepatocellucar carcinoma, testicular cancers, renal cancers, sarcomas, and neuroendocrine tumors have variable $^{18}$F-FDG uptake [4]. Prostate adenocarcinoma, the most common cancer in males, has generally low metabolic activity, rendering $^{18}$F-FDG particularly less helpful for this malignancy in the primary setting, leading to potential false negative interpretation [5–7]. As $^{18}$F-FDG undergoes physiologic excretion through the bladder hinders evaluation of both bladder and prostate malignancies. Overall, $^{18}$F-FDG has been the most used oncologic tracer, but its applicability is not universal across all malignancies, nor is its uptake specific to only neoplasm. Though aberrant tumor growth in malignancy routinely results in increased $^{18}$F-FDG avidity, it is not tumor specific other benign tissue and benign conditions can also have variable uptake of $^{18}$F-FDG (e.g. inflammation or hyperplastic bone marrow) potentially leading to false positive findings [4,7]. As bone marrow hyperplasia and inflammation are not uncommon consequences after oncologic treatment including surgery, radiation therapy, and/or chemotherapy, $^{18}$F-FDG PET has limitations particulary in post-therapeutic assessment.

### 2.2. Other radiotracers

Beyond $^{18}$F-FDG, other markers exploit other cellular mechanisms for biologic imaging with PET. Other markers have been used to assess tumor proliferation with markers of DNA synthesis. As thymidine is unique to DNA, this has been exploited with various radiotracers including $^{11}C$-thymidine—which is limited by the short half-life of $^{11}C$—as well as thymidine analogs $^{18}F$-FLT and $^{8}F$-FMAU with the longer half-life of $^{18}F$ [8]. $^{18}F$-FLT acts as a substrate of cytosolic thymidine kinase 1 (TK1), a key enzyme for salvage DNA synthesis, and $^{8}F$-FMAU is a substrate of thymidine kinase 2 (TK2), located in mitochondria, resulting in different distributions of these markers in tissue [9,10]. Although tumors tend to be less avid of $^{18}F$-FLT in comparison go $^{18}F$-FDG, tumor delineation from background tissue can be superior with $^{18}F$-FLT in regions such as the brain, mediastinum, and intestines, where normal physiologic uptake of $^{18}F$-FLT in these areas are much lower, yielding a high tumor-to-background ratio [1,11–13]. In a head-to-head comparison of $^{18}F$-FLT to $^{18}F$-FDG to assess chemotherapy response in patients with breast cancer who had imaging with both radiotracers, change in FLT uptake after one cycle of chemotherapy better predicted late changes in tumor marker levels and correlated well with eventual radiographic tumor response [14]. Though less employed in comparison to $^{18}F$-FLT, $^{18}F$-FMAU has shown ability to visualize breast, brain, lung, and prostate tumors. As $^{18}F$-FMAU shows low uptake in normal bone marrow—as opposed to $^{18}F$-FLT, which has high bone marrow uptake—$^{18}F$-FMAU is more suitable for visualization of metastatic prostate cancer.

Radiolabeled Cu-ATSM ($^{60/62/64}Cu$-ATSM) and $^{18}F$-FMISO are currently the two primary radiotracers employed for imaging tissue hypoxia—correlated with decreased sensitivity to treatment—and has been with worse clinical outcomes [15,16]. $^{60}Cu$-ATSM has been found to predict aresponse to therapy for NSCLC and predict both recurrence and survival outcomes for cervical and rectal cancers [17–19]. Clinically, pretreatment $^{18}F$-FMISO has been shown to predict survival in patients with head and neck cancer and glioblastoma multiforme [20,21].

Various amino acid radiotracers have been used, with $^{11}C$-MET (a methionine analog) the most common. It has found a niche in CNS malignancies. In malignant gliomas, decreased uptake during temozolomide therapy has shown improved time to progression; areas of uptake have shown areas at high risk of recurrence, and has helped distinguish post-radiation necrosis versus recurrent malignancy [22–24].

An additional class of radiotracers have aimed to assess hormone receptors, as receptors play an integral role in malignancies, paticulary prostate and breast cancers. $^{18}F$-FES is the most commonly used, showing correlation with estrogen receptor (ER) levels as well as response to aromatase inhibitors [25,26]. Ultimately, pretreatment uptake values have shown to predict patients who would or would not respond to therapy [25]. For prostate cancer, $^{18}F$-FDHT is an analog of $5\alpha$-dihydrotestosterone. Correlation with treatment response has not as well been shown in prostate cancer with this marker, though $^{18}F$-FDHT uptake has been associated with high PSA levels [27].

**Single-phase / Dual-phase / Dynamic PET**

Historically, PET imaging was obtained with a single static set of images obtained up to 1 hour after injection of $^{18}F$-FDG. As noted previously, a diagnostic limitation of PET imaging for oncologic diagnosis are the false positive findings secondary to inflammation quite commonly associated to therapeutic response. As $^{18}F$-FDG uptake and retention kinetics are potentially different between tumor and normal tissue inflammation, people have investigated more dynamic methods of acquiring metabolic PET data.

In a series of 21 patients with head and neck carcinomas, dual-time-point $^{18}$F-FDG PET studies helped differentiate malignancy from inflammation [28]. Standard uptake values (SUVs) of tumors were shown to increase on the second (delayed) study by mean of 12% in comparison to matched contralateral normal tissue which showed a mean decrease of 5% on delayed imaging ($p<0.05$) [28]. Inflammatory sites showed relatively stable uptake over the two scans; time interval between scans correlate with tumor SUV increase; and interval of greater than 30 minutes was recommended for separation [28].

For evaluation of pulmonary nodules, an early study of 36 patients siwht 38 pulmonary nodules, malignant or benign, underwent dual-time-point PET at 70 and 123 minutes post-injection [29]. A similar trend was seen with mean increase of tumor SUV of 20% (from 3.7 to 4.4) in malignant lesions from early to delayed scan ($P<0.01$); benign lesions showed stable and lower mean SUVs (1.1 on both early and delayed imaging) [29]. They determine a threshold of 10% increase from early to delayed imaging as the best predictor, reaching sensitivity of 100% and specificity of 89% [29]. Other data have shown similar trends of increased $^{18}$F-FDG uptake from first to second scan in malignant tissue and stable to decreased uptake in benign lesions [30].

In a study of 47 patients with suspected pancreatic cancer, patients had dual-time-point $^{18}$F-FDG PET imaging acquired 1 and 2 hours after injection; further, some patients had a third scan at the 3-hour time point after injection [31]. Twenty-two lesions were malignant, whereas 20 were benign. With a constant SUV threshold, the initial 1-hour PET was found to be 95% sensitive, missing one of 22 malignant lesions, and 83% accurate. With addition information of 2-hour PET imaging, retention characteristics of $^{18}$F-FDG increased diagnostic accuracy to 91.5%, with no decrease in false negatives [31]. The additional information provided by a 3-hour PET did not improve diagnostic accuracy beyond the dual-phase imaging obtained at the 1-hour and 2-hour time points [31].

With these potential diagnostic advantages from dual-phase PET-CT (with 2 PET scans separated by a time interval) has grown increasingly common. With the extra information provided with dual-phase imaging, people have further investigated 'dynamic PET' imaging, obtaining continuous PET data over time rather than at discrete or brief time spans, adding further breadth of data to kinetic profiles of uptake. Early work used dynamic continuous imaging to model discrete time-point imaging, showing linear change over time in patients with breast cancer. A recent study utilized dynamic PET imaging with $^{18}$F-FCho ($^{18}$F-labelled fluoromethylcholine) to assess time-activity curves of space occupying brain lesions [32]. Another recent study used a dynamic PET-CT approach to assess cervical adenopathy in patients with oral/head and neck cancer; consecutive imaging at nine time points with PET/CT were obtained from 60-115 minutes after injection [33]. At our institution, we have recently initiated an adaptive radiation therapy protocol for patients with head/neck cancer in which patients receive weekly dynamic PET imaging over approximately 90 minutes during the course of treatment.

Though PET imaging acquires three-dimensional (3D) data, as CT technology has advanced to enable four-dimensional (4D) imaging with full 3D CT image sets corresponding to various portions of a respiratory cycle, so now have 4D-PET-CTs come into clinical use, with potential to reduce image smearing, improve accuracy of PET-CT co-registration, and increase the measured SUV [34,35]. A study evaluating 57 pulmonary lesions showed particular benefit in characterizing smaller tumors, with 4D studies showing higher differences in SUVmax percent difference in comparison to 3D studies ($p<0.05$) assessment of smaller lesion lung lesions, with better characterization [36]. A recent study illustrated utility of respiratory-correlated 4D-PET-CT for target delineation of squamous cell carcinoma of the esophagus, further indicating SUV threshold of 20% or 2.5 for autocontouring the gross tumor volume (GTV) [37]. Algorithms for semiautomatic contouring have also been proposed for pulmonary lesions with minimal difference (0.1 ± 0.1 mm) on phantom studies and 0.8 ± 0.2 mm on patient tumors [38]. Four-dimensional PET/CT has been reported to facilitate planning stereotactic radiotherapy of liver metastases [39] and pulmonary tumors [40].

## 3. PET parameters

From an oncologic standpoint, PET imaging is notably quite useful in its ability to quantitate parameters associated with PET uptake. An assortment of quantitative values can be obtained from each scan and from multiple-time-point scans, as well as across different scans obtained at different time points with respect to treatment (e.g. pre-treatment versus post-treatment), providing valuable information for treating physicians.

A common measurement of PET images for clinicians is the semi-quantitative value referred to as "standardized uptake value (SUV) [41]." Standardized uptake values are calculated throughout the three-dimensional array of CT regions, with variable SUVs throughout an image. SUV provides an index of regional tracer uptake and is a function of local radioactivity concentration, injected activity, and patient's weight. $^{18}$F-FDG SUV can help differentiate tumor from tissue, and when used, corrections to calculation are recommended [42]. A common method of correction accounts for a patient's lean body mass "$SUV_{lbm}$," commonly written as "$SUV_{lbw}$" (lbw="lean body weight"), "$SUV_{lean}$," or "SUL."[43]

$$SUV_{lean} = \frac{Radioactivity\,(\mu C_i\,/\,mL)}{Dose\,(mC_i)\,/\,lean\,body\,mass\,(kg)} \tag{1}$$

$$SUV_{lean} = SUV_{lbm} = SUV_{lbw} = SUL \tag{2}$$

Within a region of interest (ROI) on a PET-CT, various PET quantitative factors can readily be obtained. The most commonly reported value from PET-CT oncologic imaging the maximum SUV value ($SUV_{max}$). $SUV_{max}$ values are measured and reported at areas concerning for malignancy (e.g. a primary tumor and associated regional lymph nodes and distant metastases as well as other highly avid areas that may represent inflammation or reactive changes). Pre-treatment $SUV_{max}$ with $^{18}$F-FDG has been reported to be prognostic for many organ sites including lung [44–46], head and neck [47], esophagus [48,49], gastroesophageal junction [49] gastric [50], pancreas [51] cervix [52], rectum [53,54], lymphoma [55], and soft tissue sarcoma [56].

Beyond $SUV_{max}$ of an ROI, the arithmetic mean SUV ($SUV_{mean}$) of voxels within the ROI have been used for oncologic assessment [57–59]. New parameters, which show promise in oncologic assessment, include the metabolic tumor volume (MTV) and total glycolytic activity (TGA) [60–63]. The MTV is defined as the tumor volume based on PET uptake and can be particularly helpful in comparison to CT-imaging when background density is similar to tumor density on CT. The boundary of MTV can be defined manually or with various parameters such as a fixed SUV threshold, percentage of $SUV_{max}$ (e.g. 38%, 50%, and 60%), and gradient. On pre-treatment imaging prior to radiotherapy the volume delineated by PET-fusion to planning CT effectively corresponds to the MTV, which is utilized for biologically-targeted radiotherapy [64–66]. Such methods have been used extensively for lung radiotherapy planning, where PET staging is recommended [67]. MTV has shown to predict overall survival in lung cancer [61], head and neck cancer [60], and esophageal cancer [68].

Total glycolytic activity (TGA), defined as the (MTV) x ($SUV_{mean}$), is the primary PET parameter that includes both both anatomic (size) as well as metabolic parameters (e.g. with $^{18}$F-FDG). In an analysis of TGA and MTV in 45 patients with oral or oropharyngeal SCC, stage, on univariate cox regression, MTV and TGA were the most associated with progression-free survival (PFS) and overall survival (OS) (p=0.002 and p=0.006, respectively), moreso than tumor grade (p=004) and SUVmax (p=0.56) [69].

$$TGA = MTV \ x \ SUVmean \tag{3}$$

Retention index (RI) is a dynamic parameter that can be calculated with dual-time-point (early and delayed) PET imaging, where RI is the difference of SUVmax on two scans divided by initial SUVmax. Rate of decline of RI during lung irradiation has shown to predict locoregional recurrence [70]. Further, in an analysis of 68 women with breast cancer, in comparison to other parameters including early and delayed $SUV_{max}$, RI showed best relation to biologic parameters including grade, Ki-67, and c-erbB-2 expression [71].

$$RI = \frac{SUV\max_{delayed} - SUV\max_{early}}{SUV\max_{early}} \tag{4}$$

From an oncologic standpoint, beyond the importance of baseline PET imaging for staging and radiotherapy planning, subsequent PET scans, whether during treatment or subsequent,

http://dx.doi.org/10.5772/57127

are used for assessment of treatment response. From such data, inter-PET analysis can be performed (e.g. comparison of a pre-treatment scan to a post-treatment scan), not to be confused with factors such as the RI which are measured across two different scans performed during two time points of a single PET (e.g. early and delayed scans). Inter-PET parameters include the difference or change in (delta, Δ) values of parameters already previously discussed as well as "percent of" (e.g. percent of baseline), percent reduction from baseline, and rate of change (velocity "VEL"). Examples of such variables comparing a new PET to a baseline PET are as indicated below, where $t$ is the time between PETs..

$$\Delta SUV\max = SUV\max_{new} - SUV\max_{baseline} \tag{5}$$

$$SUV\max_{\%Baseline} = \frac{SUV\max_{new}}{SUV\max_{baseline}} x100 \tag{6}$$

$$SUV\max_{\%reduction} = 100\% - SUV\max_{\%baseline} \tag{7}$$

$$VEl_{SUV\max} = \frac{SUV\max_{new} - SUV\max_{baseline}}{t} \tag{8}$$

## 4. Response criteria

Various methods for assessing and categorizing response of tumors based on radiographic imaging have been proposed, including the World Health Organization (WHO) criteria, the Response Evaluation Criteria in Solid Tumors (RECIST), and RECIST 1.1 [72–75]. Such criterica, depend on radiographic imaging, which may not best assess the biologic response, particularly given that metabolic response on PET routinely anatomic radiographic response on CT [76]. Accordingly, methods of categorizing response with PET have been developed, namely the European Organization for Research and Treatment of Cancer (EORTC) criteria and newer PET Response Criteria in Solid Tumors (PERCIST, version 1.0) [43,77]. A separate metric of response definitions using $^{18}$F-FDG PET has been developed for lymphoma response and used for clinical trials [78]. Definitions of criteria are delineated in Table 1, Table 2, Table 3, Table 4, and Table 5.

| RECIST 1.1 (2009) [75] (Anatomic) | EORTC (1990) [77] (Metabolic) | PERCIST (2009) [43] (Metabolic) |
|---|---|---|
| Measurable lesions have minimum size of 10 mm by CT scan,10 mm caliper measurement by clinical exam (lesions which cannot be accurately measured with calipers should be recorded as non-measurable), or 20 mm by chest X-ray. All other lesions are considered non-measurable | Tumor regions defined on pretreatment scan should be drawn on region of high $^{18}$F-FDG uptake representing viable tumor. Whole tumor uptake should also be recorded.<br>Uptake measurements should be made for mean and maximal tumor ROI counts per pixel per second calibrated as MBq/L.<br>Partial volume may affect measurement of $^{18}$F-FDG uptake.<br>Tumor size from anatomic imaging in relation to PET scanner resolution should be documented where possible. | Measurable target lesion is hottest single tumor lesion $SUV_{lbw}$ of "maximal 1.2-cm diameter volume ROI in tumor" (Peak $SUV_{lbw}$). Peak $SUV_{lbw}$ is at least 1.5-fold greater than liver $SUV_{lbw}$ mean +2 SDs (in 3-cm spherical ROI in normal right lobe of liver). If liver is abnormal, primary tumor should have uptake > 2.0 $SUV_{lbw}$ mean of blood pool in 1-cm-diameter ROI in descending thoracic aorta extended over 2-cm z-axis.<br>Uptake measurements should be made for peak and maximal single-voxel tumor $SUV_{lbw}$. Other SUV metrics, including $SUV_{lbw}$ mean at 50% or 70% of Peak SUV, can be collected as exploratory data; TLG can be collected ideally on basis of voxels more intense than 2 SDs above liver mean SUL |

RECIST, Response Evaluation Criteria in Solid Tumors, European Organization for Research and Treatment of Cancer; PERCIST, PET Response Criteria in Solid Tumors; CT, Computed Tomography, ROI: Region of interest, SD, standard deviation.

**Table 1.** Evaluation of baseline lesions

| | Target Lesions | Non-Target Lesions |
|---|---|---|
| **CR** | Disappearance of all target lesions. Any pathological lymph nodes must have reduction in short axis to <10 mm. | Disappearance of all non-target lesions and normalization of tumor marker level. All lymph nodes must be non-pathological in size (<10 mm short axis). |
| **PR** | ≥ 30% decrease in the sum of diameters of target lesions, taking as reference the baseline sum diameters. | N/A |
| **SD** | Neither sufficient shrinkage to qualify for PR nor sufficient increase to qualify for PD, taking as reference the smallest sum diameters while on study. | N/A |
| **PD** | ≥ 20% increase in the sum of diameters of target lesions, taking as reference the smallest sum on study (including the baseline sum if that is the smallest on study). In addition to the relative increase of 20%, the sum must also demonstrate an absolute increase of at least 5 mm.<br>The appearance of one or more new lesions is also considered progression. | Unequivocal progression of existing non-target lesions. The appearance of one or more new lesions is considered progression. |
| **Non-CR/ Non-PD** | N/A | Persistence of one or more non-target lesion(s) and/or maintenance of tumor marker level above the normal limits. |

Adapted from Eisenhauer *et al.* (2009) [75]. CR, Complete Response; PR, Partial Response; SD, Stable Disease; PD, Progressive Disease; N/A, Not Applicable

**Table 2.** RECIST 1.1 (Non-metabolic) response criteria

| Response | IWC[79] | IWC+PET[80] |
|---|---|---|
| CR | - no detectable clinical or radiographic evidence of disease<br>- no disease-related symptoms<br>- no biochemical abnormalities<br>- negative BMB (if positive before treatment)<br>- lymph nodes >1.5 cm at baseline regress to ≤ 1.5 cm<br>- lymph nodes 1.1-1.5 cm at baseline regress to ≤ 1.0 cm | -CR by IWC with a completely negative PET<br>- CRu, PR, or SD by IWC with a completely negative PET and negative BMB if positive prior to therapy<br>- PD by IWC with a completely negative PET and CT abnormalities (new lesion or increasing size of previous lesion) ≥ 1.5 cm (≥ 1.0 cm in the lungs) and negative BMB if positive prior to therapy |
| CRu | - same as CR but either residual lymph mass > 1.5cm transverse diameter that has regressed > 75% or indeterminate BMB | - CRu by IWC with a completely negative PET but with an indeterminate BMB |
| PR | - ≥ 50% reduction in SPD of the six largest dominant nodes or nodal masses<br>- no increase in size of spleen, liver, or other nodes<br>- no new sites of disease | - CR, CRu, or PR by IWC with a positive PET at the site of a previously involved node/nodal mass<br>- CR, CRu, PR, or SD by IWC with a positive PET outside the site of a previously involved node/nodal mass<br>- SD by IWC with a positive PET at the site of a previously involved node/nodal mass that regressed to < 1.5 cm if previously > 1.5 cm, or < 1 cm if previously 1.1-1.5 cm |
| SD | - less than PR but not PD | - SD by IWC with a positive PET at the site of a previously involved node/nodal mass |
| PD | - applies only to patients with PR or nonresponders<br>- ≥ 50% increase in the SPD from nadir of any previously identified abnormal node<br>- any new lesion | - PD by IWC with a positive PET finding corresponding to the CT abnormality (new lesion, increasing size of previous lesion)<br>- PD by IWC with a negative PET and a CT abnormality (new lesion, increasing size of previous lesion) of < 1.5 cm (< 1.0 cm in the lungs) |
| RD | - applies only to patients with CR or Cru<br>- ≥ 50% increase in size of previously involved sites or<br>- ≥ 50% increase in greatest diameter of any previously identified node > 1cm in short axis or<br>- ≥ 50% increase in the SPD of ≥ 2 nodes or<br>- any new lesion | (not defined) |

Adapted from Juweid *et al.* (2005) [79]. IWC, International Workshop Criteria; PET, positron emission tomography; CR, complete remission; CRu, unconfirmed complete response, BMB, bone marrow biopsy, CT, computed tomography; PR, Partial Response; SPD, sum of the product of the diameters; SD, stable disease; PD, progressive disease; RD, relapsed disease

**Table 3.** IWC+PET-based response definitions for lymphoma based on IWC designations and PET findings

| Response | Definition | Nodal Masses | Spleen, Liver | Bone Marrow |
|---|---|---|---|---|
| CR | Disappearance of all evidence of disease | (a) FDG-avid or PET positive prior to therapy; mass of any size permitted if PET negative<br>(b) Variably FDG-avid or PET negative; regression to normal size on CT | Not palpable, nodules disappeared | Infiltrate cleared on repeat biopsy; if indeterminate by morphology, immunohistochemistry |
| PR | Regression of measurable disease and no new sites | ≥ 50% decrease in SPD of up to 6 largest dominant masses; no increase in size of other nodes<br>(a) FDG-avid or PET positive prior to therapy; one or more PET positive at previously involved site<br>(b) Variably FDG-avid or PET negative; regression on CT | ≥ 50% decrease in SPD of nodules (for single nodule in greatest transverse diameter); no increase in size of liver or spleen | Irrelevant if positive prior to therapy; cell type should be specified |
| SD | Failure to attain CR/PR, or PD | (a) FDG-avid or PET positive prior to therapy; PET positive at prior sites of disease and no new sites on CT or PET<br>(b) Variably FDG-avid or PET negative; no change in size of previous lesions on CT | | |
| Relapsed Disease or PD | Any new lesion or increase of previously involved sites by ≥ 50% from nadir. | Appearance of a new lesion(s) > 1.5 cm in any axis, 50% increase in SPD of more than one node, or > 50% increase in longest diameter of a previously identified node >1 cm in short axis<br>Lesions PET positive if FDG-avid lymphoma or PET positive prior to therapy. | > 50% increase from nadir in the SPD of any previous lesions | New or recurrent involvement |

From Cheson *et al.* Revised Response Criteria for Malignant Lymphoma (2007) [78]. CR, Complete Remission; FDG, $^{18}$F-fluorodeoxyglucose; PET, positron emission tomography; CT, computed tomography; PR = Partial Remission, SPD = sum of the product of the diameters; SD, stable disease; PD, progressive disease.

**Table 4.** PET response definitions for clinical trials

| Response | EORTC | PERCIST 1.0 | PERCIST Comment |
|---|---|---|---|
| Metabolic CR (CMR) | Complete resolution of $^{18}$F-FDG uptake within tumor volume so that it was indistinguishable from surrounding normal tissue. | Complete resolution of $^{18}$F-FDG uptake within measurable target lesion so that it is less than mean liver activity and indistinguishable from surrounding background blood-pool levels.<br>No new $^{18}$F-FDG-avid lesions in pattern typical of cancer.<br>Disappearance of all other lesions to background blood-pool levels. | Percent reduction in $SUV_{lbw}$ should be recorded from measurable region and time (weeks) after treatment initiated<br>(i.e., CMR 290, 4).<br>If anatomic progression by RECIST, must verify with follow-up. |
| Metabolic PR (PMR) | Reduction of minimum of 15% ± 25% in tumor $^{18}$F-FDG SUV after 1 cycle of chemotherapy, and >25% after >1 treatment cycle.<br>Reduction in extent of tumor $^{18}$F-FDG uptake is not a requirement for PR. | ≥ 0.8 and ≥ 30% reduction of Peak* $^{18}$F-FDG $SUV_{lbw}$ in target measurable tumor.<br>No new lesions.<br>$SUV_{lbw}$ measurement is obtained from the most active lesion also present at baseline (even if a different lesion than measured at baseline).<br>No increase > 30% in $SUV_{lbw}$ or size of target or nontarget lesions. | Measurement is of the single most active lesion after treatment that was also present at baseline (e.g. may be a different lesion). Percent reduction in $SUV_{lbw}$ should be recorded and time in weeks after treatment initiated<br>(i.e., PMR -40, 3).<br>If anatomic progression by RECIST, must verify with follow-up.<br>Reduction in extent of tumor $^{18}$F-FDG uptake is not requiremed. |
| Metabolic SD (SMD) | Increase in tumor $^{18}$F-FDG SUV <25% or decrease of < 15% and no visible increase in extent of $^{18}$F-FDG tumor uptake (20% in longest dimension). | No CMR, PMR, or PMD. | Peak $SUV_{lbw}$ in metabolic target lesion should be recorded, as well as time (weeks) from initation of most recent therapy, in weeks<br>(i.e., SMD -15, 7). |
| Metabolic PD (PMD) | Increase in $^{18}$F-FDG tumor SUV of >25% within tumor region defined on baseline scan; visible increase in extent of $^{18}$F-FDG tumor uptake (20% in longest dimension) or appearance of new $^{18}$F-FDG uptake in metastatic lesions. | (1) >30% and >0.8 increase in $^{18}$F-FDG Peak* $SUV_{lbw}$ from baseline in pattern typical of tumor and not of infection/ treatment effect.<br>Or<br>(2) Visible increase in extent of $^{18}$F-FDG tumor uptake (75% in TGA volume with no decline in $SUV_{lbw}$<br>Or<br>(3) New $^{18}$F-FDG-avid lesions that are typical of cancer and not related to treatment effect or infection. | PD other than new visceral lesions should be confirmed on follow-up study within 1 month unless clearly associated with PD by RECIST 1.1.<br>Should report percent change in Peak $SUV_{lbw}$, time elased since treatment (weeks) and whether new lesions are present/absent and their number<br>(i.e., PMD, 135, 4, new: 5). |

Adapted from Wahl *et al.*[43]. TLG, total lesion glycolysis; CMR, complete metabolic response; PMR, partial metabolic response; PD, progressive disease; SMD, stable metabolic disease; PMD, progressive metabolic disease; CR, complete remission; PR, partial remission.

*Single-voxel $SUV_{lbw}$ (e.g. "$SUV_{max}$") is commonly used but has been reported to be less reproducible than Peak $SUV_{lbw}$, especially with very small single-voxel values. Peak $SUV_{lbw}$ represents the highest mean value of a 1.2-cm-diameter spherical volume within a lesion and reduces variability secondary to voxel-to-voxel noise. It is suggested, but not required, that lesions assessed on PERCIST be larger than the 1.5-cm-diameter volume ROI used to minimize partial-volume effects.

**Table 5.** Metabolic Objective Response Assessment with $^{18}$F-FDG PET: EORTC & PERCIST 1.0

# 4. Clinical relevance of treatment response assessment

## 4.1. Head & neck cancer – Definitive/preoperative chemoradiation

$^{18}$F-FDG PET has found a particularly significant role in treatment of head and neck cancers. It has long shown promise in its ability to prognosticate; in 37 patients from 1991-1994 with head and neck squamous cell carcinomas (HNSCC) receiving baseline $^{18}$F-FDG PET, $SUV_{max}$ showed correlation with aggressive disease and potential prediction for survival [81].

Beyond prognostication, $^{18}$F-FDG PET is now routinely used to adapt treatment management, particularly in obviating surgical neck dissection in patients with complete response to initial radiation or chemoradiation therapy. Early studies have supported observation and omission of planned dissection after definitive radiotherapy for node-positive HNSCC with complete response on CT imaging, though at least selective nodal dissection was routinely practiced for residual neck masses [82,83]. With implementation of $^{18}$F-FDG PET, its negative predictive value has further supported omission of planned neck dissection, including in patients with residual neck mass/lymphadenopathy [84–88].

In an early study by Yao *et al.* [84], 41 patients from 2000-02 with locally-advanced HNSCC received radiation therapy with or without chemotherapy as upfront treatment had pretreatment and follow-up CT and $^{18}$F-FDG PET, with follow-up imaging 2.5-6 months (usually 3-4 months) post-treatment. Those without residual lymphadenopathy were observed. Twelve of 41 had residual lymphadenopathy; all had pathological testing, four with fine needle aspiration (FNA) biopsy, and eight had neck dissection. Follow-up $^{18}$F-FDG PET correlated better than follow-up CT for residual disease, and $SUV_{max}$ cutoff of $<3.0$ had 100% negative predictive value and 80% positive predictive value, serving as a good "rule-out" test for residual disease and potential to forego planned neck dissection in favor of initial observation, thus decreasing overall toxicity [84].

In a further analysis, Yao *et al.* (2005) [85] reviewed findings in 53 patients (70 heminecks; 17 patients with bilateral disease) with N2A or higher HNSCC with complete response to radiation therapy (± chemotherapy). Forty-two had clinically positive (exam or CT) lymphadenopathy but negative PET; this group had option to pursue dissection; 17 were observed, and 4 had negative neck dissection. The remaining 7 heminecks had clinically and PET-positive lymphadenopathy, six had neck dissection, one FNA; three were positive and four were negative for residual disease. No regional recurrences had occurred after median follow-up of 26 months (range 12-57 months). Negative predictive value of PET was 100% and positive predictive value 43%. They conclude that observation is safe if both CT and PET-negative 12 weeks after treatment and potentially also if CT reveals small (e.g. <2-3 cm) but PET-negative lymphadenopathy.

Porceddu *et al.* [88] analyzed a select cohort of 39 patients with HNSCC treated with definitive radiotherapy (± chemotherapy) with (a) complete regression of the primary HNSCC, (b) clinical evidence of residual neck mass by exam or CT imaging 8 weeks after treatment, (c) a follow-up $^{18}$F-FDG PET (median 12 weeks), and (d) either pathologic confirmation of neck status or > 12 months follow-up. Seven patients had residual PET uptake in the mass and proceeded to neck dissection (five were positive). Of the 32 with no residual tumor uptake, five had neck dissection (all pathologically negative), and 27 were observed (median follow-up of 34 months). One of the 27 observed patients had recurrence, yielding 97% negative predictive value. They conclude that in patients with a residual neck mass that is PET-negative 12 weeks after definitive radiotherapy (± chemotherapy), neck dissection is not required, and patients can be safely observed.

Such studies support timing of follow-up $^{18}$F-FDG PET to be 12 weeks post-treatment [84,85,88]. High negative predictive value (91%) has been shown at 16 weeks [86] post-treatment, though early time points (e.g. 4 weeks) have shown increased false positives [87]. Metaanalyses support PET ≥ 12 weeks after completion of definitive therapy for moderately higher diagnostic accuracy. An added benefit of $^{18}$F-FDG PET at this early follow-up interval is the potential to spare neck dissection in patients who show early distant metastatic disease [88,89].

Despite lack of any randomized prospective studies, significant retrospective evidence has continued to show similar findings. Recent metaanalyses [90–92], discuss 26, 27, and 51 studies including up to 2335 patients [92], overall supporting the high negative predictive value (approximately 95%) of follow-up PET and its value in omitting planned neck dissection. Further, despite the increased costs of PET imaging, PET-guided management in patients with complete response at the primary site has shown to be the more cost effective than CT-guided management or planned neck dissection [93].

### 4.2. Rectal cancer – Preoperative chemoradiation

Similar to HNSCC, first line treatment for locally-advanced rectal cancer includes upfront chemoradiation. In this setting, however, subsequent planned surgery remains standard of care. This multimodality neoadjuvant approach has shown to decrease local recurrence and improve overall survival [94,95]. Furthermore, neoadjuvant treatment has shown to increase sphincter-preserving surgery, conferring decreased surgical morbidity and improved quality of life [96–98].

Deferring subsequent surgical intervention in this disease site has similarly been investigated. In a cohort of 71 patients with distal rectal carcinoma considered resectable prior to concurrent chemoradiation with subsequent complete clinical response treated subsequently with observation alone (no planned surgery), five-year overall and disease-free survivals were 100% and 92%, respectively.

Improving restaging methods after neoadjuvant chemotherapy provides clinicians with increased information to guide management. Radiographic imaging modalities, however, are less sensitive to assessment of pathologic response, which is better characterized by metabolic imaging with $^{18}$F-FDG PET [54,99,100].

A number of studies have attempted correlation of $^{18}$F-FDG PET with tumor downstaging and response to neoadjuvant chemoradiation [100–105]. In a study by Capirci *et al.* [100] including 81 patients with locally-advanced rectal cancer, percent reduction of $SUV_{max}$ from baseline to follow-up $^{18}$F-FDG PET at 5-6 weeks after concurrent chemoradiation was most predictive of responders (71% reduction) versus non-responders (38% reduction) based on Mandard's criteria. They propose a cutoff of 65% reduction, yielding 85% sensitivity, 80% specificity, 81% positive predictive value, 84% negative predictive value, and 81% accuracy.

Notably, surgery is routinely planned approximately 6 weeks after neoadjuvant treatment, as surgery at 6-weeks was shown to have more tumor downstaging than at 2 weeks [106]. However, further tumor response and increased survival has been noted with intervals > 7 weeks [107]. A recent similar study by Perez *et al.* (2012) [105] of 91 patients with follow-up $^{18}$F-FDG PET at 6 weeks but also again at 12 weeks showed best separation of good responders (49%) versus bad responders (51%) at 12 weeks ($SUV_{max}$ of 9.1 in bad responders vs. 4.3 in good responders, p<0.001) rather than at 6 weeks ($SUV_{max}$ of 6.4 in bad responders versus 5.8 in good responders, p=0.5). Good responders were more likely to have complete clinical response (38% vs. 7%, p=0.001) complete or near-complete pathologic response (45% vs. 16%, p=0.008) and smaller pathologic size (3.3 vs. 4.4, p=0.03). Increase from early-phase (1 hour after injection) to delayed-phase PET (3 hours after injection) at the 6 –week time point was 67% accurate of predicting good vs. bad responders. A good responder was considered anyone with $SUV_{12week} < SUV_{6week}$. They conclude that approximately half of patients will have continued improved response beyond 6 weeks, whereas approximately half will have increased metabolic activity. Dual-phase imaging at the 6-week point may help stratify the two groups, which may help guide clinicians in best timing for planned surgery.

In rectal cancer, $^{18}$F-FDG PET restaging does show promise in potentially affecting treatment management; prospective studies investigating its role in this setting are awaited.

### 4.3. Lymphoma

$^{18}$FDG-PET finds various roles in management of lymphoma. For staging in Hodgkin lymphoma (HL) and non-Hodgkin lymphoma (NHL), PET with CT (PET-CT) has been shown to improve sensitivity and specificity in evaluation of nodal and extranodal sites in comparison to contrast-enhanced CT without PET [108,109]. It has further shown to be 92% sensitive for bone marrow involvement in HL [110]. Beyond staging, PET has been used for post-chemotherapy restaging, assessing response during chemotherapy at initial diagnosis, and also during salvage treatment. In current NCCN guidelines for both HL & NHL, PET-CT has variably been incorporated into staging, restaging during chemotherapy, and restaging after chemotherapy; routine PET-CT in the surveillance setting, however, is recommended against secondary to false-positive risk [111,112].

#### Restaging

The role for PET in lymphoma is clearest in the setting of restaging, either during or subsequent to treatment. PET has a very high negative predictive value (88-100%, see Table 6) [113]. Further, after treatment, PET is superior to CT for distinguishing residual mass with versus without residual viable disease (e.g. post-treatment fibrosis) [114]. Spaepen *et al.* report on two cohorts, one with HL [115] and one with NHL [116] who were assessed with PET at baseline and after completion of chemotherapy. In the HL cohort [115] of 60 patients, 55 were PET- (PET negative) after chemotherapy and 5 were PET+ (PET positive). All 5 PET+ patients had relapse of disease. Of the PET- patients, 91% remained without recurrence after median follow-up of 32 months. Two-year PFS rates were 91% vs. 0% for PET- vs. PET+ patients (p<0.0001). Similarly, in the NHL cohort [116] of 93 patients, all 27 PET+ patients after chemotherapy had relapse (median 2.4 months), whereas 84% of the PET- patients remained in remission (median

21 months). Two-year PFS rates were 85% vs. 4% for PET- vs. PET+ patients (p<0.0001). Halasz *et al.* (2011) [117] report a summary of post-chemotherapy and interim PET results. They further report a cohort of 59 patients with NHL, receiving 36 Gy (median) consolidative in-field radiation therapy (RT) (all patients) and R-CHOP chemotherapy (58 of 59 patients). Median follow-up was 47 months. In the 66% with negative PET after chemotherapy, 3-year PFS was 97%. However, with this treatment including RT, 3-year PFS was 90% in those with positive PET after chemotherapy (p-value not reported).

| Author | Year | n | PPV (%) | NPV (%) |
|---|---|---|---|---|
| **HL** | | | | |
| Spaepen [115] | 2001 | 60 | 100 | 91% |
| Cerci [118] | 2010 | 130 | 92% | 100% |
| Engert [119] | 2012 | 728 | N/A | 95% |
| **NHL** | | | | |
| Bangerter [120] | 1998 | 89 | 90% | 98% |
| Jerusalem [114] | 1999 | 35 | 43% | 100% |
| Zinzani [121] | 1999 | 31 | 93% | 100% |
| Mikhaeel [122] | 2000 | 45 | 60% | 100% |
| Naumann [123] | 2001 | 15 | 86% | 88% |
| Spaepen [116] | 2001 | 93 | 70% | 100% |
| Gigli [124] | 2008 | 42 | 75% | 94% |
| Cashen [125] | 2011 | 50 | 80% | 92% |

Adapted from Cheson [113]. HL, Hodgkin Lymphoma; NHL, Non-Hodgkin Lymphoma; PPV, positive predictive value; NPV, negative predictive value

**Table 6.** Positive and negative predictive value of PET-CT in lymphoma staging

## Interim (during-chemotherapy) PET

More research has investigated interim (during chemotherapy) $^{18}$FDG-PET for assessment of treatment response and prognostication (see Table 7). Cerci *et al.* [126] assessed interim PET after 2 cycles of ABVD (coxorubicin, bleomycin, vinblastine, and dacarbazine) chemotherapy in 104 patients with early and advanced Hodgkin lymphoma. Negativity vs. positivity at interim PET significantly predicted event-free survival (EFS), 91% vs. 53% at 3 years for PET- vs. PET+ patients (p<0.001). On univariate analysis, interim PET was the best prognosticator of event-free survival (p<0.001), more so than stage, bulky disease, and international prognostic score (IPS) (p=0.24, p=0.15, p=0.99, respectively). It however failed to prognosticate survival (p=0.2), which was better predicted by age (cutoff 45 years, p=0.01) and IPS (0-2 vs. 3-7, p=0.04).

| Author | Year | n | FU (months) | # cycles | Interim PET Response | Outcomes | p-value |
|---|---|---|---|---|---|---|---|
| **HL** | | | | | | | |
| Hutchings [127] | 2005 | 85 | 40 | 2-3 | 74% PET-<br>11% PET+<br>15% MRU | 97% 2y PFS<br>46% 2y PFS | <0.001 |
| Hutchings [109] | 2006 | 77 | 23 | 2 | 79% PET-<br>21% PET+ | 96% 2y PFS<br>0% 2y PFS | <0.001 |
| Kostakoglu [128] | 2006 | 23 | 21 | 1 | 74% PET-<br>26% PET+ | 100% 2y PFS<br>13% 2y PFS | <0.001 |
| Zinzani [129] | 2006 | 40 | 18 | 2 | 80% PET-<br>20% PET+ | 97% PFS<br>12% PFS | <0.001 |
| Gallamini [130] | 2007 | 260 | 26 | 2 | 81% PET-<br>19% PET+ | 95% 2y PFS<br>13% 2y PFS | <0.001 |
| Markova [131] | 2009 | 50 | 25 | 4 | 72% PET-<br>28% PET+ | 100% PFS<br>28% PFS | NR |
| Cerci [126] | 2010 | 104 | 36 | 2 | 71% PET-<br>29% PET+ | 91% 3y EFS<br>53% 3y EFS | <0.001 |
| **NHL** | | | | | | | |
| Jerusalem [114] | 2000 | 28 | 18 | 3 | 82% PET-<br>18% PET+ | 62% 2y PFS<br>0% 2y PFS | <0.001 |
| Spaepen [132] | 2002 | 70 | 36 | 2-3 | 53% PET -<br>47% PET + | 16% progressed<br>100% progressed | <0.001 |
| Haioun [133] | 2005 | 90 | 24 | 2 | 60% PET -<br>40% PET + | 82% 2y EFS<br>43% 2y EFS | <0.001 |
| Mikhaell [134] | 2005 | 121 | 29 | 2-3 | 41% PET -<br>43% PET +<br>16% MRU | 88% 5y PFS<br>16% 5y PFS<br>59% 5y PFS | <0.001 |
| Ng [135] | 2007 | 45 | 31 | 1-5 | 69% PET -<br>31% PET + | 15% relapsed<br>61% relapsed | <0.001 |
| Han [136] | 2009 | 40 | 24 | 2-4 | 68% PET -<br>32% PET + | 10% progressed<br>71% progressed | NR |
| Pregno [137] | 2009 | 88 | 26 | 2-4 | 72% PET -<br>28% PET + | 85% 2y PFS<br>72% 2y PFS | 0.048 |
| Safar [138] | 2009 | 112 | 38 | 2 | 63% PET -<br>37% PET + | 84% 3y PFS<br>47% 3y PFS | <0.001 |
| Cashen [125] | 2011 | 50 | 15 | 2-3 | 52% PET -<br>48% PET + | 85% 2y PFS<br>63% 2y EFS | 0.031 |
| Zinzani [139] | 2011 | 91 | 50 | variable | 62% PET-<br>39% PET+ | 75% 4y EFS<br>18% 4y EFS | <0.001 |

HL, Hodgkin Lymphoma; NHL, Non-Hodgkin Lymphoma; PET, positron emission tomography; FU, Follow-up; n, number of patients in study with interim PET scan; EFS, event-free survival; PFS, progression-free survival; MRU, minimal residual uptake; # cycles, number of cycles of chemotherapy completed prior to interim PET; NR, not reported

**Table 7.** Prognostication of interim PET in lymphoma

**Drug salvage**

In the setting of relapsing/refractory Hodgkin lymphoma, interim PET after 2 cycles of salvage high-dose chemotherapy has been assessed. Limited retrospective data from Castagna *et al.* [125] has shown similar prognostic potential, reporting 2-year progression-free survival of 93% (PET-negative) versus 10% (PET-positive, $p<0.001$).

**PET Response-Adapted radiotherapy**

In the German Hodgkin Study Group HD15 trial (2012) [119,140] with over 2,000 patients with advanced-stage Hodgkin lymphoma, 3 BEACOPP chemotherapy regimens were compared in a non-inferiority randomized trial. Radiotherapy was implemented with a "PET-guided" adaptive approach based on post-chemotherapy response regardless of treatment arm. If a PET-positive persistent mass 2.5cm or larger was present after completion of chemotherapy (median 21 days), 30Gy local radiation therapy was administered for consolidation. Negative predictive value for post-chemotherapy PET was 94% at 12 months follow-up. In the 3 arms, five-year freedom from failure ranged from 84%-89%, and five-year survival ranged from 92-95%. Consolidative radiotherapy was not randomized and was administered to 11% of patients (compared to 71% in HD9 [141]). With such excellent outcomes with this PET-guided radiotherapy approach, the authors indicate this approach as their current standard of care. Longer follow-up and prospective clinical trials assessing need for consolidative radiotherapy are still awaited.

### 4.4. Esophageal cancer – Definitive/preoperative

The role of multimodality therapy for esophageal and gastroesophageal cancer has historically not been well defined. Resection has been considered standard treatment for patients with resectable/localized disease without strong evidence supporting neoadjuvant therapy, despite significant risk for local and distant recurrences yielding poor 5-year survival rates ranging from 15-39%[142]. Neoadjuvant treatment is increasingly becoming adopted as standard of care for locally-advanced disease, with use continuing to increase [143,144]. Multiple prospective trials did not report survival benefit with neoadjuvant chemoradiotherapy [145–147], and randomized studies supporting neoadjuvant treatment are scarce. Walsh *et al.* (1996) [148] showed increased 3-year overall survival from 6% to 32% with neoadjuvant treatment ($p<0.01$) in a study of 113 patients. In the recently published CROSS trial [149] with 366 patients, addition of neoadjuvant chemoradiation increased R0 resection (resection with negative pathologic margins) from 69% to 92% ($p<0.001$) and more than doubled median overall survival from 24 to 49 months (hazard ratio = 0.66, $p=0.003$).

In patients receiving neoadjuvant chemoradiation, a portion—29% in the Dutch CROSS study—are found to have pathologic complete response on subsequent surgery. In a single-institution review, pathologic complete response from neoadjuvant treatment was associated with higher 5-year and overall survival (48% vs. 18% and 50 months vs. 28 months, respectively) in comparison to patients without complete response [150]. With treatment response bearing significant prognostic potential, assessment of response to neoadjuvant treatment for esophageal cancer has been an area of increasing research [150–163].

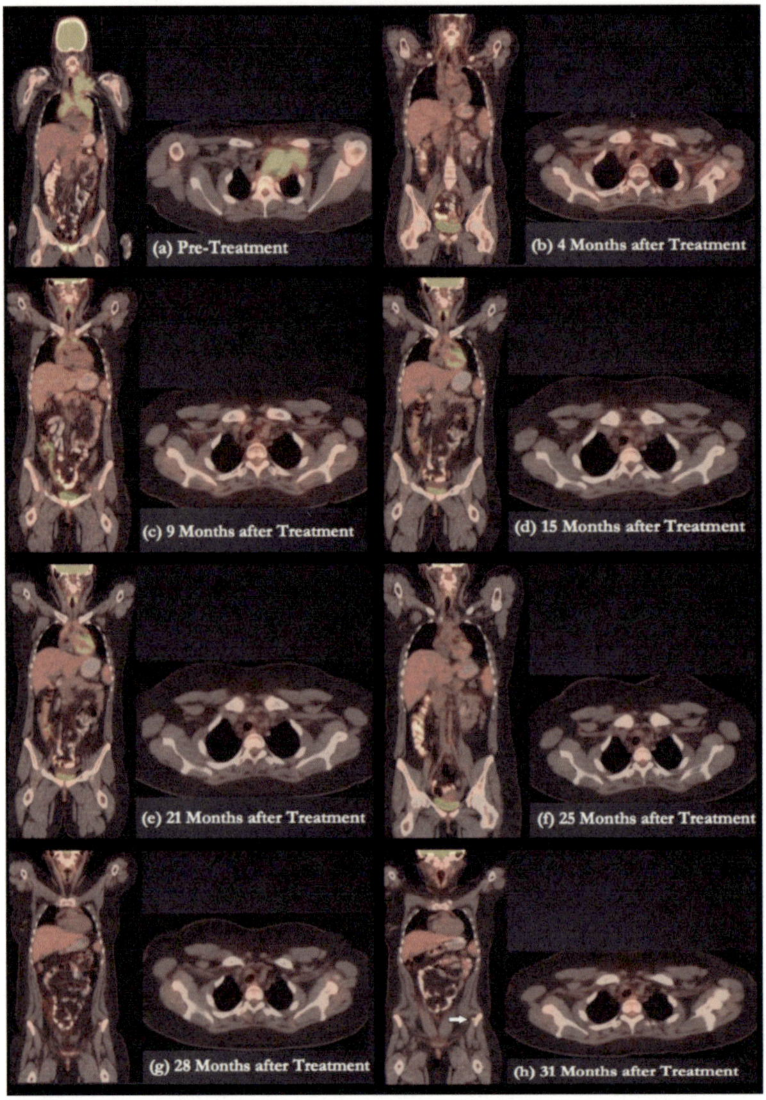


**Figure 1.** This is a 12-year-old female with a history of Stage IIB bulky nodular sclerosing Hodgkin lymphoma involving the bilateral cervical chain and mediastinum. She had achieved a complete response with 6 cycles of COPP-ABV chemotherapy. She then received a total radiation dose of 3060 cGy in 17 fractions of 180 cGy to the cervical and mediastinal lymph nodes. As seen in the serial PET/CT images (b-f above), the mediastinal and cervical lymph nodes responded well. However, by 28 months post-treatment, a left iliacus muscle lymph node became suspicious for lymphoma involvement (g – max SUV 5.0). By 31 months post-treatment, this node had increased further (h – max SUV 7.7).

In an early study by Weber *et al.* (2001) [151] in forty patients receiving neoadjuvant chemotherapy (without radiotherapy) for esophageal cancer, patients had $^{18}$FDG-PET both pretreatment and after 14 days of treatment (during chemotherapy). Metabolic response was considered decrease of 35% from baseline, which was associated with 93% sensitivity and 95%

specificity for prediction of clinical response. Responders had longer time to progression/recurrence and overall survival.

In a follow-up study [152], patients had three $^{18}$FDG-PET scans: one pretreatment, one during treatment (2 weeks after starting), then 3-4 weeks preoperatively (but after neoadjuvant treatment. Responders had more decrease at 2 weeks (44% vs. 21%, p<0.01) and preoperatively (70% vs. 51%, p=0.01). During-treatment PET had higher power than the preoperative PET treatment to predict response (area under curve (AUC) of receiver operator characteristic (ROC) 0.78 vs. 0.88), though difference was not statistically significant (p=0.40). Best cutoff for response in this cohort was 30% reduction from baseline (93% sensitive, 88% accurate), who all proceed to have R0 resection. Responders by this PET criteria had higher survival (median 38 vs. 18 months; 2-year rates 79% vs. 38%, p<0.01).

Analysis of gastroesophageal junction tumors again showed improved prognostic potential with PET using percent reduction of $SUV_{max}$ 2 weeks after treatment start (p=0.03) versus after completion of neoadjuvant treatment (p=0.09) [153]. Though percent reduction is routinely used to assess response, thresholds of decrease of $SUV_{max}$ (e.g. decrease of ≥10) from before to after neoadjuvant treatment have shown to predict significant histopathologic response [158].

More recent studies have showed other metrics as better predictors of response. In a comparison of $SUV_{max}$, MTV based on fixed threshold of 2.5 SUV, and $SUV_{mean}$ (of MTV), and TGA, MTV and TGA were both 91% sensitive in predicting histopathologic response when also using CT, but MTV increase specificity from 90% to 93%. Most predictive was TGA (AUC=0.95) followed by MTV (AUC=0.92), $SUV_{max}$ (AUC=0.84), and $SUV_{mean}$ (AUC=0.82) [159]. Further, metabolic response criteria (e.g. PERCIST) have shown better assessed response in comparison to non-metabolic methods (e.g. RECIST and WHO) [159,163].

With various studies showing prognostic potential of $^{18}$FDG-PET early during treatment, there is question as to the utility of PET to potentially facilitate treatment modification [152]. Kwee (2010) [160] performed a metaanalysis of 20 PET-response studies including 849 patients; it however showed wide ranges of sensitivity and specificity with overall AUC of 0.78. Based on the pooled data, PET was not recommended for routine clinical use to guide neoadjuvant treatment. Furthermore, in a retrospective single-institution review [164], patients treated with neoadjuvant chemotherapy followed by surgery had similar freedom from local failure (p=0.92) and overall survival (p=0.15) in comparison to patients receiving definitive chemoradiation who attained metabolic CR (SUV<3). Furthermore, in this retrospective study, though not statistically significant, rate of death in the definitive chemoradiation group was higher than in the surgical group despite worse baseline characteristics.

Similar to head and neck cancer, prospective studies are awaited to formally assess necessity of surgical management after complete metabolic response to neoadjuvant chemoradiation therapy in operable/resectable patients.

### 4.5. Non-Small Cell Lung Cancer (NSCLC)

$^{18}$FDG-PET is currently recommended by NCCN guidelines for routine staging of stage I-III NSCLC [67]. Radiotherapy planning with PET fusion has further been recommended for biologically-targeted radiotherapy in which 3D-PET fusion is implemented for tumor delineation, with PET performed with minimal delay between PET and start of treatment, given propensity for rapid disease progression [64–66,165]. Metabolic (PET) response to treatment has been shown to pre-date radiographic (CT) response. Despite increasing data showing utility of PET for assessing treatment response in NSCLC and predicting outcomes including survival, guidelines currently do not recommend PET in this setting [44,45,67,76,166–177].

In an early study of 15 patients receiving chemotherapy for IIIB-IV NSCLC, patients received weekly PET starting at initiation of chemotherapy until completion of 2 cycles (6 weeks later) [171]. Reduction of $SUV_{max}$ by 50% week 1 to week 3 was predictive of survival of > 6 months, thus facilitating prediction of response to treatment. Those with less reduction died within 6 months. In patients without early response, management may thus be altered to forego futile chemotherapy. In an early study [167] of 15 stage I-III patients receiving radiotherapy, patients received 3 PETs: one pre-treatment, one during treatment after approximately 45 Gy, and one 3 months post-treatment. Response during treatment was shown to correlate with overall response after treatment (p=0.03), and SUV during treatment correlated with SUV 3 months after (p<0.001). A number of studies with prospective PET data with cutoffs are listed in Table 8.

| Author | Year | n | Stage | Criteria | Outcome | p |
|---|---|---|---|---|---|---|
| Vansteenkiste [172] | 1985 | 15 | IIIA | 50% decrease | OS | 0.03 |
| MacManus [173] | 2003 | 73 | I-III | CMR | OS | <0.01 |
| Weber [174] | 2003 | 57 | IIIB-IV | 20% decrease | OS | <0.01 |
| Hellwig [175] | 2004 | 47 | IIB-III | SUV < 4 | OS | <0.01 |
| Eschmann [176] | 2007 | 70 | III | CMR or 80% decrease | OS | <0.01 |
| de Geus-Oei [177] | 2007 | 51 | IB-IV | 35% decrease | OS | 0.02 |
| Nahmias [171] | 2007 | 16 | IIIB-IV | 50% decrease from week 1 to week 3 | OS | <0.01 |
| Tanvetyanon [178] | 2008 | 89 | IB-IIIB | CMR | OS | NS |
| Mangona [45] | 2012 | 129 | IA-IB | At 12 months | | |
| | | | | SUV ≥ 3.9 | LF* | <0.01 |
| | | | | 60% decrease | LF* | <0.01 |
| | | | | SUV ≥ 6.0 | LF† | <0.01 |
| Mangona [70] | 2012 | 16 | IIB-IIIB | During treatment | | |
| | | | | 30% decrease | CSS | <0.01 |
| | | | | decrease ≥ 4 | LRR | <0.01 |

Adapted from Hicks *et al.* [170]. CMR, complete metabolic response; OS, overall survival; LF, local failure; CSS, cause-specific survival; LRR, locoregional recurrence; NS, not statistically significant.*100% sensitive. †100% specific.

**Table 8.** PET Cutoffs/Criteria and Outcomes in NSCLC

## SBRT

Stereotactic body radiotherapy (SBRT), employing modern techniques including 4-D treatment planning and image-guided radiotherapy (IGRT) has been shown to be an effective, cost-efficient, treatment option for definitive management of early-stage NSCLC as well as lung metastases from other organs with excellent tumor control rates; in comparison to medically-operable patients who are treated with resection, retrospective data of primarily medically-inoperable patients with poor pulmonary function suggests excellent tumor control with SBRT with rates similar to that of sublobar resection and minimal toxicity [179–191].

In a large single-institution analysis [45] of 129 consecutive NSCLC tumors treated with SBRT, 58% enrolled on a prospective phase II protocol, patients had baseline and serial follow-up PET imaging. Sixteen patients additionally had weekly on-treatment 4D-PET-CT. Median follow-up was 19 months and median time until local failure (LF) of 15 months. A total of 475 PETs were obtained. Change in SUV from pre-treatment to follow-up are seen in Figure 1 and stratified by status of LF vs. no-LF based on last follow-up. Though baseline $SUV_{max}$ was higher in the LF group (12.4 vs. 6.5, p=0.0001), difference was not significant at 1.5 and 6 months, as both groups responded. SUV at 12 months, however, was significantly higher for the LF vs. no-LF group (6.8 vs. 2.5, p=0.02). Cutoffs predictive of LF were 12-month SUV $\geq$ 3.9 (100 sensitive), 12-month SUV $\geq$ 6 (100 specific), and 12-month SUV $\geq$ 40% of baseline (see Table 8). Analysis of $SUV_{max}$ velocity showed trend for higher velocity at 12 months (+0.18 SUV/month vs. -0.03 SUV/month, p=0.058). On multivariate logistic regression, 12-month SUV was most predictive of LF (p=0.057).

## Hyperfractionated radiotherapy

In a cohort of 16 patients with locally-advanced NSCLC enrolled on a phase II protocol, patients had PET at baseline, weekly during treatment, and at follow-up [70,192] (see Figure 2). Patients received hyperfractionated radiation therapy 1.5 Gy BID with concurrent chemotherapy either as definitive treatment (n=12) or as neoadjuvant treatment (n=4) delivering RT with daily online cone-beam CT for image guidance and intensity modulated radiotherapy (IMRT) to minimize potential normal tissue toxicity [190,193,194]. After potential follow-up of 20 months (range 12-28), 7 had locoregional recurrence (LRR), and 8 died (5 of disease). Interestingly, there was trend for higher $SUV_{max}$ at baseline in those without LRR (the no-LRR group) than in those with LRR (19.0 vs. 11.9, p=0.08), an inverse relationship than expected. The rate of SUV decrease in the LRR group during RT was 1.6 per week, significantly faster than the no-LRR group (0.23 per week, p=0.02) such that SUV values were similar for both groups by the 4$^{th}$ on-treatment PET (p=0.95) (see Table 9). A during-RT decrease of less than 4 from baseline was predictive of LRR (p<0.01), and a during-RT decrease less 30% from baseline was predictive of death from disease (p<0.01). Velocity of retention index from PET1 to PET-FU predicted overall survival (+1.6%/week in those who died vs. -1.7%/week in those alive, p=0.03).

(a)

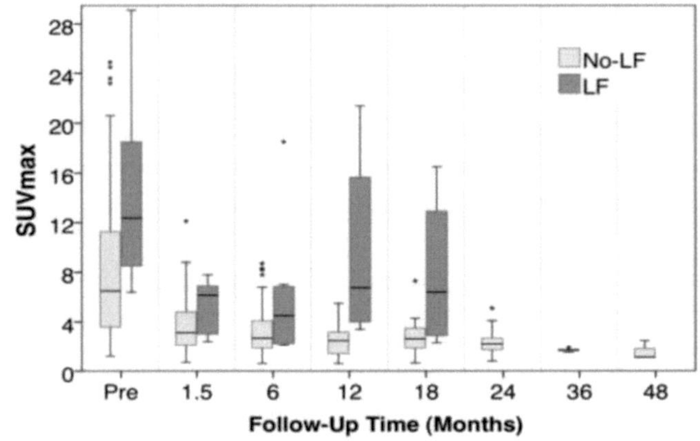


| | | Pre | 1.5 | 6 | 12 | 18 | 24 | 36 | 48 |
|---|---|---|---|---|---|---|---|---|---|
| LF | Median | 12.4 (n=10) | 6.2 (n=8) | 4.5 (n=8) | 6.8 (n=8) | 9.3 (n=5) | - | - | - |
| | IQR [25%-75%] | [8.3-19.6] | [2.8-7.2] | [2.2-6.9] | [4.0-16.8] | [2.9-18.0] | - | - | - |
| No LF | Median | 6.5 (n=119) | 3.2 (n=108) | 2.7 (n=88) | 2.5 (n=46) | 2.7 (n=20) | 2.2 (n=13) | 1.7 (n=5) | 1.1 (n=3) |
| | IQR [25%-75%] | [3.6-11.4] | [2.1-4.8] | [1.8-4.1] | [1.4-3.3] | [1.8-3.5] | [1.5-2.9] | [1.6-1.8] | [1.1-1.1] |
| $p$ | (LF vs. no-LF) | 0.001 | 0.033 | 0.203 | 0.024 | 0.097 | - | - | - |

(b)

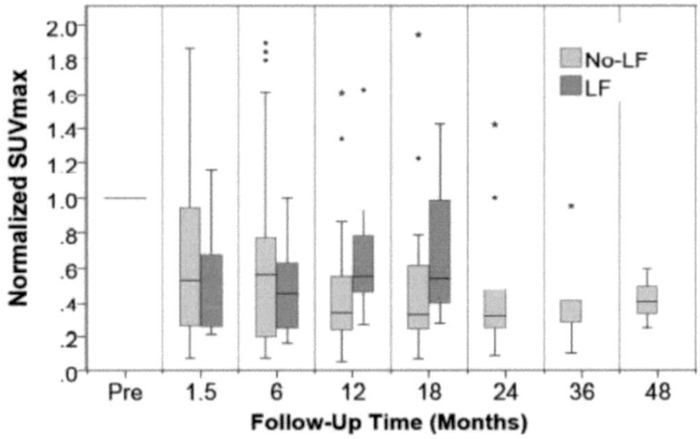


| | | Pre | 1.5 | 6 | 12 | 18 | 24 | 36 | 48 |
|---|---|---|---|---|---|---|---|---|---|
| LF | Median | 1.00 (n=10) | 0.36 (n=8) | 0.45 (n=8) | 0.55 (n=8) | 0.55 (n=5) | - | - | - |
| | IQR [25%-75%] | [1.00-1.00] | [0.23-0.75] | [0.22-0.66] | [0.46-0.85] | [0.40-1.04] | - | - | - |
| No LF | Median | 1.00 (n=119) | 0.53 (n=108) | 0.56 (n=88) | 0.33 (n=46) | 0.32 (n=20) | 0.31 (n=13) | 0.37 (n=5) | 0.41 (n=3) |
| | IQR [25%-75%] | [1.00-1.00] | [0.25-0.95] | [1.8-4.1] | [1.4-3.3] | [1.8-3.5] | [1.5-2.9] | [1.6-1.8] | [1.1-1.1] |
| $p$ | (LF vs. no-LF) | - | 0.365 | 0.501 | 0.044 | 0.875 | - | - | - |

Assessment of response for NSCLC with serial $^{18}$FDG-PET. 129 node-negative non-small-cell lung tumors were treated with stereotactic body radiation therapy (SBRT) and followed with routine follow-up imaging. SUV for tumors with eventual local failure (LF) and no local failure (no-LF) at last follow-up are compared. (a) Plot of $SUV_{max}$ vs. time, with baseline PET $SUV_{max}$ at t=0. Tumors with resulting LF show higher $SUV_{max}$ both at pre-treatment and at 12-months follow-up, though $SUV_{max}$ at 1.5 and 6 months were similar. (b) Plot of normalized $SUV_{max}$ (baseline normalized SUV = 1). Normalized $SUV_{max}$ is higher at 12 months in the LF group but similar at other time points. Values are plotted as box plots with thick black line representing the median value, lower box border the 25th percentile, upper box border the 75th percentile, and outliers with points. PET SUVs subsequent to any treatment for recurrence (e.g. chemotherapy) were excluded; thus, the no-LF group had data at longer follow-up (e.g. 24, 36, and 48 months).

**Figure 2.** SUV kinetics after stereotactic body radiotherapy for NSCLC

| | | PET0 | PET1 | PET2 | PET3 | PET4 | PET-FU | Velocity during RT |
|---|---|---|---|---|---|---|---|---|
| $SUV_{max}$ | LRR | 11.9 | 9.5 | 11.4 | 10.6 | 9.8 | 6.7 | -0.23/week |
| | no-LRR | 19.0 | 17.3 | 16.3 | 12.8 | 9.4 | 4.6 | -1.60/week |
| | *p* | *0.08* | *0.02* | *0.13* | *0.32* | *0.95* | *0.66* | *0.02* |
| $SUV_{delayed}$- $SUV_{early}$ | LRR | | 1.90 | 2.00 | 2.15 | 1.30 | 0.95 | -0.05/week |
| | no-LRR | - | 4.20 | 2.80 | 1.60 | 1.55 | 0.61 | -0.68/week |
| | *p* | | *0.02* | *0.15* | *0.82* | *0.55* | *0.82* | *0.15* |
| Retention Index | LRR | | 23.3% | 22.5% | 22.8% | 14.3% | 18.4% | -0.8%/week |
| | no-LRR | - | 27.1% | 19.8% | 18.5% | 15.3% | 17.6% | -3.4%/week |
| | *p* | | *0.92* | *0.88* | *0.16* | *0.57* | *0.76* | *0.04* |

Patients had PET-CT before treatment for staging/planning (PET0), weekly during treatment (PET1, PET2, PET3, and PET4), and at 6-12 weeks follow-up (PET-FU); RT, Radiation Therapy; LRR, locoregional recurrence; no-LRR, no locoregional recurrence at last follow-up.

**Table 9.** On-treatment SUV kinetics of locally-advanced NSCLC treated with concurrent chemoradiation

PET shows prognostic potential in this disease site from prior to treatment to early in treatment, to later in follow-up. It further holds potential for adjusting management (e.g. discontinuing ineffective chemotherapy, potentially modifying radiation therapy during treatment, and predicting delayed local failure for potential earlier biopsy/intervention). We await further prospective PET data and clinical trials to best define the role of PET in assessment of treatment in NSCLC.

## 5. Future directions

As PET is used for staging and radiotherapy prior to treatment for a number of organ sites, PET further has potential for restaging and replanning radiotherapy during the course of therapy. Beyond mid-treatment prognostication, this facilitates potential treatment modification. For radiotherapy re-planning, potential changes are include modification of target volumes based on anatomic changes from treatment, modification of boost volumes, and potentially adjustment of prescription dose based on response (e.g. higher dose for poor responders vs. less dose for good responders). Such investigations are currently ongoing in clinical protocols.

In treatment of locally-advanced head and neck squamous cell carcinomas, our institution has initiated a prospective, non-randomized trial evaluating the utility of such an adaptive approach focusing on target volume adaptation. Patients receiving 70 Gy IMRT in 35 daily fractions (7 week duration) with concurrent cisplatin or cetuximab are eligible. $^{18}$FDG-PET-CT is utilized for treatment planning. Repeat PET-CTs and diagnostic CTs are obtained after

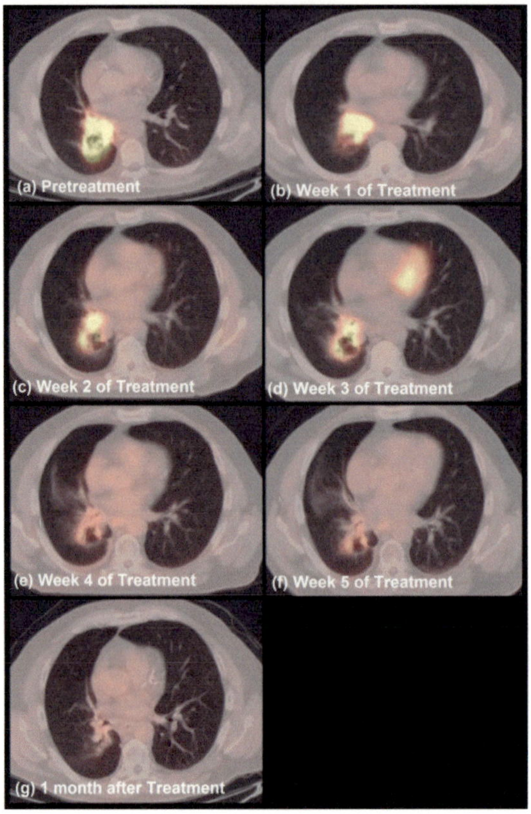


1.5 Gy twice daily with concurrent Taxotere. He had a complete metabolic response to treatment evident at first follow-up PET 1-month after treatment. SUV values (early → delayed): (a) Pre: 29.4 → 36.9; (b) Week 1: 17.8 → 23.6; (c) Week 2: 13.3 → 16.0; (d) Week 3: 15.7 → 17.0; (e) Week 4: 4.6 → 5.8; (f) Week 5: 4.2 → 5.3; (g) 1 month follow-up: 2.0 → 2.2

**Figure 3.** This is a 68-year-old male who presented with dyspnea and hemoptysis. Workup revealed a stage IIIB (T4, N2, M0) squamous cell carcinoma of the right lower lobe, 7cm in size invading the mediastinum. He received hyperfractionated intensity-modulated radiotherapy, 66 Gy in 1.5 Gy fractions twice daily.

fractions 10 and 22 for the purpose of treatment adaptation. Three different treatment plans will be created, one for fractions 1-12 (based on pre-treatment PET-CT), one for fractions 13-24 (based on PET-CT after fraction 10), and one for fractions 25-35 (based on PET-CT after fraction 22). Such an adaptive approach may help decrease dose delivered to normal tissue as tumors decrease in size during treatment, potentially decreasing toxicity. On this protocol, patients also obtain weekly PET-CTs for assessment of treatment response, though prescription dose is not modified in this study.

For non-small cell lung cancer, investigators have further used on-treatment PET to facilitate PET-adaptive replanning, with PET-adaptive dose escalation incorporated into a currently-enrolling Radition Therapy Oncology Group (RTOG) Protocol, RTOG 1106 [195,196]. All

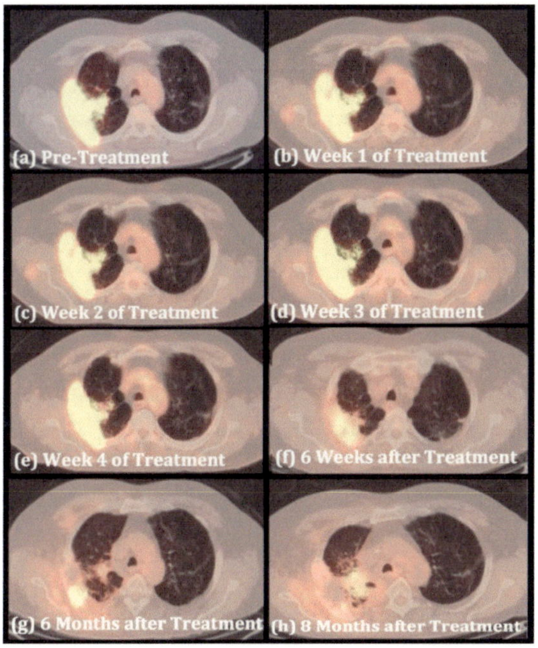


SUV values (early → delayed): (a) Pre: 23.4 → 28.7; (b) Week 1: 14.8 → 16.0; (c) Week 2: 11.0 → 12.7; (d) Week 3: 11.0 → 12.8; (e) Week 4: 12.1 → 15.; (f) 6-week FU: 6.5 → 8.; (g) 6-month FU: 12.5 → 15.7; (h) 8-month FU: 4.9 → 6.3

**Figure 4.** This is a 66-year-old male who presented with right shoulder pain. Workup revealed a clinical stage IIIA (T3 N1 M0) squamous cell carcinoma of the right upper lobe of the lobe with chest wall invasion causing destruction of ribs 2-4. He received hyperfractionated intensity-modulated radiotherapy 72Gy, 1.5 Gy twice daily, with concurrent and maintenance taxotere for 4 months. SUV nadir occurred at 6 weeks with evident local progression at 6 months.

patients on this protocol will have $^{18}$FDG-PET; however, a subset are planned to also have $^{18}$F-MISO-PET at staging.

As such radiotracers beyond $^{18}$F-FDG show particular promise, further results of clinical trials implementing these are awaited.

## 6. Conclusion

Over the past 20 years, the body of data assessing treatment response with PET has grown significant. Assessing treatment response with PET can yield highly prognostic information. Such information, however, may have no end-effect on management. As clinicians, many of our PET-based decisions are based on retrospective and prospective data without comparison of management options based on PET results. Such results are significantly hypothesis-generating. The high negative predictive value of PET in various organ sites may increase comfort of clinicians when considering omitting potentially unnecessary interventions (e.g. neck dissection after complete metabolic response of locally-advanced head and neck cancer to chemoradiation, esophagectomy after complete metabolic response to chemoradiotion, or consolidative radiotherapy after complete metabolic response in Hodgkin lymphoma). High-level evidence to justify such treatment-adapting decisions based on PET are currently lacking, thus we caution application of such data as justification for modifying standard of care. We strongly encourage PET-adaptive management under the guise of clinical trials at this time, as the role of PET in oncology continues to best be defined.

## Acknowledgements

Special thanks to Dr. Katie Traylor, Rob Ceruti, and Matthew Johnson of Nuclear Medicine for their assistance with PET figures presented in this chapter.

## Author details

Inga S. Grills[1,2] and Victor S. Mangona[1]

1 Department of Radiation Oncology, Beaumont Cancer Institute, Beaumont Health System, Royal Oak, Michigan, USA

2 Oakland University William Beaumont School of Medicine, Rochester, Michigan, USA

## References

[1] Dunphy MPS, Lewis JS. Radiopharmaceuticals in preclinical and clinical development for monitoring of therapy with PET. J. Nucl. Med. 2009 May;50 Suppl 1:106S–21S.

[2] Conti PS, Lilien DL, Hawley K, Keppler J, Grafton ST, Bading JR. PET and [$^{18}$F]-FDG in oncology: a clinical update. Nucl. Med. Biol. 1996 Aug;23(6):717–35.

[3] Bos R, van Der Hoeven JJM, van Der Wall E, van Der Groep P, van Diest PJ, Comans EFI, et al. Biologic correlates of (18)fluorodeoxyglucose uptake in human breast cancer measured by positron emission tomography. J. Clin. Oncol. 2002 Jan 15;20(2):379–87.

[4] Juweid ME, Cheson BD. Positron-emission tomography and assessment of cancer therapy. N. Engl. J. Med. 2006 Feb 2;354(5):496–507.

[5] Siegel R, Naishadham D, Jemal A. Cancer statistics, 2012. CA Cancer J Clin. 2012 Feb; 62(1):10–29.

[6] Lee ST, Lawrentschuk N, Scott AM. PET in prostate and bladder tumors. Semin Nucl Med. 2012 Jul;42(4):231–46.

[7] Long NM, Smith CS. Causes and imaging features of false positives and false negatives on F-PET/CT in oncologic imaging. Insights Imaging. 2011 Dec;2(6):679–98.

[8] Bading JR, Shields AF. Imaging of cell proliferation: status and prospects. J. Nucl. Med. 2008 Jun;49 Suppl 2:64S–80S.

[9] Juweid ME, Stroobants S, Hoekstra OS, Mottaghy FM, Dietlein M, Guermazi A, et al. Use of positron emission tomography for response assessment of lymphoma: consensus of the Imaging Subcommittee of International Harmonization Project in Lymphoma. J. Clin. Oncol. 2007 Feb 10;25(5):571–8.

[10] Tehrani OS, Douglas KA, Lawhorn-Crews JM, Shields AF. Tracking cellular stress with labeled FMAU reflects changes in mitochondrial TK2. Eur. J. Nucl. Med. Mol. Imaging. 2008 Aug;35(8):1480–8.

[11] Kasper B, Egerer G, Gronkowski M, Haufe S, Lehnert T, Eisenhut M, et al. Functional diagnosis of residual lymphomas after radiochemotherapy with positron emission tomography comparing FDG- and FLT-PET. Leuk. Lymphoma. 2007 Apr;48(4):746–53.

[12] Smyczek-Gargya B, Fersis N, Dittmann H, Vogel U, Reischl G, Machulla H-J, et al. PET with [$^{18}$F]fluorothymidine for imaging of primary breast cancer: a pilot study. Eur. J. Nucl. Med. Mol. Imaging. 2004 May;31(5):720–4.

[13] Dittmann H, Dohmen BM, Paulsen F, Eichhorn K, Eschmann SM, Horger M, et al. [$^{18}$F]FLT PET for diagnosis and staging of thoracic tumours. Eur. J. Nucl. Med. Mol. Imaging. 2003 Oct;30(10):1407–12.

[14] Pio BS, Park CK, Pietras R, Hsueh W-A, Satyamurthy N, Pegram MD, et al. Usefulness of 3′-[F-18]fluoro-3′-deoxythymidine with positron emission tomography in predicting breast cancer response to therapy. Mol Imaging Biol. 2006 Feb;8(1):36–42.

[15] Graeber TG, Osmanian C, Jacks T, Housman DE, Koch CJ, Lowe SW, et al. Hypoxia-mediated selection of cells with diminished apoptotic potential in solid tumours. Nature. 1996 Jan 4;379(6560):88–91.

[16] Hockel M, Schlenger K, Aral B, Mitze M, Schaffer U, Vaupel P. Association between tumor hypoxia and malignant progression in advanced cancer of the uterine cervix. Cancer Res. 1996 Oct 1;56(19):4509–15.

[17] Dehdashti F, Grigsby PW, Mintun MA, Lewis JS, Siegel BA, Welch MJ. Assessing tumor hypoxia in cervical cancer by positron emission tomography with 60Cu-ATSM: relationship to therapeutic response-a preliminary report. Int. J. Radiat. Oncol. Biol. Phys. 2003 Apr 1;55(5):1233–8.

[18] Dietz DW, Dehdashti F, Grigsby PW, Malyapa RS, Myerson RJ, Picus J, et al. Tumor hypoxia detected by positron emission tomography with 60Cu-ATSM as a predictor

of response and survival in patients undergoing Neoadjuvant chemoradiotherapy for rectal carcinoma: a pilot study. Dis. Colon Rectum. 2008 Nov;51(11):1641–8.

[19] Dehdashti F, Mintun MA, Lewis JS, Bradley J, Govindan R, Laforest R, et al. In vivo assessment of tumor hypoxia in lung cancer with 60Cu-ATSM. Eur. J. Nucl. Med. Mol. Imaging. 2003 Jun;30(6):844–50.

[20] Rajendran JG, Schwartz DL, O'Sullivan J, Peterson LM, Ng P, Scharnhorst J, et al. Tumor hypoxia imaging with [F-18] fluoromisonidazole positron emission tomography in head and neck cancer. Clinical Cancer Research. 2006;12(18):5435–41.

[21] Spence AM, Muzi M, Swanson KR, O'Sullivan F, Rockhill JK, Rajendran JG, et al. Regional hypoxia in glioblastoma multiforme quantified with [$^{18}$F] fluoromisonidazole positron emission tomography before radiotherapy: correlation with time to progression and survival. Clinical Cancer Research. 2008;14(9):2623–30.

[22] Galldiks N, Kracht LW, Burghaus L, Thomas A, Jacobs AH, Heiss W-D, et al. Use of 11C-methionine PET to monitor the effects of temozolomide chemotherapy in malignant gliomas. Eur. J. Nucl. Med. Mol. Imaging. 2006 May;33(5):516–24.

[23] Lee IH, Piert M, Gomez-Hassan D, Junck L, Rogers L, Hayman J, et al. Association of 11C-methionine PET uptake with site of failure after concurrent temozolomide and radiation for primary glioblastoma multiforme. Int. J. Radiat. Oncol. Biol. Phys. 2009 Feb 1;73(2):479–85.

[24] Terakawa Y, Tsuyuguchi N, Iwai Y, Yamanaka K, Higashiyama S, Takami T, et al. Diagnostic accuracy of 11C-methionine PET for differentiation of recurrent brain tumors from radiation necrosis after radiotherapy. J. Nucl. Med. 2008 May;49(5):694–9.

[25] Dehdashti F, Mortimer JE, Trinkaus K, Naughton MJ, Ellis M, Katzenellenbogen JA, et al. PET-based estradiol challenge as a predictive biomarker of response to endocrine therapy in women with estrogen-receptor-positive breast cancer. Breast cancer research and treatment. 2009;113(3):509–17.

[26] Peterson LM, Mankoff DA, Lawton T, Yagle K, Schubert EK, Stekhova S, et al. Quantitative imaging of estrogen receptor expression in breast cancer with PET and $^{18}$F-fluoroestradiol. Journal of Nuclear Medicine. 2008;49(3):367–74.

[27] Dehdashti F, Picus J, Michalski JM, Dence CS, Siegel BA, Katzenellenbogen JA, et al. Positron tomographic assessment of androgen receptors in prostatic carcinoma. European journal of nuclear medicine and molecular imaging. 2005;32(3):344–50.

[28] Hustinx R, Smith RJ, Benard F, Rosenthal DI, Machtay M, Farber LA, et al. Dual time point fluorine-18 fluorodeoxyglucose positron emission tomography: a potential method to differentiate malignancy from inflammation and normal tissue in the head and neck. European Journal of Nuclear Medicine and Molecular Imaging. 1999;26(10):1345–8.

[29] Matthies A, Hickeson M, Cuchiara A, Alavi A. Dual Time Point $^{18}$F-FDG PET for the Evaluation of Pulmonary Nodules. J Nucl Med. 2002 Jul 1;43(7):871–5.

[30] Zhuang H, Pourdehnad M, Lambright ES, Yamamoto AJ, Lanuti M, Li P, et al. Dual Time Point $^{18}$F-FDG PET Imaging for Differentiating Malignant from Inflammatory Processes. J Nucl Med. 2001 Sep 1;42(9):1412–7.

[31] Nakamoto Y, Higashi T, Sakahara H, Tamaki N, Kogire M, Doi R, et al. Delayed $^{18}$F-fluoro-2-deoxy-D-glucose positron emission tomography scan for differentiation between malignant and benign lesions in the pancreas. Cancer. 2000;89(12):2547–54.

[32] Mertens K, Bolcaen J, Ham H, Deblaere K, Van den Broecke C, Boterberg T, et al. The optimal timing for imaging brain tumours and other brain lesions with $^{18}$F-labelled fluoromethylcholine: a dynamic positron emission tomography study. Nucl Med Commun. 2012 Sep;33(9):954–9.

[33] Carlson ER, Schaefferkoetter J, Townsend D, McCoy JM, Campbell PD Jr, Long M. The Use of Multiple Time Point Dynamic Positron Emission Tomography/Computed Tomography in Patients With Oral/Head and Neck Cancer Does Not Predictably Identify Metastatic Cervical Lymph Nodes. Journal of oral and maxillofacial surgery: official journal of the American Association of Oral and Maxillofacial Surgeons [Internet]. 2012 Jun 26 [cited 2012 Sep 28]; Available from: http://www.ncbi.nlm.nih.gov/pubmed/22742956

[34] Nehmeh SA, Erdi YE, Pan T, Pevsner A, Rosenzweig KE, Yorke E, et al. Four-dimensional (4D) PET/CT imaging of the thorax. Med Phys. 2004 Dec;31(12):3179–86.

[35] Nehmeh SA, Erdi YE, Pan T, Yorke E, Mageras GS, Rosenzweig KE, et al. Quantitation of respiratory motion during 4D-PET/CT acquisition. Med Phys. 2004 Jun;31(6): 1333–8.

[36] García Vicente AM, Castrejón AS, León Martín AA, García BG, Pilkington Woll JP, Muñoz AP. Value of 4-dimensional $^{18}$F-FDG PET/CT in the classification of pulmonary lesions. J Nucl Med Technol. 2011 Jun;39(2):91–9.

[37] Wang Y-C, Hsieh T-C, Yu C-Y, Yen K-Y, Chen S-W, Yang S-N, et al. The clinical application of 4D $^{18}$F-FDG PET/CT on gross tumor volume delineation for radiotherapy planning in esophageal squamous cell cancer. J. Radiat. Res. 2012 Jul 1;53(4):594–600.

[38] Mancosu P, Danna M, Bettinardi V, Aquilina MA, Lobefalo F, Cozzi L, et al. Semiautomatic method to identify the best phase for gated RT in lung region by 4D-PET/CT acquisitions. Med Phys. 2011 Jan;38(1):354–62.

[39] Bundschuh RA, Andratschke N, Dinges J, Duma MN, Astner ST, Brügel M, et al. Respiratory gated [$^{18}$F]FDG PET/CT for target volume delineation in stereotactic radiation treatment of liver metastases. Strahlenther Onkol. 2012 Jul;188(7):592–8.

[40] Aristophanous M, Berbeco RI, Killoran JH, Yap JT, Sher DJ, Allen AM, et al. Clinical utility of 4D FDG-PET/CT scans in radiation treatment planning. Int. J. Radiat. Oncol. Biol. Phys. 2012 Jan 1;82(1):e99–105.

[41] Lucignani G, Paganelli G, Bombardieri E. The use of standardized uptake values for assessing FDG uptake with PET in oncology: a clinical perspective. Nucl Med Commun. 2004 Jul;25(7):651–6.

[42] Huang SC. Anatomy of SUV. Standardized uptake value. Nucl. Med. Biol. 2000 Oct; 27(7):643–6.

[43] Wahl RL, Jacene H, Kasamon Y, Lodge MA. From RECIST to PERCIST: Evolving Considerations for PET response criteria in solid tumors. J. Nucl. Med. 2009 May;50 Suppl 1:122S–50S.

[44] Mangona V, Grills I, Wong C, McGee M, Stone B, Hung B, et al. Can Standardized Uptake Value (SUV) Predict Local Failure after Stereotactic or Hyperfractionated Lung Radiotherapy (RT) for Non-small Cell Lung Cancer (NSCLC)? An Evaluation of SUV Kinetics. International Journal of Radiation Oncology* Biology* Physics. 2011;81(2):S167–S168.

[45] Mangona VS, Kestin LL, Yan D, Stone BM, Gustafson BR, Wong CYO, et al. Can $^{18}$FDG-PET Predict Local Failure after Stereotactic Body Radiotherapy (SBRT) for Non-Small Cell Lung Cancer (NSCLC)? An Analysis of PET Kinetics. American Journal of Clinical Oncology. 2012;(00):3.

[46] Xiang Z-L, Erasmus J, Komaki R, Cox JD, Chang JY. FDG uptake correlates with recurrence and survival after treatment of unresectable stage III non-small cell lung cancer with high-dose proton therapy and chemotherapy. Radiat Oncol. 2012;7:144.

[47] Kim G, Kim YS, Han EJ, Yoo IR, Song J-H, Lee S-N, et al. FDG-PET/CT as prognostic factor and surveillance tool for postoperative radiation recurrence in locally advanced head and neck cancer. Radiation Oncol J. 2011 Dec;29(4):243–51.

[48] Chan DSY, Fielding P, Roberts SA, Reid TD, Ellis-Owen R, Lewis WG. Prognostic significance of 18-FDG PET/CT and EUS-defined tumour characteristics in patients with oesophageal cancer. Clin Radiol [Internet]. 2012 Sep 13 [cited 2012 Sep 29]; Available from: http://www.ncbi.nlm.nih.gov/pubmed/22981727

[49] Rizk NP, Tang L, Adusumilli PS, Bains MS, Akhurst TJ, Ilson D, et al. Predictive Value of Initial PET-SUVmax in Patients with Locally Advanced Esophageal and Gastroesophageal Junction Adenocarcinoma. Journal of Thoracic Oncology. 2009 Jul;4(7): 875–9.

[50] Lee JW, Lee SM, Lee M-S, Shin HC. Role of (18)F-FDG PET/CT in the prediction of gastric cancer recurrence after curative surgical resection. Eur. J. Nucl. Med. Mol. Imaging. 2012 Sep;39(9):1425–34.

[51] Schellenberg D, Quon A, Minn AY, Graves EE, Kunz P, Ford JM, et al. $^{18}$Fluorodeoxyglucose PET Is Prognostic of Progression-Free and Overall Survival in Locally Ad-

vanced Pancreas Cancer Treated With Stereotactic Radiotherapy. International Journal of Radiation Oncology*Biology*Physics. 2010 Aug;77(5):1420–5.

[52] Kidd EA, El Naqa I, Siegel BA, Dehdashti F, Grigsby PW. FDG-PET-based prognostic nomograms for locally advanced cervical cancer. Gynecol. Oncol. 2012 Oct;127(1): 136–40.

[53] Capirci C, Rubello D, Chierichetti F, Crepaldi G, Fanti S, Mandoliti G, et al. Long-Term Prognostic Value of $^{18}$F-FDG PET in Patients with Locally Advanced Rectal Cancer Previously Treated with Neoadjuvant Radiochemotherapy. AJR. 2006 Aug 1;187(2):W202–W208.

[54] Kalff V, Duong C, Drummond EG, Matthews JP, Hicks RJ. Findings on $^{18}$F-FDG PET Scans After Neoadjuvant Chemoradiation Provides Prognostic Stratification in Patients with Locally Advanced Rectal Carcinoma Subsequently Treated by Radical Surgery. J Nucl Med. 2006 Jan 1;47(1):14–22.

[55] Cazaentre T, Morschhauser F, Vermandel M, Betrouni N, Prangère T, Steinling M, et al. Pre-therapy <sup>18</sup>F-FDG PET quantitative parameters help in predicting the response to radioimmunotherapy in non-Hodgkin lymphoma. European Journal of Nuclear Medicine and Molecular Imaging. 2010;37(3):494–504.

[56] Schwarzbach MHM, Hinz U, Dimitrakopoulou-Strauss A, Willeke F, Cardona S, Mechtersheimer G, et al. Prognostic Significance of Preoperative [18-F] Fluorodeoxyglucose (FDG) Positron Emission Tomography (PET) Imaging in Patients With Resectable Soft Tissue Sarcomas. Ann Surg. 2005 Feb;241(2):286–94.

[57] Ho K-C, Lin G, Wang J-J, Lai C-H, Chang C-J, Yen T-C. Correlation of apparent diffusion coefficients measured by 3T diffusion-weighted MRI and SUV from FDG PET/CT in primary cervical cancer. European Journal of Nuclear Medicine and Molecular Imaging. 2009;36(2):200–8.

[58] Beaulieu S, Kinahan P, Tseng J, Dunnwald LK, Schubert EK, Pham P, et al. SUV Varies with Time After Injection in $^{18}$F-FDG PET of Breast Cancer: Characterization and Method to Adjust for Time Differences. J Nucl Med. 2003 Jul 1;44(7):1044–50.

[59] Berriolo-Riedinger A, Touzery C, Riedinger J-M, Toubeau M, Coudert B, Arnould L, et al. [$^{18}$F]FDG-PET predicts complete pathological response of breast cancer to neoadjuvant chemotherapy. European Journal of Nuclear Medicine and Molecular Imaging. 2007;34(12):1915–24.

[60] Seol YM, Kwon BR, Song MK, Choi YJ, Shin HJ, Chung JS, et al. Measurement of tumor volume by PET to evaluate prognosis in patients with head and neck cancer treated by chemo-radiation therapy. Acta Oncol. 2010;49(2):201–8.

[61] Lee P, Weerasuriya DK, Lavori PW, Quon A, Hara W, Maxim PG, et al. Metabolic tumor burden predicts for disease progression and death in lung cancer. Int. J. Radiat. Oncol. Biol. Phys. 2007 Oct 1;69(2):328–33.

[62] Hadiprodjo D, Ryan T, Truong M-T, Mercier G, Subramaniam RM. Parotid gland tumors: preliminary data for the value of FDG PET/CT diagnostic parameters. AJR Am J Roentgenol. 2012 Feb;198(2):W185–190.

[63] Hatt M, Visvikis D, Albarghach NM, Tixier F, Pradier O, Cheze-le Rest C. Prognostic value of $^{18}$F-FDG PET image-based parameters in oesophageal cancer and impact of tumour delineation methodology. Eur. J. Nucl. Med. Mol. Imaging. 2011 Jul;38(7): 1191–202.

[64] Werner-Wasik M, Nelson AD, Choi W, Arai Y, Faulhaber PF, Kang P, et al. What is the best way to contour lung tumors on PET scans? Multiobserver validation of a gradient-based method using a NSCLC digital PET phantom. Int. J. Radiat. Oncol. Biol. Phys. 2012 Mar 1;82(3):1164–71.

[65] Black QC, Grills IS, Kestin LL, Wong C-YO, Wong JW, Martinez AA, et al. Defining a radiotherapy target with positron emission tomography. International Journal of Radiation Oncology*Biology*Physics. 2004 Nov;60(4):1272–82.

[66] Grills IS, Yan D, Black QC, Wong C-YO, Martinez AA, Kestin LL. Clinical implications of defining the gross tumor volume with combination of CT and $^{18}$FDG-positron emission tomography in non-small-cell lung cancer. Int. J. Radiat. Oncol. Biol. Phys. 2007 Mar 1;67(3):709–19.

[67] Ettinger D. NCCN Clinical Practice Guidelines in Oncology (NCCN Guidelines®) Non-Small Cell Lung Cancer Version 3.2012 [Internet]. National Comprehensive Cancer Network, Inc.; 2012 [cited 2012 Sep 29]. Available from: http://www.nccn.org/professionals/physician_gls/pdf/nscl.pdf

[68] Jayachandran P, Pai RK, Quon A, Graves E, Krakow TE, La T, et al. Postchemoradiotherapy positron emission tomography predicts pathologic response and survival in patients with esophageal cancer. Int. J. Radiat. Oncol. Biol. Phys. 2012 Oct 1;84(2): 471–7.

[69] Dibble EH, Alvarez ACL, Truong M-T, Mercier G, Cook EF, Subramaniam RM. $^{18}$F-FDG metabolic tumor volume and total glycolytic activity of oral cavity and oropharyngeal squamous cell cancer: adding value to clinical staging. J. Nucl. Med. 2012 May;53(5):709–15.

[70] Mangona V, Kestin L, Wong C, McGee M, Hung B, Lurie M, et al. SUV Kinetics of Weekly $^{18}$FDG-PET During Radiotherapy Predict Eventual Outcome in Locally-Advanced Non-Small Cell Lung Cancer (NSCLC). International Journal of Radiation Oncology* Biology* Physics. 2012 Nov 1;84(3S):S103–S104.

[71] García Vicente AM, Castrejón ÁS, Relea Calatayud F, Muñoz AP, León Martín AA, López-Muñiz IC, et al. $^{18}$F-FDG retention index and biologic prognostic parameters in breast cancer. Clin Nucl Med. 2012 May;37(5):460–6.

[72] Moertel CG, Hanley JA. The effect of measuring error on the results of therapeutic trials in advanced cancer. Cancer. 1976 Jul;38(1):388–94.

[73] Miller AB, Hoogstraten B, Staquet M, Winkler A. Reporting results of cancer treatment. Cancer. 1981 Jan 1;47(1):207–14.

[74] Therasse P, Arbuck SG, Eisenhauer EA, Wanders J, Kaplan RS, Rubinstein L, et al. New guidelines to evaluate the response to treatment in solid tumors. European Organization for Research and Treatment of Cancer, National Cancer Institute of the United States, National Cancer Institute of Canada. J. Natl. Cancer Inst. 2000 Feb 2;92(3):205–16.

[75] Eisenhauer EA, Therasse P, Bogaerts J, Schwartz LH, Sargent D, Ford R, et al. New response evaluation criteria in solid tumours: revised RECIST guideline (version 1.1). Eur. J. Cancer. 2009 Jan;45(2):228–47.

[76] Mohammed N, Grills IS, Wong C-YO, Galerani AP, Chao K, Welsh R, et al. Radiographic and metabolic response rates following image-guided stereotactic radiotherapy for lung tumors. Radiother Oncol. 2011 Apr;99(1):18–22.

[77] Young H, Baum R, Cremerius U, Herholz K, Hoekstra O, Lammertsma AA, et al. Measurement of clinical and subclinical tumour response using [$^{18}$F]-fluorodeoxyglucose and positron emission tomography: review and 1999 EORTC recommendations. European Organization for Research and Treatment of Cancer (EORTC) PET Study Group. Eur. J. Cancer. 1999 Dec;35(13):1773–82.

[78] Cheson BD, Pfistner B, Juweid ME, Gascoyne RD, Specht L, Horning SJ, et al. Revised response criteria for malignant lymphoma. J. Clin. Oncol. 2007 Feb 10;25(5): 579–86.

[79] Cheson BD, Horning SJ, Coiffier B, Shipp MA, Fisher RI, Connors JM, et al. Report of an international workshop to standardize response criteria for non-Hodgkin's lymphomas. NCI Sponsored International Working Group. J. Clin. Oncol. 1999 Apr;17(4): 1244.

[80] Juweid ME, Wiseman GA, Vose JM, Ritchie JM, Menda Y, Wooldridge JE, et al. Response assessment of aggressive non-Hodgkin's lymphoma by integrated International Workshop Criteria and fluorine-18-fluorodeoxyglucose positron emission tomography. J. Clin. Oncol. 2005 Jul 20;23(21):4652–61.

[81] Minn H, Lapela M, Klemi PJ, Grénman R, Leskinen S, Lindholm P, et al. Prediction of survival with fluorine-18-fluoro-deoxyglucose and PET in head and neck cancer. J. Nucl. Med. 1997 Dec;38(12):1907–11.

[82] Peters LJ, Weber RS, Morrison WH, Byers RM, Garden AS, Goepfert H. Neck surgery in patients with primary oropharyngeal cancer treated by radiotherapy. Head Neck. 1996 Dec;18(6):552–9.

[83] Johnson CR, Silverman LN, Clay LB, Schmidt-Ullrich R. Radiotherapeutic management of bulky cervical lymphadenopathy in squamous cell carcinoma of the head

and neck: is postradiotherapy neck dissection necessary? Radiat Oncol Investig. 1998;6(1):52–7.

[84] Yao M, Graham MM, Hoffman HT, Smith RB, Funk GF, Graham SM, et al. The role of post-radiation therapy FDG PET in prediction of necessity for post-radiation therapy neck dissection in locally advanced head-and-neck squamous cell carcinoma. Int. J. Radiat. Oncol. Biol. Phys. 2004 Jul 15;59(4):1001–10.

[85] Yao M, Smith RB, Graham MM, Hoffman HT, Tan H, Funk GF, et al. The role of FDG PET in management of neck metastasis from head-and-neck cancer after definitive radiation treatment. Int. J. Radiat. Oncol. Biol. Phys. 2005 Nov 15;63(4):991–9.

[86] Kubota K, Yokoyama J, Yamaguchi K, Ono S, Qureshy A, Itoh M, et al. FDG-PET delayed imaging for the detection of head and neck cancer recurrence after radio-chemotherapy: comparison with MRI/CT. Eur. J. Nucl. Med. Mol. Imaging. 2004 Apr; 31(4):590–5.

[87] Rogers JW, Greven KM, McGuirt WF, Keyes JW Jr, Williams DW 3rd, Watson NE, et al. Can post-RT neck dissection be omitted for patients with head-and-neck cancer who have a negative PET scan after definitive radiation therapy? Int. J. Radiat. Oncol. Biol. Phys. 2004 Mar 1;58(3):694–7.

[88] Porceddu SV, Jarmolowski E, Hicks RJ, Ware R, Weih L, Rischin D, et al. Utility of positron emission tomography for the detection of disease in residual neck nodes after (chemo)radiotherapy in head and neck cancer. Head & Neck. 2005;27(3):175–81.

[89] Fogarty GB, Peters LJ, Stewart J, Scott C, Rischin D, Hicks RJ. The usefulness of fluorine 18-labelled deoxyglucose positron emission tomography in the investigation of patients with cervical lymphadenopathy from an unknown primary tumor. Head Neck. 2003 Feb;25(2):138–45.

[90] Isles MG, McConkey C, Mehanna HM. A systematic review and meta-analysis of the role of positron emission tomography in the follow up of head and neck squamous cell carcinoma following radiotherapy or chemoradiotherapy. Clin Otolaryngol. 2008 Jun;33(3):210–22.

[91] Ferlito A, Corry J, Silver CE, Shaha AR, Thomas Robbins K, Rinaldo A. Planned neck dissection for patients with complete response to chemoradiotherapy: a concept approaching obsolescence. Head Neck. 2010 Feb;32(2):253–61.

[92] Gupta T, Master Z, Kannan S, Agarwal JP, Ghsoh-Laskar S, Rangarajan V, et al. Diagnostic performance of post-treatment FDG PET or FDG PET/CT imaging in head and neck cancer: a systematic review and meta-analysis. Eur. J. Nucl. Med. Mol. Imaging. 2011 Nov;38(11):2083–95.

[93] Pryor DI, Porceddu SV, Scuffham PA, Whitty JA, Thomas PA, Burmeister BH. Economic analysis of FDG-PET-guided management of the neck after primary chemora-

diotherapy for node-positive head and neck squamous cell carcinoma. Head Neck. 2012 Sep 18;

[94] Adjuvant radiotherapy for rectal cancer: a systematic overview of 8,507 patients from 22 randomised trials. Lancet. 2001 Oct 20;358(9290):1291–304.

[95] Improved survival with preoperative radiotherapy in resectable rectal cancer. Swedish Rectal Cancer Trial. N. Engl. J. Med. 1997 Apr 3;336(14):980–7.

[96] Sauer R, Becker H, Hohenberger W, Rödel C, Wittekind C, Fietkau R, et al. Preoperative versus postoperative chemoradiotherapy for rectal cancer. N. Engl. J. Med. 2004 Oct 21;351(17):1731–40.

[97] Janjan NA, Abbruzzese J, Pazdur R, Khoo VS, Cleary K, Dubrow R, et al. Prognostic implications of response to preoperative infusional chemoradiation in locally advanced rectal cancer. Radiother Oncol. 1999 May;51(2):153–60.

[98] Janjan NA, Khoo VS, Abbruzzese J, Pazdur R, Dubrow R, Cleary KR, et al. Tumor downstaging and sphincter preservation with preoperative chemoradiation in locally advanced rectal cancer: the M. D. Anderson Cancer Center experience. Int. J. Radiat. Oncol. Biol. Phys. 1999 Jul 15;44(5):1027–38.

[99] Hoffmann K-T, Rau B, Wust P, Stroszczynski C, Hünerbein M, Schneider U, et al. Restaging of locally advanced carcinoma of the rectum with MR imaging after preoperative radio-chemotherapy plus regional hyperthermia. Strahlenther Onkol. 2002 Jul; 178(7):386–92.

[100] Capirci C, Rampin L, Erba PA, Galeotti F, Crepaldi G, Banti E, et al. Sequential FDG-PET/CT reliably predicts response of locally advanced rectal cancer to neo-adjuvant chemo-radiation therapy. Eur. J. Nucl. Med. Mol. Imaging. 2007 Oct;34(10):1583–93.

[101] Calvo FA, Domper M, Matute R, Martínez-Lázaro R, Arranz JA, Desco M, et al. $^{18}$F-FDG positron emission tomography staging and restaging in rectal cancer treated with preoperative chemoradiation. Int. J. Radiat. Oncol. Biol. Phys. 2004 Feb 1;58(2): 528–35.

[102] Capirci C, Rubello D, Pasini F, Galeotti F, Bianchini E, Del Favero G, et al. The role of dual-time combined 18-fluorodeoxyglucose positron emission tomography and computed tomography in the staging and restaging workup of locally advanced rectal cancer, treated with preoperative chemoradiation therapy and radical surgery. Int. J. Radiat. Oncol. Biol. Phys. 2009 Aug 1;74(5):1461–9.

[103] Kristiansen C, Loft A, Berthelsen AK, Graff J, Lindebjerg J, Bisgaard C, et al. PET/CT and histopathologic response to preoperative chemoradiation therapy in locally advanced rectal cancer. Dis. Colon Rectum. 2008 Jan;51(1):21–5.

[104] Guillem JG, Moore HG, Akhurst T, Klimstra DS, Ruo L, Mazumdar M, et al. Sequential preoperative fluorodeoxyglucose-positron emission tomography assessment of

response to preoperative chemoradiation: a means for determining longterm outcomes of rectal cancer. J. Am. Coll. Surg. 2004 Jul;199(1):1–7.

[105] Perez RO, Habr-Gama A, São Julião GP, Gama-Rodrigues J, Sousa AHS Jr, Campos FG, et al. Optimal Timing for Assessment of Tumor Response to Neoadjuvant Chemoradiation in Patients With Rectal Cancer: Do All Patients Benefit From Waiting Longer Than 6 Weeks? International journal of radiation oncology, biology, physics. 2012 May 12;

[106] Francois Y, Nemoz CJ, Baulieux J, Vignal J, Grandjean JP, Partensky C, et al. Influence of the interval between preoperative radiation therapy and surgery on downstaging and on the rate of sphincter-sparing surgery for rectal cancer: the Lyon R90-01 randomized trial. J. Clin. Oncol. 1999 Aug;17(8):2396.

[107] Tulchinsky H, Shmueli E, Figer A, Klausner JM, Rabau M. An interval >7 weeks between neoadjuvant therapy and surgery improves pathologic complete response and disease-free survival in patients with locally advanced rectal cancer. Ann. Surg. Oncol. 2008 Oct;15(10):2661–7.

[108] Schaefer NG, Hany TF, Taverna C, Seifert B, Stumpe KDM, von Schulthess GK, et al. Non-Hodgkin lymphoma and Hodgkin disease: coregistered FDG PET and CT at staging and restaging--do we need contrast-enhanced CT? Radiology. 2004 Sep; 232(3):823–9.

[109] 109. Hutchings M, Loft A, Hansen M, Pedersen LM, Berthelsen AK, Keiding S, et al. Position emission tomography with or without computed tomography in the primary staging of Hodgkin's lymphoma. Haematologica. 2006 Jan 1;91(4):482–9.

[110] Pakos EE, Fotopoulos AD, Ioannidis JPA. $^{18}$F-FDG PET for Evaluation of Bone Marrow Infiltration in Staging of Lymphoma: A Meta-Analysis. J Nucl Med. 2005 Jun 1;46(6):958–63.

[111] Hoppe RT. NCCN Clinical Practice Guidelines in Oncology (NCCN Guidelines®) Hodgkin Lymphoma Version 2.2012 [Internet]. National Comprehensive Cancer Network, Inc.; 2012 [cited 2012 Oct 14]. Available from: http://www.nccn.org/professionals/physician_gls/pdf/hodgkins.pdf

[112] Zelenetz AD. NCCN Clinical Practice Guidelines in Oncology (NCCN Guidelines®) Non-Hodgkin's Lymphoma Version 3.2012 [Internet]. National Comprehensive Cancer Network, Inc.; 2012 [cited 2012 Oct 14]. Available from: http://www.nccn.org/professionals/physician_gls/pdf/nhl.pdf

[113] Cheson BD. Role of functional imaging in the management of lymphoma. J. Clin. Oncol. 2011 May 10;29(14):1844–54.

[114] Jerusalem G, Beguin Y, Fassotte MF, Najjar F, Paulus P, Rigo P, et al. Whole-body positron emission tomography using $^{18}$F-fluorodeoxyglucose for posttreatment evaluation in Hodgkin's disease and non-Hodgkin's lymphoma has higher diagnostic

and prognostic value than classical computed tomography scan imaging. Blood. 1999 Jul 15;94(2):429–33.

[115] Spaepen K, Stroobants S, Dupont P, Thomas J, Vandenberghe P, Balzarini J, et al. Can positron emission tomography with [18F]-fluorodeoxyglucose after first-line treatment distinguish Hodgkin's disease patients who need additional therapy from others in whom additional therapy would mean avoidable toxicity? British Journal of Haematology. 2001;115(2):272–8.

[116] Spaepen K, Stroobants S, Dupont P, Van Steenweghen S, Thomas J, Vandenberghe P, et al. Prognostic value of positron emission tomography (PET) with fluorine-18 fluorodeoxyglucose ([18F]FDG) after first-line chemotherapy in non-Hodgkin's lymphoma: is [18F]FDG-PET a valid alternative to conventional diagnostic methods? J. Clin. Oncol. 2001 Jan 15;19(2):414–9.

[117] Halasz LM, Jacene HA, Catalano PJ, Van den Abbeele AD, Lacasce A, Mauch PM, et al. Combined Modality Treatment for PET-Positive Non-Hodgkin Lymphoma: Favorable Outcomes of Combined Modality Treatment for Patients With Non-Hodgkin Lymphoma and Positive Interim or Postchemotherapy FDG-PET. Int. J. Radiat. Oncol. Biol. Phys. 2012 Aug 1;83(5):e647–654.

[118] Cerci JJ, Trindade E, Pracchia LF, Pitella FA, Linardi CCG, Soares J Jr, et al. Cost effectiveness of positron emission tomography in patients with Hodgkin's lymphoma in unconfirmed complete remission or partial remission after first-line therapy. J. Clin. Oncol. 2010 Mar 10;28(8):1415–21.

[119] Engert A, Haverkamp H, Kobe C, Markova J, Renner C, Ho A, et al. Reduced-intensity chemotherapy and PET-guided radiotherapy in patients with advanced stage Hodgkin's lymphoma (HD15 trial): a randomised, open-label, phase 3 non-inferiority trial. Lancet. 2012 May 12;379(9828):1791–9.

[120] Bangerter M, Moog F, Buchmann I, Kotzerke J, Griesshammer M, Hafner M, et al. Whole-body 2-[18F]-fluoro-2-deoxy-D-glucose positron emission tomography (FDG-PET) for accurate staging of Hodgkin's disease. Ann. Oncol. 1998 Oct;9(10):1117–22.

[121] Zinzani PL, Magagnoli M, Chierichetti F, Zompatori M, Garraffa G, Bendandi M, et al. The role of positron emission tomography (PET) in the management of lymphoma patients. Ann. Oncol. 1999 Oct;10(10):1181–4.

[122] Mikhaeel NG, Timothy AR, Hain SF, O'Doherty MJ. 18-FDG-PET for the assessment of residual masses on CT following treatment of lymphomas. Ann. Oncol. 2000;11 Suppl 1:147–50.

[123] Naumann R, Vaic A, Beuthien-Baumann B, Bredow J, Kropp J, Kittner T, et al. Prognostic value of positron emission tomography in the evaluation of post-treatment residual mass in patients with Hodgkin's disease and non-Hodgkin's lymphoma. Br. J. Haematol. 2001 Dec;115(4):793–800.

[124] Gigli F, Nassi L, Negri M, others. Interim 18f [FDG] positron emission tomography in patients with diffuse large B-cell lymphoma. Blood. 2008;112:1234.

[125] Cashen AF, Dehdashti F, Luo J, Homb A, Siegel BA, Bartlett NL. $^{18}$F-FDG PET/CT for early response assessment in diffuse large B-cell lymphoma: poor predictive value of international harmonization project interpretation. J. Nucl. Med. 2011 Mar;52(3):386–92.

[126] Cerci JJ, Pracchia LF, Linardi CCG, Pitella FA, Delbeke D, Izaki M, et al. $^{18}$F-FDG PET after 2 cycles of ABVD predicts event-free survival in early and advanced Hodgkin lymphoma. J. Nucl. Med. 2010 Sep;51(9):1337–43.

[127] Hutchings M, Mikhaeel NG, Fields PA, Nunan T, Timothy AR. Prognostic value of interim FDG-PET after two or three cycles of chemotherapy in Hodgkin lymphoma. Ann. Oncol. 2005 Jul;16(7):1160–8.

[128] Kostakoglu L, Goldsmith SJ, Leonard JP, Christos P, Furman RR, Atasever T, et al. FDG-PET after 1 cycle of therapy predicts outcome in diffuse large cell lymphoma and classic Hodgkin disease. Cancer. 2006 Dec 1;107(11):2678–87.

[129] Zinzani PL, Tani M, Fanti S, Alinari L, Musuraca G, Marchi E, et al. Early positron emission tomography (PET) restaging: a predictive final response in Hodgkin's disease patients. Ann. Oncol. 2006 Aug;17(8):1296–300.

[130] Gallamini A, Hutchings M, Rigacci L, Specht L, Merli F, Hansen M, et al. Early interim 2-[$^{18}$F]fluoro-2-deoxy-D-glucose positron emission tomography is prognostically superior to international prognostic score in advanced-stage Hodgkin's lymphoma: a report from a joint Italian-Danish study. J. Clin. Oncol. 2007 Aug 20;25(24):3746–52.

[131] Markova J, Kobe C, Skopalova M, Klaskova K, Dedeckova K, Plütschow A, et al. FDG-PET for assessment of early treatment response after four cycles of chemotherapy in patients with advanced-stage Hodgkin's lymphoma has a high negative predictive value. Ann. Oncol. 2009 Jul;20(7):1270–4.

[132] Spaepen K, Stroobants S, Dupont P, Vandenberghe P, Thomas J, de Groot T, et al. Early restaging positron emission tomography with ( 18)F-fluorodeoxyglucose predicts outcome in patients with aggressive non-Hodgkin's lymphoma. Ann. Oncol. 2002 Sep;13(9):1356–63.

[133] Haioun C, Itti E, Rahmouni A, Brice P, Rain J-D, Belhadj K, et al. [$^{18}$F]fluoro-2-deoxy-D-glucose positron emission tomography (FDG-PET) in aggressive lymphoma: an early prognostic tool for predicting patient outcome. Blood. 2005 Aug 15;106(4):1376–81.

[134] Mikhaeel NG, Hutchings M, Fields PA, O'Doherty MJ, Timothy AR. FDG-PET after two to three cycles of chemotherapy predicts progression-free and overall survival in high-grade non-Hodgkin lymphoma. Ann. Oncol. 2005 Sep;16(9):1514–23.

[135] Ng AP, Wirth A, Seymour JF, Lee M, Hogg A, Januszewicz H, et al. Early therapeutic response assessment by (18)FDG-positron emission tomography during chemothera-

py in patients with diffuse large B-cell lymphoma: isolated residual positivity involving bone is not usually a predictor of subsequent treatment failure. Leuk. Lymphoma. 2007 Mar;48(3):596–600.

[136] Han HS, Escalón MP, Hsiao B, Serafini A, Lossos IS. High incidence of false-positive PET scans in patients with aggressive non-Hodgkin's lymphoma treated with rituximab-containing regimens. Ann. Oncol. 2009 Feb;20(2):309–18.

[137] Pregno P, Chiappella A, Bellò M, Botto B, Ferrero S, Franceschetti S, et al. Interim 18-FDG-PET/CT failed to predict the outcome in diffuse large B-cell lymphoma patients treated at the diagnosis with rituximab-CHOP. Blood. 2012 Mar 1;119(9):2066–73.

[138] Safar V, Dupuis J, Itti E, Jardin F, Fruchart C, Bardet S, et al. Interim [$^{18}$F]fluorodeoxyglucose positron emission tomography scan in diffuse large B-cell lymphoma treated with anthracycline-based chemotherapy plus rituximab. J. Clin. Oncol. 2012 Jan 10;30(2):184–90.

[139] Zinzani PL, Gandolfi L, Broccoli A, Argnani L, Fanti S, Pellegrini C, et al. Midtreatment $^{18}$F-fluorodeoxyglucose positron-emission tomography in aggressive non-Hodgkin lymphoma. Cancer. 2011 Mar 1;117(5):1010–8.

[140] Kobe C, Dietlein M, Franklin J, Markova J, Lohri A, Amthauer H, et al. Positron emission tomography has a high negative predictive value for progression or early relapse for patients with residual disease after first-line chemotherapy in advanced-stage Hodgkin lymphoma. Blood. 2008 Nov 15;112(10):3989–94.

[141] Engert A, Diehl V, Franklin J, Lohri A, Dörken B, Ludwig W-D, et al. Escalated-dose BEACOPP in the treatment of patients with advanced-stage Hodgkin's lymphoma: 10 years of follow-up of the GHSG HD9 study. J. Clin. Oncol. 2009 Sep 20;27(27): 4548–54.

[142] Refaely Y, Krasna MJ. Multimodality therapy for esophageal cancer. Surg. Clin. North Am. 2002 Aug;82(4):729–46.

[143] Stahl M, Budach W, Meyer H-J, Cervantes A. Esophageal cancer: Clinical Practice Guidelines for diagnosis, treatment and follow-up. Ann. Oncol. 2010 May;21 Suppl 5:v46–49.

[144] Merkow RP, Bilimoria KY, McCarter MD, Chow WB, Ko CY, Bentrem DJ. Use of multimodality neoadjuvant therapy for esophageal cancer in the United States: assessment of 987 hospitals. Ann. Surg. Oncol. 2012 Feb;19(2):357–64.

[145] Bosset JF, Gignoux M, Triboulet JP, Tiret E, Mantion G, Elias D, et al. Chemoradiotherapy followed by surgery compared with surgery alone in squamous-cell cancer of the esophagus. N. Engl. J. Med. 1997 Jul 17;337(3):161–7.

[146] Urba SG, Orringer MB, Turrisi A, Iannettoni M, Forastiere A, Strawderman M. Randomized trial of preoperative chemoradiation versus surgery alone in patients with locoregional esophageal carcinoma. J. Clin. Oncol. 2001 Jan 15;19(2):305–13.

[147] Le Prise E, Etienne PL, Meunier B, Maddern G, Ben Hassel M, Gedouin D, et al. A randomized study of chemotherapy, radiation therapy, and surgery versus surgery for localized squamous cell carcinoma of the esophagus. Cancer. 1994 Apr 1;73(7): 1779–84.

[148] Walsh TN, Noonan N, Hollywood D, Kelly A, Keeling N, Hennessy TP. A comparison of multimodal therapy and surgery for esophageal adenocarcinoma. N. Engl. J. Med. 1996 Aug 15;335(7):462–7.

[149] van Hagen P, Hulshof MCCM, van Lanschot JJB, Steyerberg EW, Henegouwen MI van B, Wijnhoven BPL, et al. Preoperative Chemoradiotherapy for Esophageal or Junctional Cancer. New England Journal of Medicine. 2012;366(22):2074–84.

[150] Berger AC, Farma J, Scott WJ, Freedman G, Weiner L, Cheng JD, et al. Complete Response to Neoadjuvant Chemoradiotherapy in Esophageal Carcinoma Is Associated With Significantly Improved Survival. JCO. 2005 Jul 1;23(19):4330–7.

[151] Weber WA, Ott K, Becker K, Dittler HJ, Helmberger H, Avril NE, et al. Prediction of response to preoperative chemotherapy in adenocarcinomas of the esophagogastric junction by metabolic imaging. J. Clin. Oncol. 2001 Jun 15;19(12):3058–65.

[152] Wieder HA, Brücher BLDM, Zimmermann F, Becker K, Lordick F, Beer A, et al. Time Course of Tumor Metabolic Activity During Chemoradiotherapy of Esophageal Squamous Cell Carcinoma and Response to Treatment. JCO. 2004 Mar 1;22(5):900–8.

[153] Wieder HA, Ott K, Lordick F, Becker K, Stahl A, Herrmann K, et al. Prediction of tumor response by FDG-PET: comparison of the accuracy of single and sequential studies in patients with adenocarcinomas of the esophagogastric junction. Eur. J. Nucl. Med. Mol. Imaging. 2007 Dec;34(12):1925–32.

[154] Downey RJ, Akhurst T, Ilson D, Ginsberg R, Bains MS, Gonen M, et al. Whole Body $^{18}$FDG-PET and the Response of Esophageal Cancer to Induction Therapy: Results of a Prospective Trial. JCO. 2003 Feb 1;21(3):428–32.

[155] Kostakoglu L, Goldsmith SJ. PET in the Assessment of Therapy Response in Patients with Carcinoma of the Head and Neck and of the Esophagus*. J Nucl Med. 2004 Jan 1;45(1):56–68.

[156] Weber WA. Use of PET for Monitoring Cancer Therapy and for Predicting Outcome. J Nucl Med. 2005 Jun 1;46(6):983–95.

[157] Chao KS. Functional imaging for early prediction of response to chemoradiotherapy: 3′-deoxy-3′-$^{18}$F-fluorothymidine positron emission tomography-A clinical application model of esophageal cancer. Seminars in oncology [Internet]. 2006 [cited 2012 Oct 7]. Available from: http://cat.inist.fr/?aModele=afficheN&cpsidt=18445320

[158] Levine EA, Farmer MR, Clark P, Mishra G, Ho C, Geisinger KR, et al. Predictive Value of 18-Fluoro-Deoxy-Glucose-Positron Emission Tomography ($^{18}$F-FDG-PET) in the

Identification of Responders to Chemoradiation Therapy for the Treatment of Locally Advanced Esophageal Cancer. Ann Surg. 2006 Apr;243(4):472–8.

[159] Roedl JB, Colen RR, Holalkere NS, Fischman AJ, Choi NC, Blake MA. Adenocarcinomas of the esophagus: Response to chemoradiotherapy is associated with decrease of metabolic tumor volume as measured on PET–CT. Radiotherapy and Oncology. 2008 Dec;89(3):278–86.

[160] Kwee RM. Prediction of Tumor Response to Neoadjuvant Therapy in Patients with Esophageal Cancer with Use of $^{18}$F FDG PET: A Systematic Review1. Radiology. 2010 Mar 1;254(3):707–17.

[161] Kauppi JT, Oksala N, Salo JA, Helin H, Karhumäki L, Kemppainen J, et al. Locally advanced esophageal adenocarcinoma: Response to neoadjuvant chemotherapy and survival predicted by [$^{18}$F] FDG-PET/CT. Acta Oncologica. 2012 May;51(5):636–44.

[162] Ishihara R, Yamamoto S, Iishi H, Nagai K, Matui F, Kawada N, et al. Predicting the effects of chemoradiotherapy for squamous cell carcinoma of the esophagus by induction chemotherapy response assessed by positron emission tomography: toward PET-response-guided selection of chemoradiotherapy or esophagectomy. Int. J. Clin. Oncol. 2012 Jun;17(3):225–32.

[163] Yanagawa M, Tatsumi M, Miyata H, Morii E, Tomiyama N, Watabe T, et al. Evaluation of response to neoadjuvant chemotherapy for esophageal cancer: PET response criteria in solid tumors versus response evaluation criteria in solid tumors. J. Nucl. Med. 2012 Jun;53(6):872–80.

[164] Monjazeb AM, Riedlinger G, Aklilu M, Geisinger KR, Mishra G, Isom S, et al. Outcomes of patients with esophageal cancer staged with [$^{18}$F]fluorodeoxyglucose positron emission tomography (FDG-PET): can postchemoradiotherapy FDG-PET predict the utility of resection? J. Clin. Oncol. 2010 Nov 1;28(31):4714–21.

[165] Mohammed N, Kestin LL, Grills IS, Battu M, Fitch DL, Wong C-YO, et al. Rapid disease progression with delay in treatment of non-small-cell lung cancer. Int. J. Radiat. Oncol. Biol. Phys. 2011 Feb 1;79(2):466–72.

[166] Edet-Sanson A, Dubray B, Doyeux K, Back A, Hapdey S, Modzelewski R, et al. Serial assessment of FDG-PET FDG uptake and functional volume during radiotherapy (RT) in patients with non-small cell lung cancer (NSCLC). Radiotherapy and Oncology. 2012 Feb;102(2):251–7.

[167] Kong F-MS, Frey KA, Quint LE, Haken RKT, Hayman JA, Kessler M, et al. A Pilot Study of [$^{18}$F]Fluorodeoxyglucose Positron Emission Tomography Scans During and After Radiation-Based Therapy in Patients With Non–Small-Cell Lung Cancer. JCO. 2007 Jul 20;25(21):3116–23.

[168] van Baardwijk A, Bosmans G, Dekker A, van Kroonenburgh M, Boersma L, Wanders S, et al. Time trends in the maximal uptake of FDG on PET scan during thoracic radi-

otherapy. A prospective study in locally advanced non-small cell lung cancer (NSCLC) patients. Radiotherapy and Oncology. 2007 Feb;82(2):145–52.

[169] Vera P, Bohn P, Edet-Sanson A, Salles A, Hapdey S, Gardin I, et al. Simultaneous positron emission tomography (PET) assessment of metabolism with $^{18}$F-fluoro-2-deoxy-d-glucose (FDG), proliferation with $^{18}$F-fluoro-thymidine (FLT), and hypoxia with 18fluoro-misonidazole (F-miso) before and during radiotherapy in patients with non-small-cell lung cancer (NSCLC): A pilot study. Radiotherapy and Oncology. 2011 Jan;98(1):109–16.

[170] Hicks RJ. Role of $^{18}$F-FDG PET in Assessment of Response in Non-Small Cell Lung Cancer. Journal of Nuclear Medicine. 2009 Apr 20;50(Suppl_1):31S–42S.

[171] Nahmias C, Hanna WT, Wahl LM, Long MJ, Hubner KF, Townsend DW. Time Course of Early Response to Chemotherapy in Non–Small Cell Lung Cancer Patients with $^{18}$F-FDG PET/CT. J Nucl Med. 2007 May 1;48(5):744–51.

[172] Vansteenkiste JF, Stroobants SG, Leyn PRD, Dupont PJ, Verbeken EK. Potential use of FDG-PET scan after induction chemotherapy in surgically staged IIIa–N2 non-small-cell lung cancer: A prospective pilot study. Ann Oncol. 1998 Nov 1;9(11):1193–8.

[173] Manus MPM, Hicks RJ, Matthews JP, McKenzie A, Rischin D, Salminen EK, et al. Positron Emission Tomography Is Superior to Computed Tomography Scanning for Response-Assessment After Radical Radiotherapy or Chemoradiotherapy in Patients With Non–Small-Cell Lung Cancer. JCO. 2003 Apr 1;21(7):1285–92.

[174] Weber WA, Petersen V, Schmidt B, Tyndale-Hines L, Link T, Peschel C, et al. Positron emission tomography in non-small-cell lung cancer: prediction of response to chemotherapy by quantitative assessment of glucose use. J. Clin. Oncol. 2003 Jul 15;21(14):2651–7.

[175] Hellwig D, Graeter TP, Ukena D, Georg T, Kirsch C-M, Schäfers H-J. Value of F-18-fluorodeoxyglucose positron emission tomography after induction therapy of locally advanced bronchogenic carcinoma. J. Thorac. Cardiovasc. Surg. 2004 Dec;128(6):892–9.

[176] Eschmann SM, Friedel G, Paulsen F, Reimold M, Hehr T, Budach W, et al. $^{18}$F-FDG PET for assessment of therapy response and preoperative re-evaluation after neoadjuvant radio-chemotherapy in stage III non-small cell lung cancer. Eur. J. Nucl. Med. Mol. Imaging. 2007 Apr;34(4):463–71.

[177] de Geus-Oei L-F, van der Heijden HFM, Visser EP, Hermsen R, van Hoorn BA, Timmer-Bonte JNH, et al. Chemotherapy response evaluation with $^{18}$F-FDG PET in patients with non-small cell lung cancer. J. Nucl. Med. 2007 Oct;48(10):1592–8.

[178] Tanvetyanon T, Eikman EA, Sommers E, Robinson L, Boulware D, Bepler G. Computed tomography response, but not positron emission tomography scan response,

predicts survival after neoadjuvant chemotherapy for resectable non-small-cell lung cancer. J. Clin. Oncol. 2008 Oct 1;26(28):4610–6.

[179] Baschnagel A, Mangona VS, Robertson J, Ye H, Kestin L, Grills I. Lung metastases treated with image-guided stereotactic body radiation therapy. International Journal of Radiation Oncology Biology Physics. 2010;78(3):5.

[180] Grills IS, Hope AJ, Guckenberger M, Kestin LL, Werner-Wasik M, Yan D, et al. A Collaborative Analysis of Stereotactic Lung Radiotherapy Outcomes for Early-Stage Non-Small-Cell Lung Cancer Using Daily Online Cone-Beam Computed Tomography Image-Guided Radiotherapy. Journal of thoracic oncology: official publication of the International Association for the Study of Lung Cancer [Internet]. 2012 Jul 26 [cited 2012 Aug 14]; Available from: http://www.ncbi.nlm.nih.gov/pubmed/22843086

[181] Grills IS, Mangona VS, Welsh R, Chmielewski G, McInerney E, Martin S, et al. Outcomes after stereotactic lung radiotherapy or wedge resection for stage I non-small-cell lung cancer. J. Clin. Oncol. 2010 Feb 20;28(6):928–35.

[182] Welsh R, Grills I, Deraniyagala R, Kestin L, Baschnagel A, Mangona V, et al. Lobectomy, Wedge Resection, or Stereotactic Radiotherapy (SBRT) for Stage I Non-small Cell Lung Cancer: Which Treatment Yields the Best Outcome? International Journal of Radiation Oncology* Biology* Physics. 2010;78(3):S180–S180.

[183] Onishi H, Shirato H, Nagata Y, Hiraoka M, Fujino M, Gomi K, et al. Stereotactic body radiotherapy (SBRT) for operable stage I non-small-cell lung cancer: can SBRT be comparable to surgery? Int. J. Radiat. Oncol. Biol. Phys. 2011 Dec 1;81(5):1352–8.

[184] Timmerman R, Paulus R, Galvin J, Michalski J, Straube W, Bradley J, et al. Stereotactic body radiation therapy for inoperable early stage lung cancer. JAMA. 2010 Mar 17;303(11):1070–6.

[185] Guckenberger M, Kestin LL, Hope AJ, Belderbos J, Werner-Wasik M, Yan D, et al. Is there a lower limit of pretreatment pulmonary function for safe and effective stereotactic body radiotherapy for early-stage non-small cell lung cancer? J Thorac Oncol. 2012 Mar;7(3):542–51.

[186] Ohri N, Werner-Wasik M, Grills IS, Belderbos J, Hope A, Yan D, et al. Modeling local control after hypofractionated stereotactic body radiation therapy for stage I non-small cell lung cancer: a report from the elekta collaborative lung research group. Int. J. Radiat. Oncol. Biol. Phys. 2012 Nov 1;84(3):e379–384.

[187] Lanni TB Jr, Grills IS, Kestin LL, Robertson JM. Stereotactic radiotherapy reduces treatment cost while improving overall survival and local control over standard fractionated radiation therapy for medically inoperable non-small-cell lung cancer. Am. J. Clin. Oncol. 2011 Oct;34(5):494–8.

[188] Stone B, Grills I, Mangona V, Ye H, Martin S, Wloch J, et al. Changes in Pulmonary Function Following Imaged Guided Stereotactic Radiotherapy of the Lung. International Journal of Radiation Oncology* Biology* Physics. 2011;81(2):S611.

[189] Mangona V, Grills I, Yan D, McInerney E, Martin S, Kestin L, et al. Predictors of Pulmonary and Other Thoracic Complications after Lung Stereotactic Body Radiotherapy (SBRT) for Primary or Metastatic Lung Tumors: Dose–volume Analysis. International Journal of Radiation Oncology* Biology* Physics. 2009;75(3):S161–S161.

[190] Grills IS, Hugo G, Kestin LL, Galerani AP, Chao KK, Wloch J, et al. Image-Guided Radiotherapy via Daily Online Cone-Beam CT Substantially Reduces Margin Requirements for Stereotactic Lung Radiotherapy. International Journal of Radiation Oncology*Biology*Physics. 2008 Mar;70(4):1045–56.

[191] Galerani AP, Grills I, Hugo G, Kestin L, Mohammed N, Chao KK, et al. Dosimetric impact of online correction via cone-beam CT-based image guidance for stereotactic lung radiotherapy. Int. J. Radiat. Oncol. Biol. Phys. 2010 Dec 1;78(5):1571–8.

[192] McGee M, Grills I, Mangona V, Ionascu D, Margolis J, Welsh R, et al. Feasibility, Toxicity, and Early Outcomes for Dose-escalated 4D Adaptive Image-guided Radiotherapy (IGRT) for Non-small Cell Lung Cancer (NSCLC). International Journal of Radiation Oncology* Biology* Physics. 2011;81(2):S165–S166.

[193] Shaitelman S, Grills I, Liang J, Zhuang L, Mangona V, Yan D, et al. A Comprehensive Dose-Volume Analysis of Predictors of Pneumonitis and Esophagitis Following Radiotherapy for Non-Small Cell Lung Cancer (NSCLC). Esophagus. 2009;10:5.

[194] Grills IS, Mangona VS. Intensity-Modulated Radiation Therapy and Volumetric-Modulated Arc Therapy for Lung Cancer. Advances in Radiation Oncology in Lung Cancer. 2011;691–713.

[195] Kong F-M. Using FDG-PET During Radiation Therapy in Non-Small Cell Lung Cancer (HUM15709) [Internet]. Available from: http://clinicaltrials.gov/ct2/show/NCT01190527

[196] Kong F-M (Spring). RTOG 1106/ACRIN 6697 Randomized Phase Ii Trial of Individualized Adaptive Radiotherapy Using During-Treatment FDG-PET/CT And Modern Technology in Locally Advanced Non-Small Cell Lung Cancer (Nsclc) [Internet]. 2012 [cited 2012 Oct 16]. Available from: http://www.rtog.org/ClinicalTrials/ProtocolTable/StudyDetails.aspx?study=1106

Chapter 9

# PET-CT in Anal Cancer: Indications and Limits

Massimiliano Mistrangelo and Adriana Lesca

Additional information is available at the end of the chapter

http://dx.doi.org/10.5772/57121

## 1. Introduction

Perianal and anal canal malignancies are uncommon. The anal canal is a small area, rather complex for the presence of different histological features and for the lymphatic spread [1].

In the IUCC, American Joint Committee on Cancer (AJCC) and World Health Organization (WHO) staging systems the anal canal is described as the last part of the gastrointestinal tract extending from the anal ring at the level of the puborectalis muscle (where the rectum enters the pelvic floor), to the perianal tissue that is the junction of the hair- bearing skin and the non-keratinizing squamous epithelium of the distal anal canal.

As cited tumors of the anal canal can present different histological features. These guidelines refer to squamous cell carcinoma (including the so called cloacogenic variant) which constitutes 80% of all lesions of this area and derives from transitional and squamous cell epithelium. In some pathology literature squamous cell carcinoma of the anal canal is also described according to additional histopathologic feature such as keratinization, presence of mucin and abundance of basement mebrane-like material.

Less common are adenocarcinoma and mucinous adenocarcinoma of the anal glands or of fistula tracts that must be distinguished from very low rectal cancers. Other uncommon neoplasms of the anal canal include small cell carcinoma, carcinoid and other neuroendocrine tumors, malignant melanoma, squamous cell papilloma, papillary hidradenoma, keratoacanthoma, mesenchymal and neurogenic tumors, lymphoma, leiomyosarcoma, and secondary tumors.

Tumors originating from the anal margin should be staged as skin cancer: they can be squamous cell cancer, basal cell cancer, Bowen's or Paget's disease.

This is an important distinction as skin cancers rarely involve lymph nodes or lead to distant metastases [2-4].

INTECH
open science | open minds

© 2013 Mistrangelo and Lesca; licensee InTech. This is a paper distributed under the terms of the Creative Commons Attribution License (http://creativecommons.org/licenses/by/3.0), which permits unrestricted use, distribution, and reproduction in any medium, provided the original work is properly cited.

## 2. Incidence

Anal cancer remains a rare disease but its incidence is increasing [5], mainly in association with human papillomaviruses (HPV) infection. An estimated 5820 new cases (2140 men and 3680 women) were estimated to occur in the United States in 2011, accounting for approximately 2.1% of digestive system cancers. It has been estimated that 770 deaths due to anal cancer will occurr in U.S. alone in 2011 [6].

In western Europe the average annual incidence of anal carcinoma is 1 to 3 cases per 100,000 with a female prevalence (two to four times that of men [7]) and a highest incidence during the sixth and seventh decades of life [8]. The annual incidence incidence can be up to 35 per 100,000 in men who practice anal-receptive sexual intercourse, and those who are human immunodeficiency virus (HIV)-positive have twice the risk of those who are not [7].

In particular, squamous cell carcinoma (the other names, epidermoid or spinocellular, are no longer used) is the most common histological type of anal carcinoma and constitutes up to the 80% of all malignant anal tumours [9].

## 3. Etiology

Chromosome 11 deletions (11q22) or the short arm of chromosome 3 (3p22), environmental factors such as cigarette smoking, sexual orientation and a high number of sexual partners, anoreceptive intercourse, male homosexuality, viral infections of the anogenital area (human papillomavirus (HPV) virus type 16 and 18) and immunodeficiency, are all considered as causative factors of anal cancer [8, 10-11].

The introduction of antiretroviral drugs have improved the life expectancy of HIV- positive patients. This has contributed to increasing the incidence of anal cancer in this population.

HPV infection (type 16 in about 87% of cases [12]) and anogenital warts are closely associated with anal cancer. Anal canal lesions are more often HPV positive than perianal lesions. Ninety-five percent of anal canal cancer in women and 83% in men is HPV- positive while cancer located at the anal margin are HPV- positive in only 80% of women and 28% of men [12]. Because of this high association with anal cancer HPV is considered to be the most important causative factor much like in cases of cervical cancer [13-16].

In particular, HPV is involved in the pathogenesis of anal intraepithelial neoplasia (AIN) which progresses from dysplasia to invasive cancer. HPV type 16 seems to be associated with a higher risk of malignant transformation [17].

Other viral infections such as herpes simplex virus (HSV) have been studied but are considered to play only a marginal role in disease progression.

After solid organ transplant, patients receive chronic immunosuppressive therapy, so they are exposed to higher risk of various squamous cell carcinoma, such as of the anal canal [11]. Moreover, the use of corticosteroids can increase the risk of developing anal cancer [18].

Several studies made a connection between cigarette smoking and risk of developing anal cancer, and this risk diminished after smoking cessation [19].

## 4. Clinical manifestations

Macroscopically the squamous anal cancer appears as a small ulceration or fissure, exophytic, with indurated margins and irregular thickening [20]. Sometimes large lesions are observed.

Symptoms are rectal bleeding, rectal pain, tenesmus or mass sensation, but about 20% of patients are asymptomatic at the time of diagnosis [6].

## 5. Treatment

Prior to the mid-1980s, the treatment of choice for anal cancer was abdominoperineal resection (APR). The 5-year survival rate after APR for anal cancer was 40-70%, with worse outcomes for those with larger tumors and nodal metastases. In the 1920s and 1930s inguinal node dissection was included in the surgical management of these patients, and it was generally reserved for those patients with clinically enlarged (though not necessarily involved) inguinal nodes [21]. By the 1950s it had became clear that the morbidity associated with lymph node dissection was much greater than any survival benefit, so the procedure was gradually abandoned [22]. In 1974 Nigro proposed a multimodality treatment combining radiation and chemotherapy which has since then become the standard treatment with surgery reserved for salvage treatment following local failure [23]. Local control rates of 60-90% over all stages are achievable, with sphincter preservation in about 65% of cases. The prognosis after combined radiochemotherapy for anal cancer may be influenced by several factors: high tumor stage and regional nodal involvement; tumor site in the anal canal; inguinal lymph node involvement in anal canal carcinoma. Synchronous inguinal metastases occur in 10-25% of patients [24] and constitute an independent prognostic factor for local failure and overall mortality according to a multivariate analysis in a phase 3 EORTC trial [25]. Metachronous metastases have been reported in 5-25% of patients [10].

Adverse effects of chemoradiation therapy can be mucositis, diarrhea, skin desquamation and erytema, mielosuppression, ulcers, fistulae, necrosis, and stenosis [19]. Surgery treatment is reserved for salvage theraphy, in subjects with persistent or recurrent disease [19, 26-28]. The elective treatment of metastatic disease (often hepatic nodules), is chemotherapy; therapeutic plans include cisplatin and 5-FU, carboplatin, doxorubicin and semustine [29-32].

## 6. Diagnosis

Clinical workup in the staging of anal cancer comprises digital rectal examination, anoscopy with biopsy of suspicious lesions, palpation of inguinal lymph nodes, tumor marker assay, chest X-ray, rigid proctoscopy, total colonoscopy, rectal endosonography, contrast-enhanced diagnostic computed tomography (CT) and/or magnetic resonance imaging (MRI).

In effect, physical examination, biopsy of the tumor and endorectal ultrasonography can help in determining the tumor depth and the invasion of perirectal limph nodes; instead, palpation of the groin, CT and MRI can give important information about inguinal and iliac lymph node involvement and the evidence of distant visceral metastasis. In recent years, fluorodeoxyglucose-positron emission tomography (18F-FDG-PET/CT) has rapidly gained a expanding role in oncology, with mounting evidence for its effectiveness in the staging and management of various types of tumors.

## 7. PET-CT and tumor

2-deoxy-2[F-18]fluoro-D-glucose (FDG) Positron Emission Tomography (PET) scan is a medical examination currently approved and used in the staging work-up of primary cancers of several sites, such as lung, head and neck, oesophagus, breast, colorectum, melanoma, the Hodgkin's disease and non-Hodgkin's limphomas.

High rates of glycolysis are found in many malignant tumor cells and high uptake of FDG is usually associated with a high expression of glucose transporters. Many tumors are avid of FDG and PET/CT scan can help in staging the primary cancer, in choosing the best side for biopsy, in evaluating the treatment response, in searching other synchronous tumors, in suspect recurrence of tumor with markers increasing, and in planning radiation treatment. We must remember that increased FDG uptake is not specific for neoplasm but inflammatory processes may also show increased uptake, so that abscesses, tuberculosis, inflammations, fungal infections, inflammation related to radiation treatment can concentrate radioglucose, causing false positive results [33].

Evaluation of PET images can be performed visually or semiquantitatively, using the Standardized Uptake Value (SUV). Semiquantitative evaluation offers a more objective way of reporting lesion than visual image interpretation and is useful for comparing lesion activity in consecutive studies. However, visual interpretation is equally effective for one-time diagnosis [33].

## 8. PET-CT and anal cancer

Since 2005, the use of PET-CT in anal cancer has been described [34-54]. As suggested by Grigsby et al., the advantage of FDG-PET/CT is that it can address all three staging criteria of the TNM system in a single whole-body imaging procedure: demonstrate the extent of the primary tumor; detect lymph node metastases; and reveal any sites of distant metastases [55]. The 2007 National Comprehensive Cancer Network treatment guidelines included PET/CT as a part of the standard pre-treatment workup of patients diagnosed with anal carcinoma [56]. The new version 2.2012 consider PET-CT scan for work up, even if its use for staging or treatment planning has not been validated [57]. The Authors suggest that PET-CT actually does not replace a diagnostic CT scan [57].

## 9. Detection of primary neoplam

Evidence from published data indicates that PET/CT is clearly superior to CT in visualizing the biopsy-proven primary tumor, although the lack of sensitivity did not affect treatment. Analyzing the Literature PET-CT detected the primary anal tumor in 59-100% of cases, while CT scan only in 47-75%. In almost all large series are included some patients, who previously were submitted to surgical removal of the anal cancer but with histologically confirmed positive surgical margins. In these cases PET-CT resulted negative (false negative). When we exclude these patients by the review, the percentage of the detection of the primary neoplasm with PET-CT arises to 87.5-100% of cases. This suggests that both PET/CT and CT were unable to detect residual tumor after surgical excision.

Results are repoted in Table 1 [34-54]. Figures 1 and 2 present two cases of PET-CT positive for anal cancer.

| Author, year | Patients (Total) | Detection | Previous surgery | Excluding previous surgery | Detection CT scan |
|---|---|---|---|---|---|
| **Trautmann, 2005** | 21 | 21/21 (100%) | 0 | 21/21 (100%) | n.r. |
| **Cotter, 2006** | 41 | 31/41 (75.6%) | 7 | 31/34 (91%) | 20/34 (59%) |
| **Piperkova, 2006** | 1 | 1/1 (100%) | 0 | 1/1 (100%) | 1/1 (100%) |
| **Anderson, 2007** | 3 | 3/3 (100%) | 0 | 3/3 (100%) | n.r. |
| **Joon, 2007*** | 48 | 40/48 (83.3%) | 7 | 40/41 (97.5%) | 24/41 (58.5%) |
| **Schwarz, 2008** | 53 | n.r. | n.r. | n.r. | n.r. |
| **Nguyen, 2008*** | 48 | 40/48 (83.3%) | 7 | 40/41 (97.5%) | 22/38 (58%) |
| **Iagaru, 2009** | 8 | 7/8 (87.5%) | 0 | 7/8 (87.5%) | n.r. |
| **de Winton, 2009** | 61 | 45/61 (73.7%) | 16 | 45/45 (100%) | n.r. |
| **Forrest, 2009** | 39 | 38/39 (97%) | 0 | 38/39 (97%) | 22/39 (56%) |
| **Renaud, 2009** | 20 | 20/20 (100%) | n.r. | 20/20 (100%) | n.r. |
| **Kidd, 2010** | 77 | n.r. | n.r. | n.r. | n.r. |
| **Krengli, 2010** | 27 | 26/27 (96.3%) | n.r. | 26/27 | n.r. |
| **Bannas, 2010** | 22 | 15/17 (88%) | n.r. | 15/17 (88%) | 8/22 (47%) |
| **Engledow, 2010** | 40 | 40/40 (100%) | n.r. | 40/40 (100%) | n.r. |

| Author, year | Patients (Total) | Detection | Previous surgery | Excluding previous surgery | Detection CT scan |
|---|---|---|---|---|---|
| **Vercellino, 2011** | 22 | 13/22 (59%) | 8 | 13/14 (92.8%) | n.r. |
| **Sveistrup, 2012** | 91 | 89/91 (97%) | 4 | 87/87 (100%) | n.r. |
| **Mistrangelo, 2012** | 53 | 47/53 (88.7%) | 5 | 47/48 (97.9%) | 30/40 (75%) |
| **Wells, 2012** | 30 | 28/30 (93%) | 2 | 28/28 (100%) | n.r. |
| **Bhuva, 2012** | 43 | 40/43 (93%) | n.r. | n.r. | n.r. |

PS: * The 2 papers were published separately considering the same series.

n.r.: Not Reported

**Table 1.** Detection of primary neoplasm.

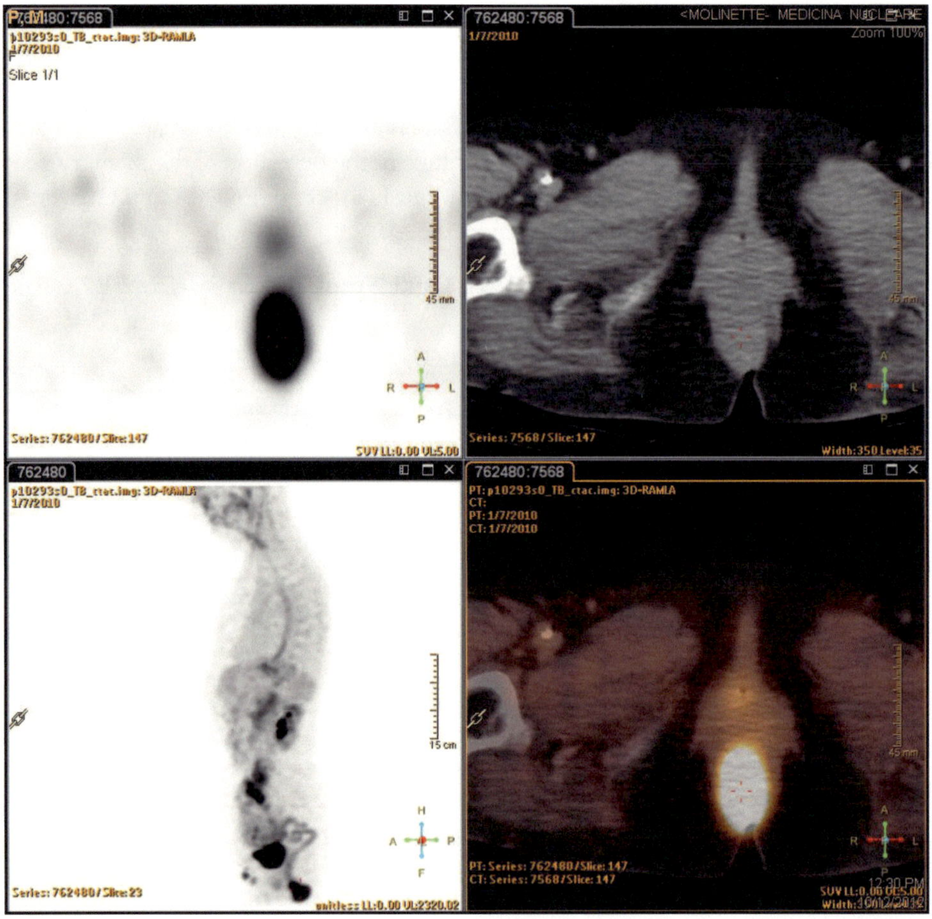


**Figure 1.** PET-CT positive for anal cancer.

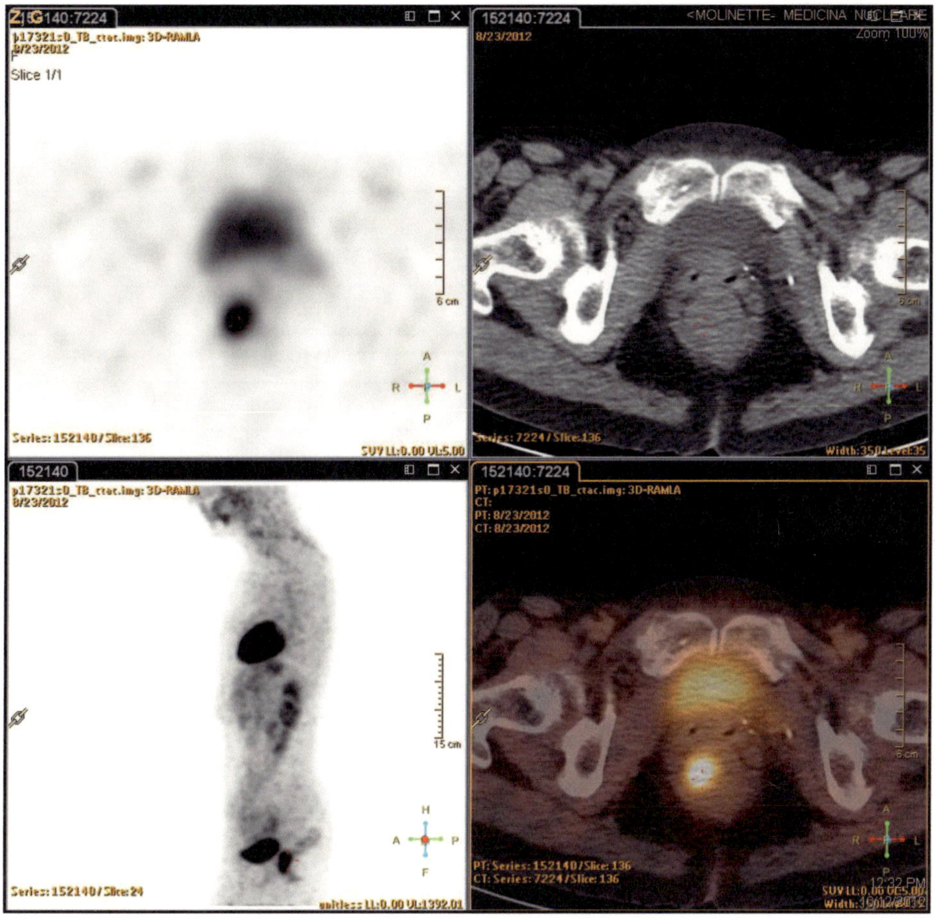

**Figure 2.** PET-CT positive for anal cancer.

## 10. Detection of perirectal and pelvic nodes

Perirectal and/or pelvic nodes were revealed by PET-CT in 4.5-67% and by CT-scan in 13.6-49% of patients. In all the reported series, except the one of Bannas and Coll [47], PET-CT evidentiated more perirectal and pelvic nodes vs CT-scan

Results are repoted in Table 2 [34-54]. Figure 3 present a case of PET-CT positive for perirectal lymph nodes metastases.

| Author, year | Patients (Total) | Incidence PET-CT | Incidence CT scan |
|---|---|---|---|
| Trautmann, 2005 | 21 | 9/21 (42.8%) | n.r. |
| Cotter, 2006 | 41 | 9/41 (22%) | 8/41 (20%) |
| Piperkova, 2006 | 1 | 1/1 (100%) | n.r. |
| Anderson, 2007 | 3 | 1/3 (33.3%) | n.r. |
| Schwarz, 2008 | 53 | n.r. | n.r. |
| Nguyen, 2008 | 48 | 9/48 (19%) | 7/38 (18%) |
| Iagaru, 2009 | 8 | 2/8 (20%) | n.r. |
| de Winton, 2009 | 61 | 41/61 (67%) | 30/61 (49%). |
| Forrest, 2009 | 39 | n.r. | n.r. |
| Renaud, 2009 | 20 | 12/20 (60%) | n.r. |
| Kidd, 2010 | 77 | 8/77 (10.4%) | n.r. |
| Krengli, 2010 | 27 | n.r. | n.r. |
| Bannas, 2010 | 22 | 2/17 (11.7%) | 3/22 (13.6%) |
| Engledow, 2010 | 40 | n.r. | n.r. |
| Vercellino, 2011 | 22 | 1/22 (4.5%) | n.r. |
| Sveistrup, 2012 | 91 | 28/91 (30.7%) | n.r. |
| Mistrangelo, 2012 | 53 | 14/53 (26.4%) | 7/40 (17.5%) |
| Wells, 2012 | 30 | n.r. | n.r. |
| Bhuva, 2012 | 43 | n.r. | n.r. |

n.r.: Not Reported

**Table 2.** Incidence of perirectal and pelvic metastases in lymph nodes

## 11. Detection of inguinal lymph nodes

PET/CT was positive for inguinal metastases in 0-37% of patients, while CT scan in 7.4-41% of them. Mistrangelo et Al [49] compared PET-CT with sentinel lymph node biopsy (SNB) of inguinal nodes in 41 cases. Their findings showed that SNB confirmed the presence of inguinal metastases in only 8 cases, with 4 of 41 patients (9.7%) false positive and 2 of 41 patients (4.9%) false negative. Comparison between SNB and CT findings (34 patients) showed that SNB identified 4 of 34 patients (11.7%) false positive and 4 of 34 patients (11.7%) false negative patients. This is the only paper, to our knowledge, that compares the 2 techniques.

http://dx.doi.org/10.5772/57121

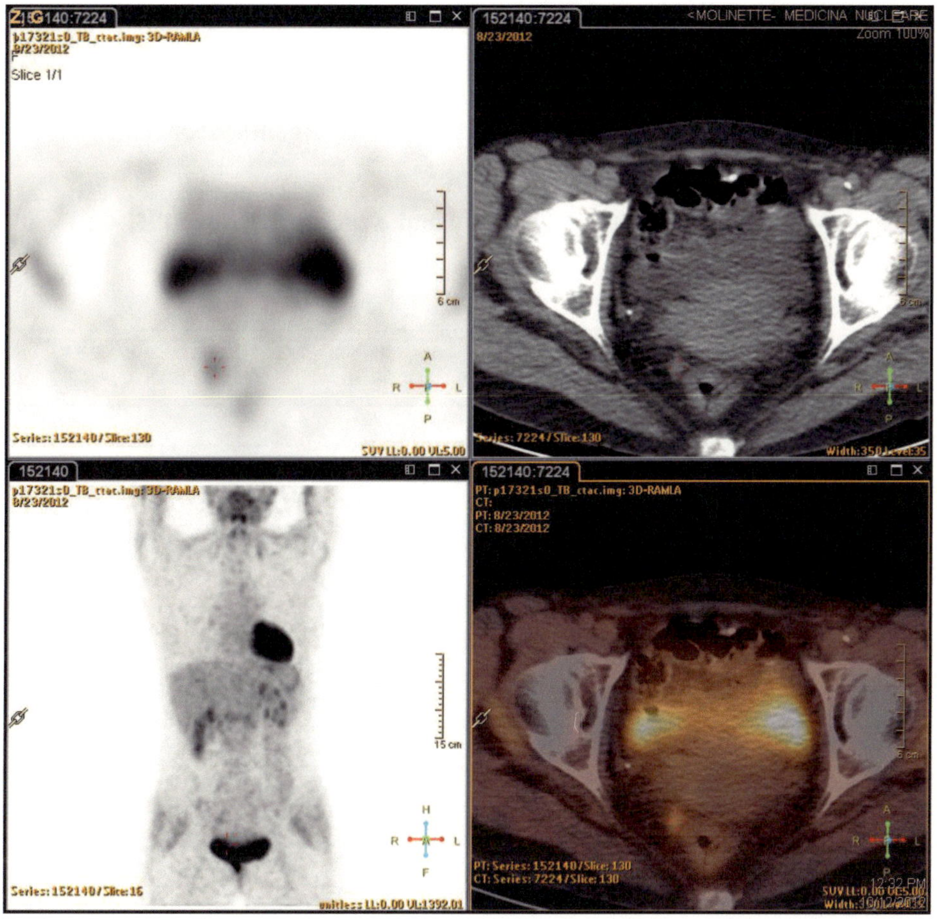


**Figure 3.** PET-CT positive for perirectal lymph nodes metastases.

Cotter and colleagues compared CT and physical examination to 18F-FDG PET/CT in the staging of carcinoma of anal canal, particularly of the inguinal nodal involvement [35]. They enrolled 41 consecutive patients with biopsy proved anal cancer and studied them with physical examination, CT scan and PET-CT scan. PET-CT scans described nodal groin positivities in 15 patients (37%); CT documented abnormal nodes in 9 subjects (22%). Particularly, 20% of CT-negative groins were PET positive, leading to upstaging in 8 of the 32 patients (25%). Furthermore, 3 of 13 CT-positive groins were PET-negative (23%) [35]. About 23% of clinically negative groins were PET-positive, leading to upstaging in 9 of the 32 subjects without clinical inguinal nodal involvement. Moreover, about 17% of inguinal stations negative by both CT and physical exam were PET-positive, allowing for upstaging in each of these cases. Ten of 18 inguinal stations (56%) positive by either physical examination or CT, but not both, were positive by PET. Moreover, all four groins positive by both CT and physical examination were positive by PET [35]. Autors concluded that PET-CT documented more abnormal inguinal nodes than CT or physical examination and they explained that cancer nodal metastases occur in node <5 mm in size, below the limit of detection by CT or physical exam; instead, FDG-PET scan detects pathological sites by differential glucose intake rather than limph node morphology; so that, PET is able in detecting little nodal metastases, but no micrometastases.

Results are repoted in Table 3 [34-54]. Figures 4 and 5 present a case of PET-CT positive for inguinal lymph nodes metastases.

| Author, year | Patients (Total) | Incidence PET-CT | Incidence CT scan |
|---|---|---|---|
| **Trautmann, 2005** | 21 | 0/21 (0%) | n.r. |
| **Cotter, 2006** | 41 | 15/41 (37%) | 9/41 (22%) |
| **Piperkova, 2006** | 1 | 0/1 (0%) | n.r. |
| **Anderson, 2007** | 3 | 0/3 (0%) | n.r. |
| **Joon, 2007*** | 48 | n.r. | n.r. |
| **Schwarz, 2008** | 53 | n.r. | n.r. |
| **Nguyen, 2008*** | 48 | 8/48 (16.6%) | n.r. |
| **Iagaru, 2009** | 8 | 1/8 (12.5%) | n.r. |
| **de Winton, 2009** | 61 | 6/61 (10%) | 9/61 (15%). |
| **Forrest, 2009** | 39 | n.r. | n.r. |
| **Renaud, 2009** | 20 | 5/20 (25%) | 4/20 (20%) |
| **Kidd, 2010** | 77 | 6/77 (7.8%) | n.r. |
| **Krengli, 2010** | 27 | 3/27 (11.1%) | 2/27 (7.4%) |
| **Bannas, 2010** | 22 | 6/22 (27%) | 9/22 (41%) |
| **Engledow, 2010** | 40 | 9/40 (22.5%) | 0/40 (0%) |
| **Vercellino, 2011** | 22 | 3/22 (13.6%) | n.r. |
| **Sveistrup, 2012** | 91 | 41/91 (45%) | n.r. |
| **Mistrangelo, 2012** | 53 | 12/53 (22.6%) | 8/40 (20%) |
| **Wells, 2012** | 30 | n.r. | n.r. |
| **Bhuva, 2012** | 43 | 7/43 (16.3%) | n.r. |

PS: * The 2 papers were published separately considering the same series.

n.r.: Not Reported

**Table 3.** Incidence of metastases in inguinal lymph nodes

http://dx.doi.org/10.5772/57121

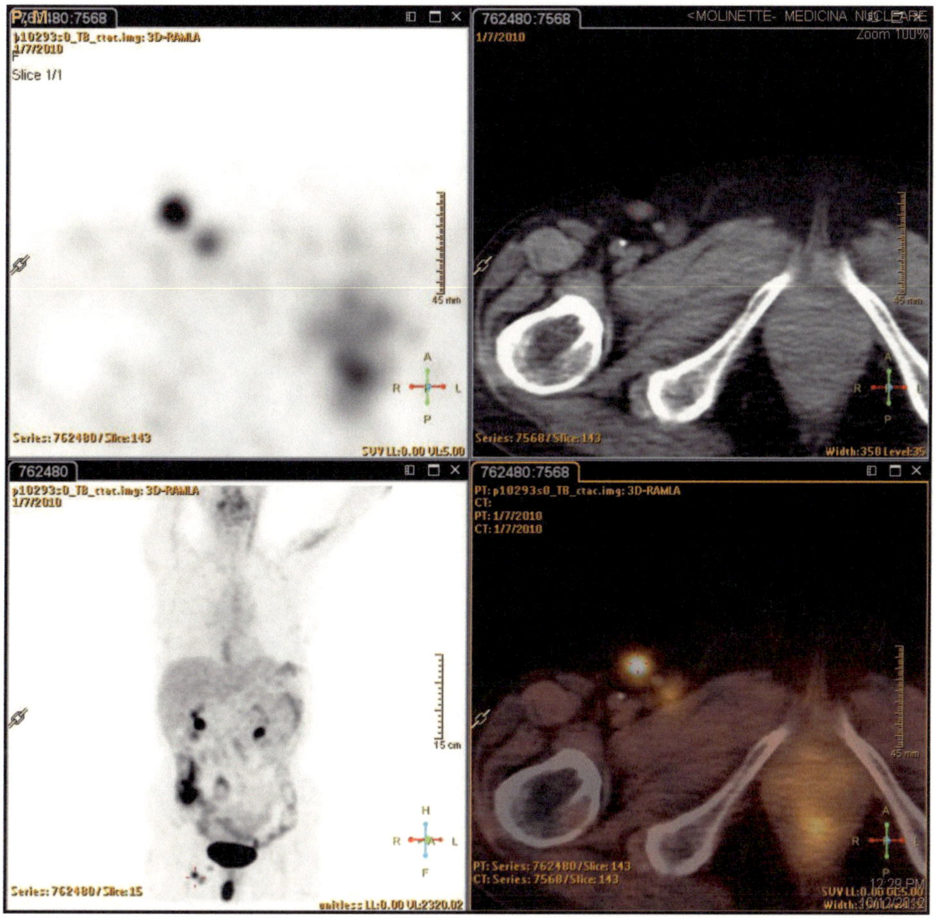


**Figure 4.** PET-CT positive for inguinal lymph nodes metastases.

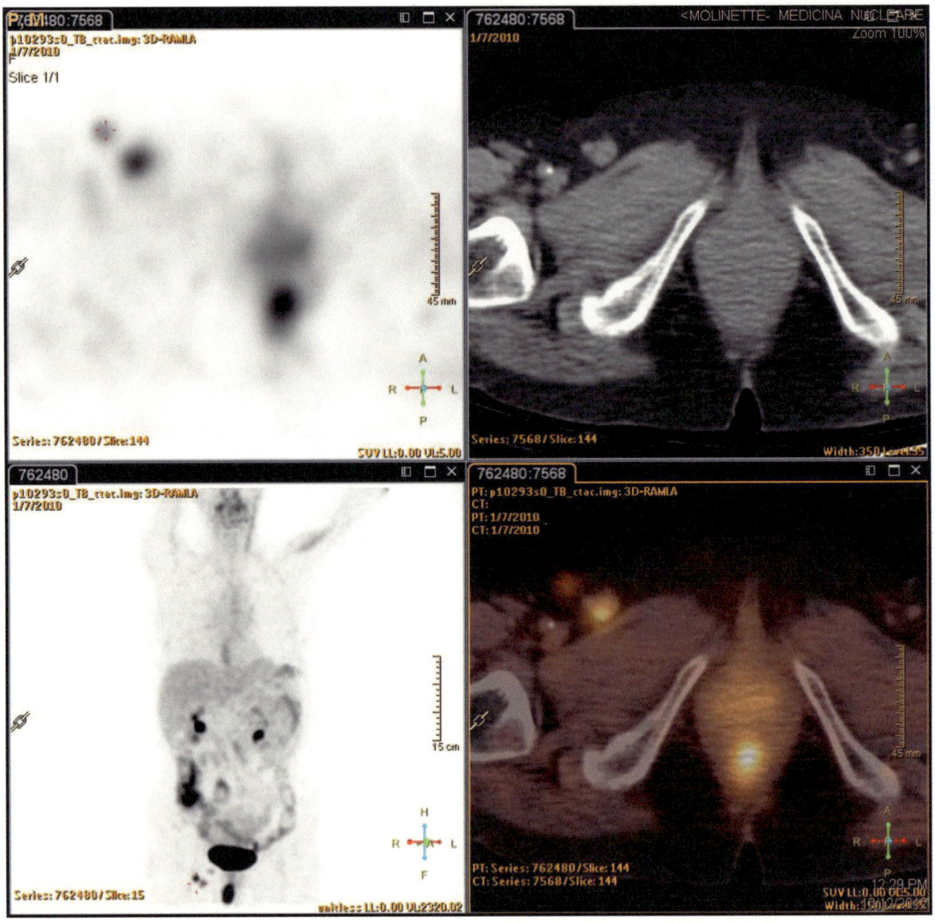


**Figure 5.** PET-CT positive for inguinal lymph nodes metastases.

## 12. Pre-treatment final staging

In the published series tumors were staged according to the American Joint Committee on Cancer staging system [22]. PET/CT upstaged 9-100% and dowstaged 0-25% of patients studied. The radiation fields changed in 3.7-33.3% of cases.

Results are repoted in Table 4 [34-54].

| Author, year | Patients (Total) | Upstaging | Downstaging | Invariate | Change RT planes |
|---|---|---|---|---|---|
| **Trautmann, 2005** | 21 | 10% | n.r. | 90% | n.r. |
| **Cotter, 2006** | 41 | 17% | n.r. | 83% | n.r. |
| **Piperkova, 2006** | 1 | 100% | 0 | 0 | n.r. |
| **Anderson, 2007** | 3 | 33.3% | n.r. | 66.6% | 33.3% |
| **Joon, 2007*** | 48 | 17% | 6% | 77% | 19% |
| **Schwarz, 2008** | 53 | n.r. | n.r. | n.r. | n.r. |
| **Nguyen, 2008*** | 48 | 17% | 6% | 77% | 19% |
| **Iagaru, 2009** | 8 | n.r. | n.r. | n.r. | n.r. |
| **de Winton, 2009** | 61 | 15% | 8% | 77% | 13% |
| **Forrest, 2009** | 39 | n.r. | n.r. | n.r. | n.r. |
| **Renaud, 2009** | 20 | 15% | n.r. | 85% | n.r. |
| **Kidd, 2010** | 77 | n.r. | n.r. | n.r. | n.r. |
| **Krengli, 2010** | 27 | 18.5% | 0% | 81.5% | 3.7% |
| **Bannas, 2010** | 22 | 9% | 18% | 73% | 23% |
| **Engledow, 2010** | 40 | n.r. | n.r. | n.r. | 12.5% |
| **Vercellino, 2011** | 22 | n.r. | n.r. | n.r. | 20% |
| **Sveistrup, 2012** | 91 | 14% | n.r. | 86% | 17% |
| **Mistrangelo, 2012** | 53 | 37.5% | 25% | 37.5% | 12.6% |
| **Wells, 2012** | 30 | 17% | 19% | 65% | 29% |
| **Bhuva, 2012** | 43 | 30.2% | 11.6% | 58.2% | n.r. |

PS: * The 2 papers were published separately considering the same series.

n.r.: Not Reported

**Table 4.** Upstaging and downstaging of PET-CT respect CT scan

| Author, year | Patients (Total) | Recurrences at PET-CT | FP | FN |
|---|---|---|---|---|
| **Trautmann, 2005** | 21 | 12/18 (66.6%) | 9/12 (75%) | 2/6 (33.3%) |
| **Mistrangelo, 2012** | 53 | 10/43 (23.2%) | 6/10 (60%) | 0/33 (0%) |

**Table 5.** Follow up at 1 month

| Author, year | Patients (Total) | Recurrences at PET-CT | FP | FN |
|---|---|---|---|---|
| Schwarz, 2008 | 53 | 9/53 (17%) | 2/9 (22.2%) | n.r. |
| Nguyen, 2008 | 48 | 5/25 (20%) | 3/5 (60%) | n.r. |
| Iagaru, 2009 | 8 | 1/6 (16.6%). | n.r. | n.r. |
| Forrest, 2009 | 39 | 13/39 (33.3%) | 4/13 (30.7%) | n.r. |
| Renaud, 2009 | 20 | 6/11 (54.5%) | 2/6 (33.3%) | 0/5 (0%) |
| Kidd, 2010 | 77 | 14/59 (14%) | n.r. | n.r. |
| Vercellino, 2011 | 22 | 18/36 (50%) | 4/18 (22.2%) | 1/18 (5.5%) |
| Mistrangelo, 2012 | 53 | 8/40 (4.6%) | 5/8 (62.5%) | 0/32 (0%) |

n.r.: Not Reported

**Table 6.** Follow up at 3 months

### 12.1. Follow-up

Few papers report the results of follow up in patients submitted to combined radiochemotherapy for anal cancer with PET-CT. Moreover PET-CTs of follow up were scheduled differently. This aspect does not permit an adequate comparison between various series.

### 12.2. Follow-up at 1 month

Only two papers reported the results of follow up with PET/CT performed 1 month after the end of combined radiochemotherapy [34, 49]. Recurrences are reported respectively in 66.6 and 23.2% of cases. When follow up is analyzed Trautmann [34] reported 75% of false positive (FP) and 33.3% of false negative (FN), while Mistrangelo [49] revealed 60% of FP and none FN. The follow up period was over 18 months in the first study, and 20.3 months in the other one.

Mistrangelo et Al compared also the results of PET-CT with anal biopsy: in the detection of persistence of disease, PET/CT had a sensitivity of 66.6%, a specificity of 92.5%, a positive predictive value (PPV) of 40% and a negative predictive value (NPV) of 97.4%, while anal biopsy had a sensitivity of 100%, a specificity of 97.5%, a PPV of 75% and a NPV of 100% [49].

### 12.3. Follow-up at 3 months

The value of PET-CT performed 3 months after combined radiochemotherapy for anal cancer was analyzed in only 8 papers. Recurrences were reported in 4.6-54.5% of cases [39-41, 43-45, 49-50]. False positive were reported in 22.2-62.5%, while FN in 0-5.5% of cases.

Mistrangelo et Al compared results with anal biopsy: in the detection of recurrence of disease, PET/CT had a sensitivity of 100%, a specificity of 97.4%, a PPV of 66% and a NPV of 100%. Anal biopsy had a sensitivity of 100%, a specificity of 100%, a PPV of 100% and a NPV of 100% [49].

## 13. Discussion

Anal cancer is a relatively uncommon tumor, but its incidence increased over the last decades. Accurate clinical staging is important for prognostic information, for planning the radiotherapy target volume and for defining therapeutic dose. An accurate evaluation of disease extent can help to individualized radiotherapy planning, ensuring the accurate coverage of disease and sparing of organs at risk. If inguinal node metastasis are known, the radiation plan must include a radiation boost to the groin, but these increased radiation doses are associated with acute and late toxicity, like chronic lymph oedema and femoral neck fracture [47].

Since 2005, the use of PET/CT in anal cancer has been described [34-55], but a medline research about the use of PET/CT and anal cancer management shows a relatively little amount of studies. As suggested by Grigsby et al., the advantage of FDG-PET/CT is that it can address all three staging criteria of the TNM system in a single whole-body imaging procedure: demonstrate the extent of the primary tumor, detect lymph node metastases, and reveal any sites of distant metastases [55]. The 2007 National Comprehensive Cancer Network treatment guidelines included PET/CT as a part of the standard pre-treatment workup of patients diagnosed with anal carcinoma [56]. The new version 2.2012 consider PET-CT scan for work up, even if its use for staging or treatment planning has not been validated [57]. The Authors suggest that PET-CT actually does not replace a diagnostic CT scan [57].

Otherwise accurate staging of anal cancer followed by optimal planning of combined radio-chemotherapy treatment can extend patient survival. Anatomical imaging techniques such as CT and MRI cannot evaluate tumor biology and behavior. PET/CT imaging is increasingly used to stage different malignant diseases [59]. The advantage of PET/CT fusion imaging resides in its ability to correlate findings from anatomic and functional imaging modalities, lending it a more important role than diagnostic CT alone in the selection of proper treatment [36]. Moreover, therapy-induced changes in tumors are related to changes in 18F-FDG uptake, and treatment response can be efficiently monitored by PET/CT also considering the standardized uptake value (SUV) of 18F-FDG.

Evidence from published data and our study [41] indicates that PET/CT is clearly superior to CT in visualizing the biopsy-proven primary tumor (87.5-100% vs 47-75%), although the lack of sensitivity did not affect treatment. Otherwise both PET/CT and CT were unable to detect residual tumor after surgical excision.

Considering the results of staging anal cancer with PET-CT respect other classical staging tools, pre-treatment PET/CT upstaged 9-37.5% and downstaged 0-25% of patients with anal cancer

[34-54]. PET/CT at diagnosis can also be used for radiation therapy treatment planning as it clearly defines sites of metabolically active tumor [47].

Radiation treatment fields changed in 3.7-33.3% of patients [37-38, 40, 42, 46-52]. Only Vercellino et al. [50] reported no change in treatment fields in their series of 44 patients.

In the majority of studies, upstaging was related to a suggested better staging of metastases in perirectal, pelvic and inguinal lymph nodes. As it defines nodal and metastatic disease, PET imaging can improve the staging of anal cancer [40].

Mai and Coll assumed that PET positive lymph nodes in a setting of anal cancer as defined by SUV uptake raise the likelihood of lymph node involvement, which would warrant more aggressive treatment in patients with PET positive nodes [60].

The sensitivity of CT for detecting nodal metastases in the pelvic and inguinal region is limited to 40-68% [25]. By contrast, PET/CT showed a higher specificity (80-90%) and sensitivity (70-90%) in the detection of nodal and distant metastases for several tumor types like non-small-cell lung cancer and head and neck cancer [25]. Also in gynecologic cancer, PET can have a specificity of 90-95%.

Cotter et al. [35] reported that PET/CT upstages inguinal nodes in 17% of patients. They also found a higher rate of PET/CT positive for inguinal metastases in HIV-seropositive versus HIV-seronegative patients (44% vs. 16%), while other Authors observed only a marginal difference in positive inguinal metastases between these two patient subgroups (28.5% vs. 25%) [49].

Otherwise some 5% of inguinal lymph node metastases detected with PET/CT are FP at fine-needle aspiration cytology (FNAC) [48] and up to 57% at histological confirmation of samples from sentinel node biopsy (SNB) [61]. Iagaru [41] and Engledow [48] reported that inguinal lymph nodes positive at PET/CT were negative at FNAC in 50% and at SNB in 5% of cases. Therefore, positive lymph nodes identified by PET/CT should be adequately studied with biopsy before changing radiotherapy plans. In this connection, the high incidence of inguinal metastases found on imaging as compared with conventional staging tools should warn against unnecessary inguinal radiotherapy. Inguinal staging with SNB may explain the lower percentage of change in radiotherapy fields in ours series compared to others.

PET/CT was recently considered also for follow-up of patients undergoing radio- and chemotherapy treatment in anal cancer. Kidd et al. [45] reported that a higher $SUV_{max}$ was associated with lymph node involvement at diagnosis. These patients were also at higher risk of persistent disease on their post-treatment PET, if the study was performed less than 4 months after completing therapy. The authors go on to suggest that $SUV_{max}$ for FDG represents a potential new biomarker for anal cancer prognosis, as it is significantly associated with lymph node involvement at diagnosis, treatment response, and disease-free survival [45].

Post-treatment PET/CT is indicated to determine response to therapy and it is highly predictive of long-term clinical outcomes [55]. It can also be used to evaluate sites of recurrent disease. Few studies have examined clinical response to therapy, and clinical workup differs widely.

http://dx.doi.org/10.5772/57121

Piperkova et al. suggested that PET/CT in anal cancer accurately identifies treatment response [36]. Schwarz et al. [39] reported that posttherapy FDG response was the most significant predictor of progression-free survival (P=0.0003) and that it was more predictive of the treatment outcome than either pre-treatment tumor size (P=0.08) or nodal status (P=0.40). Persistent disease is indeed a predictor of poor clinical outcome [39].

Mistrangelo et Al [49] reported that PET/CT assessment at 1 month had a sensitivity of 66.6%, a specificity of 92.5%, a PPV of 40% and a NPV of 97.4% for detecting persistence of anal disease. These data are not comparable to previous observations. Only Trautmann et al. [34] reported on the results of PET/CT assessment at 1 month (persistence of disease of 66.6% of cases), suggesting that PET/CT at 1 month after the end of therapy is of little value in predicting the durability of response.

In contrast, anal biopsy at 1-month follow-up had higher sensitivity and specificity than PET/CT, even if assessment with biopsy of non-progressive residual tumor at 1 month after treatment may be misleading as shortly after radiation nonviable cancer cell may look morphologically intact [62].

Considering these aspects biopsy for a non-progressive residual tumor at 1 month after treatment shoud not be taken as this can lead to unnecessary abdominoperineal excision. These patients should be closely observed.

Mistrangelo et Al reported that PET/CT assessment at 3 months had a sensitivity of 100%, a specificity of 97.4%, a PPV of 66% and a NPV of 100%; anal biopsy had the same sensitivity but a better specificity than PET/CT [49]. Vercellino and Coll [50] reported thet sensitivity, specificity and negative predictive value of PET-CT for the detection of recurrent locoregional disease is 93%, 81% and 94% respectively, resulting in an impact on management in 20%.

## 14. Conclusions

The role of PET-CT in the evaluation of anal cancer is evolving. PET/CT detect the primary tumor more often than CT, but neither tool is indicated to reveal persistent disease after surgery. PET/CT proved useful in initial staging perirectal/pelvic or inguinal lymph nodes. PET/CT can document also unknown metastases, changing the disease stadiation. However, upstaging related to lymph nodes metastases might have been overestimated, as up to 31% of inguinal metastases identified by PET/CT are reportedly false positive, but metabolic imaging can descover little nodal metastases, too little for CT and clinical evaluation. Currently, inguinal lymph nodes are better staged by sentinel node biopsy. PET/CT assessment at 1-month follow-up had lower sensitivity and specificity than anal biopsy.

PET/CT assessment at 3 months more accurately evaluated the persistence or the recurrence of anal disease and thus allowed for better follow up when combined with anal biopsy.

## Author details

Massimiliano Mistrangelo[1*] and Adriana Lesca[2]

*Address all correspondence to: mistrangelo@katamail.com

1 Digestive and Colorectal Surgical Department, Centre of Minimal Invasive Surgery, University of Turin, Città della Salute e della Scienza Hospital, Italy

2 Department of Nuclear Medicine, Città della Salute e della Scienza Hospital, Italy

## References

[1] Nivatvongs S. Perianal and Anal Canal Neoplasms. In Principles and Practice of Surgery for the Colon, Rectum and Anus. Ed. Quality Medical Publishing, Inc. St Louis Missouri. 1999: 447-471.

[2] Morson BC, Sobin LH. Histological typing of intestinal tumours. In International Histological Classification of Tumors, No 15. Geneva: World Health Organization 1976.

[3] Cummings BJ, Keane TJ, OSullivan B, Wong CS, Catton CN. Epidermoid anal cancer: treatment by radiation alone or by radiation and 5-fluorouracil with and without mitomycin C. Int J Rad Oncol Biol Phys 1991; 21:1115–25.

[4] Greene FL, Page DL, Fleming ID et Al eds. American Joint Committee on Cancer: AJCC Cancer Staging Manual. 6th ed, New York, NY, USA: Springer 2001; 157-164.

[5] Ries LAG., Harkins D., Krapcho M., et al. Edwards BK. (eds). SEER Cancer Statistics Review, 1975-2003. Baltimore, MD: National Cancer Institute, 2005: 1-103.

[6] Siegel R., Ward E., Brawley O., Jemal A. Cancer statistics, 2011. The impact of eliminating socioeconomic and racial disparities on premature cancer deaths. CA Cancer J Clin 2011; 61: 212-236.

[7] Clark MA, Hartley A, Geh JI. Cancer of the anal canal. Lancet Oncol 2004; 5:149-157.

[8] Klas J, Rothenberger D, Wong WD, Madoff R. Malignant tumors of the anal canal. The spectrum of disease, treatment and outcome. Cancer 1999; 85:1686-1693.

[9] Minsky BD, Hoffman JP, Kelsen DP. Cancer of the anal region. In: DeVita Jr VT, Hellman S, Rosenberg SA, eds. Cancer: Principles & Practice of Oncology, Sixth Edition. Philadelphia: Lippincott-Williams & Wilkins, 2001: 1319-1342.

[10] Deans GT, McAleer JJA, Spence RAJ. Malignant anal tumours. Br J Surg 1994; 81: 500-508.

[11] Ryan D, Compton C, Mayer R. Carcinoma of the anal canal. N Engl J Med 2000; 342:792–800.

[12] Frisch M, Fenger C, van den Brule AJ, et al. Variants of squamous cell carcinoma of the anal canal and perianal skin and their relation to human papilloma viruses. Cancer Res Feb 1999; 1;59:753-7.

[13] Holmes F, Borek D, Owen-Kummer M, et al. Anal cancer in women. Gastroenterology 1988; 95:107–11.

[14] Ryan DP, Mayer RJ. Anal carcinoma: histology, staging, epidemiology, treatment. Curr Opin Oncol 2000; 12: 345–52.

[15] Beckmann AM, Daling JR, Sherman KJ, et al. Human papillomavirus infection and anal cancer. Int J Cancer 1989; 43:1042-49.

[16] Williams GR, Talbot IC. Anal carcinoma: a histological review. Histopathology 1994; 25:507–16.

[17] Palmer JG, Scholefield JH, Coates PJ, et al. Anal cancer and human papillomaviruses. Dis Colon Rectum 1989; 32:1016–22.

[18] Daling JR, Madeleine MM, Johnson LG ct al. Human papillomavirus, smoking, and sexual pratices in the etiology of anal cancer. Cancer 2004;101:270-280.

[19] Hope E. Uronis, Johanna C Bendell. Anal Cancer: an overview. The Oncologist 2007;12:524-534.

[20] Salmo E., Haboubi N. Anal Cancer: Pathology, Staging and Evidence-based minimum data set. Colorectal Dis 2011; 13 (Suppl 1): 11-20.

[21] Stearns MW., Urmacher C., Sternberg SS. Cancer of the anal canal. Cur Probl Cancer 1980; 4: 1-44.

[22] Golden GT., Horsley JS. Surgical management of epidermoid carcinoma of the anus. Am J Surg 1976; 131: 275-280.

[23] Nigro N.D., Vaitkeicus V.K., Basil Considine B.: Combined therapy for cancer of the anal canal: a preliminary report. Dis Colon Rectum 1974; 17 (3): 354-356.

[24] Gerard J-P, Chapet O., Samiei F., Morignat E., Isaac S., Paulin C., Romestaing P., Favrel V., Mornex F., Bobin J-Y.: Management of inguinal lymph node metastases in patients with carcinoma of the anal canal. Experience in a series of 270 patients treated in Lyon and review of the Literature. Cancer 2001; 92: 77-84.

[25] Bartelink H., Roelofsen F., Eschwege F., et al. Concomitant radiotherapy and chemotherapy is superior to radiotherapy alone in the treatment of locally advanced anal cancer: results of a phase III randomized trial of the European Organization for Research and Treatment of Cancer Radiotherapy and Gastrointestinal Cooperative Groups. J Clin Oncol 1997; 15 (5): 2040-2049.

[26] Al B. Benson III, J Pablo Arnoletti et al. Anal Carcinoma, Version 2.2012: Featured Uptades to the NCCN Guidelines. J Nat Compr Canc Netw 2012;10:449-454

[27] Czito BG, Willet CG, Current management of anal cancer. Curr Oncol Rep 2009;11(3): 186-92.

[28] Cotter SE., Perry W Grigsby et al. FDG-PET/CT in the evaluation of anal carcinoma. Int J Radiation Onc Biol Phys 2006; 65 (3): 720-725.

[29] Jaiyesimi IA, Pazdur R. Cisplatin and 5-fluorouracil as salvage therapy for recurrent metastatic squamous cell carcinoma of the anal canal. Am J Clin Oncol 1993;16:563-540.

[30] Evans TR, Mansi JL Glees JP. Response of metastatic anal carcinama to single agent carboplatin. Clin Oncol (R Coll Radiol) 1993;5:57-58.

[31] Fisher WB, Herbst KD, Sims JE et al. Metastatic cloacogenic carcinoma of the anus: sequential responses to adriamycin and cis-dichlorodiammineplatinum (II). Cancer Treat Rep 1978;62:91-97.

[32] Zimm S, Wampler GL. Response of metastatic cloacogenic carcinoma to treatment with semustine. Cancer 1981;48:2575-2576.

[33] Walk PE, Bailey DL et al Positron Emission Tomography - Basic science and clinical practice. Ed. Springer.

[34] Trautmann TG, Zuger JH. Positron emission tomography for pre-treatment staging and posttreatment evaluation in cancer of the anal canal. Mol Imaging Biol 2005; 7: 309-313.

[35] Cotter SE., Grigsby PW, Siegel BA, Dehdashti F., Malyapa RS., Fleshman JW., Birnbaum EH., Wang X., Abbey E., Tan B., Kodner IJ., Hunt SR., Lowney JK., Mutch MG., Dietz DW., Myerson RJ. FDG-PET/CT in the evaluation of anal carcinoma. Int J Radiat Oncol Biol Phys 2006; 65: 720-725.

[36] Piperkova E., Raphael B., Altinyay M., et al. Impact of PET/CT on initial staging, restaging and treatment management of anal cancer: a clinical case with literature review. J BUON 2006; 11: 523-527.

[37] Anderson C., Koshy M., Staley C., et al. PET-CT fusion in radiation management of patients with anorectal tumors. Int J Radiation Oncology Biol Phys 2007; 69 (1): 155-162.

[38] Joon Dl., Nguyen B., Khoo V., Joon ML., See A., Kai C., Chao M., Wada M., Feigen M., Quong G. PET in anal cancer: Its role in staging and evaluation after chemoradiation. Int J Radiation Oncology Biol Phys 2007; 69 (3): S296.

[39] Schwarz JK., Siegel BA., Dehdashti F., Myerson RJ., Fleshman JW., Grigsby PW. Tumor response and survival predicted by post therapy FDG-PET/CT in anal cancer. Int J Radiation Oncol Biol Phys 2008; 71 (1): 180-186.

[40] Nguyen BT., Joon DL., Khoo V., Quong G., Chao M., Wada M., Joon ML., See A., Feigen M., Rykers K., Kai C., Zupan E., Scott A. Assessing the impact of FDG-PET in the management of anal cancer. Radiother Oncol 2008; 87: 376-382.

[41] Iagaru A., Kundu R., Jadvar H., Nagle D. Evaluation by 18 F-FDG-PET of patients with anal squamous cell carcinoma. Hell J Nucl Med 2009; 12 (1): 26-29.

[42] de Winton E., Heriot AG., Ng M., Hicks RJ., Hogg A., Milner A., Leong T., Fay M., Mackay J., Drummond E., Ngan SY. The impact of 18-fluorodeoxyglucose positron emission tomography on the staging, management and outcome of anal cancer. Br J Cancer 2009; 100: 693-700.

[43] Forrest W. FDG-PET/CT trumps CT in detecting anal carcinoma. AuntMinnie.com 2009.

[44] Renaud S., Guillermand S., Eberlé-Pouzeratte MC., Lemanski C., Faurous P., Artus J-C. Apport de la tomographie par émission de positrons au $^{18}$F-fluorodéoxyglucose (TEP-FDG) dans la prise en charge du cancer du canal anal. Med Nucl 2009; 33: 415-424.

[45] Kidd E., Dehdashti F., Siegel BA., Grigsby PW. Anal cancer maximum F-18 fluorodeoxyglucose uptake on positron emission tomography is correlated with prognosis. Radiother Oncol. 2010; 95; 288-291.

[46] Krengli M., Milia ME., Turri L.,Mones M., Bassi MC., Cannillo B., Deantonio L., Sacchetti G., Brambilla M., Inglese E. FDG-PET/CT imaging for staging and target volume delineation in conformal radiotherapy of anal carcinoma. Radiat Oncol 2010; 5: 10.

[47] Bannas P., Weber C., Adam G., Frenzel T., Derlin T., Mester J., Klutmann S. Contrast-enhanced [$^{18}$F]Fluorodeoxyglucose-positron emission tomography/computed tomography for staging and radiotherapy planning in patients with anal cancer. Int J Radiation Oncol Biol. Phys. 2011; 81: 445-451.

[48] Engledow AH., Skipworth JRA., Blackman G., Groves A., Bomanji J., Warren SJ., Ell PL., Boulos PB. The role of $^{18}$FDG PETCT in the clinical management of anal squamous cell carcinoma. Colorectal Dis 2011; 13: 532-537.

[49] Mistrangelo M., Pelosi E., Bellò M., Ricardi U., Milanesi E., Cassoni P., Baccega M. Filippini C., Racca P., Lesca A., Munoz FH., Fora G., Skanjeti A., Cravero F., Morino M. Role of positron emission Tomography-computed tomography in the management of anal cancer. Int J Radiat Oncol Biol Phys 2012; Sep 1: 84 (1): 66-72.

[50] Vercellino L., Montravers F., de Paredes V., Huchet V., Kerrou K., Bauer P., Touboul E., Talbot J-N. Impact of FDG PET/CT in the staging and the follow up of anal carcinoma. Int J Colorectal Dis 2011; 26: 201-210.

[51] Sveistrup J., Loft A., Berthelsen AK., Henriksen BM., Nielsen MB., Engelholm SA. Positron Emission Tomography/Computed Tomography in the staging and treatment of anal cancer. Int J Radiat Oncol Biol Phys 2012; 83: 134-141.

[52] Wells IT., Fox BM. PET/CT in anal cancer – is it worth doing? Clinical Radiol 2012; 67: 535-540.

[53] Bhuva NJ., Glynne-Jones R., Sonoda L., Wong W-L., Harrison MK. To PET or not to PET? That is the question. Staging in anal cancer. Ann Oncol 2012; 23 (8): 2078-2082.

[54] Saboo SS., Zukotynski K., Shinagare AB., Krajewski KM., Ramaiya N. Anal carcinoma: FDG PET/CT in staging, response evaluation, and follow up. Abdom Imaging 2012; Sept 26 [Epub ahead of print], doi: 10.1007/s00261-012-9958-3.

[55] Grigsby PW. FDG-PET/CT: New horizons in anal cancer. Gastroenterol Clin Biol 2009; 33 (5): 456-458.

[56] Engstrom PF, Arnoletti JP, Benson AB 3rd, et al. NCCN clinical practice guidelines in oncology. Anal carcinoma. J Natl Compr Canc Netw 2010; 8 (1): 106-120.

[57] Benson AB 3rd, Arnoletti JP, Bekaii-Saab T. et Al. NCCN Clinical Practice Guidelines in Oncology: Anal Carcinoma. Version 2.2012: featured updates to the National Comprehensive Cancer Network guidelines. J Natl Compr Canc Netw 2012; 10: 449-454.

[58] American Joint Commission on Cancer. Anal Canal. In AJCC Cancer Staging Manual 6th Ed. New York: Springer; 2002: 125-130.

[59] Ell PJ. PET/CT in oncology: a major technology for cancer. Chang Gung Med J. 2005; 28: 274-283.

[60] Mai SK., Welzel G., Hermann B., et al. Can the radiation dose to CT-enlarged but FDG-PET-negative inguinal lymph nodes in anal cancer be reduced? Strahlenther Onkol 2009; 185: 254-259.

[61] Mistrangelo M., Pelosi E., Bellò M., Castellano I., Cassoni P., Ricardi U., Munoz F., Racca P., Contu V., Beltramo G., Morino M., Mussa A. Comparison of positron emission tomography scanning and sentinel node biopsy in the detection of inguinal node metastases in patients with anal cancer. Int J Radiation Oncol Biol Phys 2010; 77 (1): 73-78.

[62] Suit HD, Gallager HS. Intact tumor cells in irradiated tissue. Arch Pathol 1964; 78: 648-651.

Chapter 10

# Early Prediction of Tumor Response: A Future Strategy for Optimizing Cancer Treatment

Shigeto Ueda and Toshiaki Saeki

Additional information is available at the end of the chapter

http://dx.doi.org/10.5772/57120

## 1. Introduction

Positron emission tomography (PET) with $^{18}$F-fluorodeoxyglucose (FDG) is successfully capable of imaging glucose metabolism of the tumor cells. Tumor glucose metabolism using FDG-PET has a potential to distinguish viable cancer cells from those in suspension or necrotic components because the degree of tumor FDG uptake is closely associated with its proliferation activity. There is cumulative evidence showing that reduction in FDG uptake value on the early phase after the initiation of chemotherapy more reliably predicts a favorable outcome of patients with breast cancer. Therefore, FDG-PET could help to individualize treatment and to avoid potentially ineffective chemotherapies. In this article, we discuss and illustrate the role and limitations of FDG-PET in the management of neoadjuvant chemotherapy in breast cancer.

## 2. Tumor metabolic response

FDG-PET has proven useful in the management of various cancers [1]. FDG-PET is known to play an important role in the detection of distant metastasis and recurrence [2, 3]. In addition, it provides quantitative information on tumor glucose metabolic activity, allowing the measurement of metabolic changes and cancer activity shortly after initiation of therapy and before tumor volume reduction [4]. This functional imaging tool may also be useful in predicting tumor response to therapy and optimizing individual treatment [5].

Tumor response to therapy is traditionally assessed by comparison of tumor size before and after treatment, which is determined using anatomical imaging devices such as ultrasonography and computed tomography (CT) on the basis of the Response Evaluation Criteria in Solid

INTECH
open science | open minds

© 2013 Ueda and Saeki; licensee InTech. This is a paper distributed under the terms of the Creative Commons Attribution License (http://creativecommons.org/licenses/by/3.0), which permits unrestricted use, distribution, and reproduction in any medium, provided the original work is properly cited.

Tumors (RECIST) [6]. Although RECIST has been widely adopted, tumor response must be evaluated for several months until surgery and it does not always reflect the pathological response because of difficulties in distinguishing residual cancer cells from necrotic lesions, fibrosis, or benign masses.

Because of limitations in applying the RECIST criteria using anatomic imaging alone, Wahl et al. proposed a draft framework called the PET Response Criteria in Solid Tumors (PERCIST) [7]. The proposed PERCIST criteria are being used in several current clinical studies. As far as early response assessment with FDG-PET is concerned, clinical studies involving patients with Hodgkin lymphoma and aggressive non-Hodgkin lymphoma have demonstrated that the assessment of changes in FDG uptake on PET imaging after 2 or 3 cycles of chemotherapy was superior for predicting patient prognosis compared with the assessment of morphological changes on computed tomography (CT) [8]. This method was shown to be at least as reliable as definitive response assessment at the end of therapy [8]. In a European multicenter trial monitoring chemotherapy response and survival in 260 patients with lymphoma, an early decrease in FDG uptake on PET after 2 cycles of chemotherapy was significantly correlated with progression-free survival [9]. For other types of cancers, including breast cancer [10], non-small cell lung cancer [11], esophageal cancer [12] [13], gastric cancer [14], and colorectal cancer [15], several clinical studies revealed evidence of the emerging role of FDG-PET in predicting both post-therapeutic clinicopathological response and patient survival.

In our institute, a discrepancy was observed between tumor morphological changes and tumor metabolic activity in a patient treated with neoadjuvant chemotherapy for primary breast cancer. FDG-PET was performed at the onset of chemotherapy, at the midpoint of chemotherapy, and prior to surgery. The primary tumor appeared to grow rapidly after the start of neoadjuvant chemotherapy despite the gradual reduction in glucose accumulation (Figure 1). Postoperative pathological analysis revealed that the lesion was replaced with scar tissue in addition to the presence of massive bleeding and small residual cancer cell nests. In this case, FDG-PET was able to provide more accurate and clinically beneficial information compared with CT.

Clinical studies conducted worldwide have repeatedly revealed the predictive value of FDG-PET in patients with advanced breast cancer treated by chemotherapy. As early as 1993, Wahl et al. studied 11 patients with locally advanced breast cancer before and after 1 cycle of chemotherapy. A significant difference was observed in tumor FDG influx rate (K) from baseline levels between responders and nonresponders (sensitivity: 100%, specificity: 100%) [16]. In 1996, Bassa et al. conducted a retrospective study of 13 patients with breast cancer for whom FDG-PET scans were performed prior to chemotherapy, at the end of the first cycle, at the midpoint of chemotherapy, and before surgery. The mean standardized uptake value (SUV) of the tumor after the first cycle of chemotherapy was significantly lower than the baseline value ($p < 0.01$) [17]. In 2000, reports of clinical studies from two separate institutes showed the usefulness of FDG-PET in the early evaluation of tumor metabolic response to chemotherapy. Schelling et al. demonstrated the ability of FDG-PET to differentiate between responders and nonresponders after the first course of chemotherapy (sensitivity: 100%,

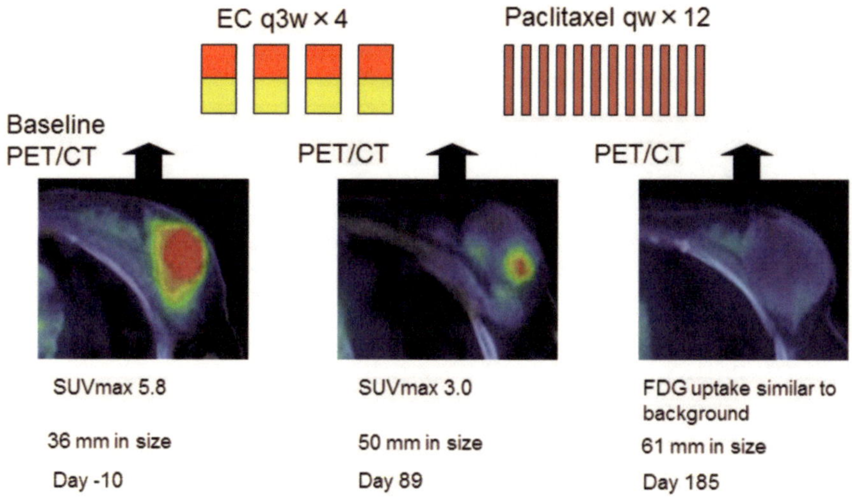


SUVmax decreased from 5.8 to 3.0 at the midpoint of treatment and returned to baseline levels prior to surgery. In contrast, the tumor diameter increased from 36 mm to 50 mm at the midpoint of treatment and to 61 mm prior to surgery.
FDG: fluoro-D-glucose; PET: positron emission tomography; CT: computed tomography
SUVmax: maximal standardized uptake value; EC: epirubicin and cyclophosphamide.

**Figure 1.** Transversal slices of FDG-PET/CT of a breast lesion before treatment (left), at the completion of the EC regimen (middle), and at the completion of the paclitaxel regimen (right).

specificity: 85%) [18]. Smith et al. also successfully utilized FDG-PET for predicting tumor response after the first cycle of chemotherapy (sensitivity: 90%, specificity: 74%) [19].

Our team investigated the maximum changes in SUV (SUVmax) in 32 primary breast cancer lesions in 30 patients. The patients were treated with neoadjuvant chemotherapy comprising 4 cycles of epirubicine and cyclophosphamide on a triweekly basis and sequential weekly cycles of taxane for 12 weeks [20]. Figure 2 shows representative tumor images on FDG-PET performed at baseline, after one cycle of chemotherapy, after four cycles of chemotherapy, and prior to surgery. The serial images on the upper row show a tumor in which a pathological complete response (pCR) can be observed. The middle row depicts a tumor exhibiting a pathological partial response (pPR), and the lower row illustrates pathological progressive disease (pPD). SUV decreased dramatically in the pCR tumor after one cycle of chemotherapy, after which metabolic activity ceased. SUV change in the pPR tumor was lower than that in the pCR tumor after one cycle of chemotherapy, but SUV gradually diminished during further chemotherapeutic treatment. The pPD tumor showed no significant changes in SUV after treatment. In terms of the optimal threshold of a 40% decrease in SUV, the rate of pathological response in terms of pCR or near pCR was higher (71.4%) in metabolic responders than in nonresponders (12.5%). The sensitivity, specificity, positive predictive value (PPV), and negative predictive value (NPV) were 63%, 92%, 71%, and 88%, respectively.

In 2008, Schwarz–Dose et al. performed the first prospective multicenter trial to evaluate the effectiveness of FDG-PET in predicting early pathological response during chemotherapeutic

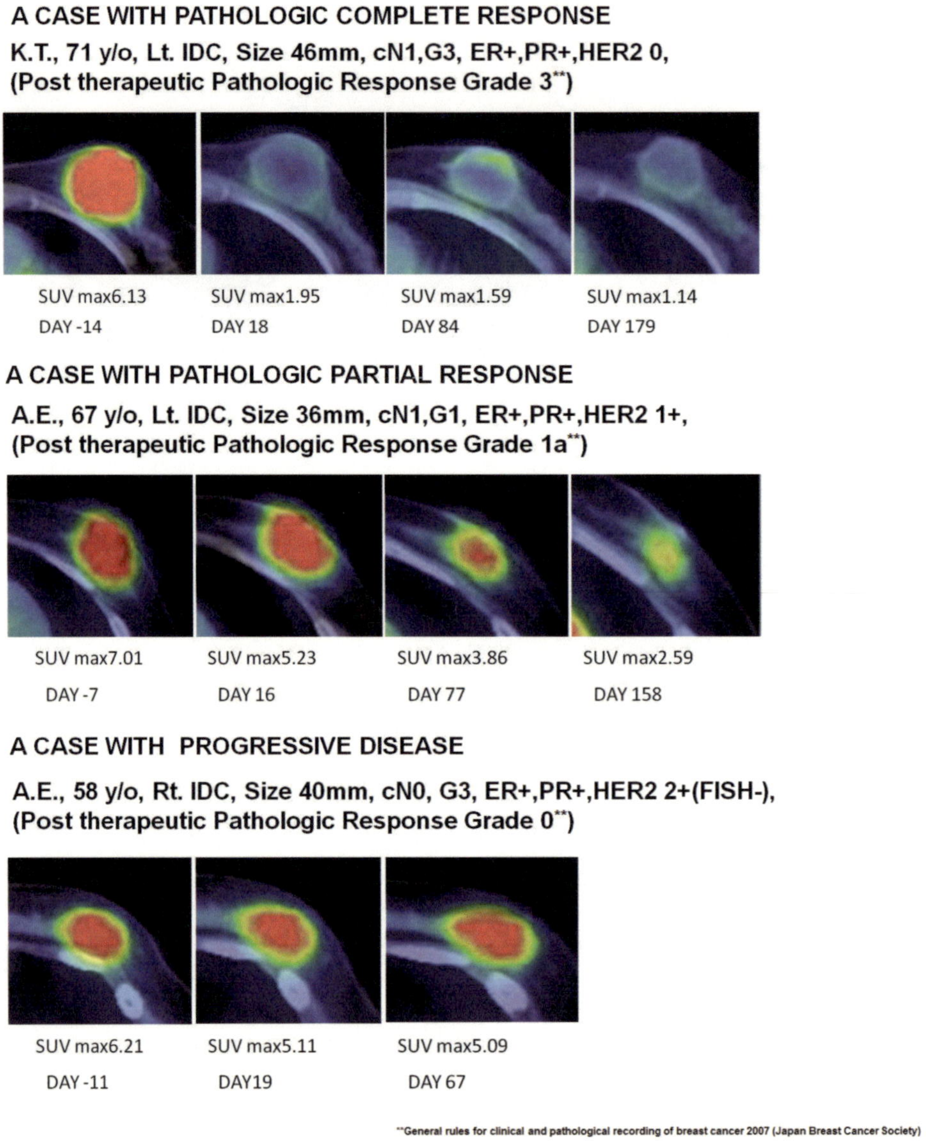


pCR: pathological complete response; pPR: pathological partial response; pPD: pathological progressive disease; FDG: fluoro-D-glucose; PET: positron emission tomography; CT: computed tomography; EC: epirubicin and cyclophosphamide

**Figure 2.** Axial FDG-PET/CT images of a pCR tumor (upper row), a pPR tumor (middle row), and a pPD tumor (lower row). Sequential FDG-PET scans were performed at baseline (left), after 1 cycle of chemotherapy (second from the left), after completion of the EC regimen (third from the left), and at the completion of chemotherapy (right).

treatment in 104 patients with locally advanced breast cancer [10]. In that report, when a 40% decrease in SUV occurred in the first cycle after initiation of chemotherapy compared with baseline values, FDG-PET predicted pCR and pathological macroscopic residual disease at a high rate, with a sensitivity of 73%, specificity of 63%, PPV of 36%, and NPV of 90% [10]. Other representative studies published in the literature since 2000 are listed in Table 1 [21-25].

In 2011, a meta-analysis in this field summarized 16 articles including a total of 920 patients with breast cancer [26]. To predict histopathological response in primary lesions, the pooled sensitivity, specificity, PPV, NPV, and diagnostic odds ratios were calculated. The results for these parameters were 84% [95% confidence interval (CI), 78%–88%], 66% (95% CI, 62%–70%), 50% (95% CI, 44%–55%), 91% (95% CI, 87%–94%), and 11.90 (95% CI, 6.33%–22.36%), respectively. Although the checkpoints of FDG-PET administration in these trials differed, a subset analysis showed that early response of glucose metabolism after the first or second cycle of chemotherapy provided a significantly better indicator of accuracy compared with a later response (third cycle or later). The subset analysis results showed in Table1. These data indicate that changes in SUV during the first 1–3 cycles of chemotherapy are better indicators of clinical outcome compared with changes during the later cycles.

| Authors | Year | Study Type | stage | Population | The timing of PETscans | Early assessment | Endpoint | Cutoff | Se | Sp | PPV | NPV | Accuracy |
|---|---|---|---|---|---|---|---|---|---|---|---|---|---|
| Martoni, et al.[22] | 2010 | one center | LABC | 34 | Baseline,after 2 cycles, 4 cycles, at the end | after 2 cycles | pCR+pMRD | 50% in ΔSUV | 100 | 30 | 27 | 100 | 44 |
| Ueda, et al.[20] | 2010 | one center | LABC | 32 | Baseline, after 1 cycyle, after 4 cycles, at the end | after 1 cycle | pCR+less than 3% disappearance of tumor | 40% in ΔSUV | 63 | 92 | 71 | 88 | 84 |
| Kumar, et al.[21] | 2009 | one center | LABC | 23 | Baseline, after 2 cycle | after 2 cycles | pCR+pMRD | 50% in ΔSUV | 93 | 75 | | | 87 |
| Schwarz-Dose, et al.[10] | 2008 | multiple centers | LABC | 104 | baseline, after 1 cycle, after 2 cycle | after 1 cycle | pCR+pMRD | 45% in ΔSUV | 73 | 63 | 36 | 90 | 65 |
| McDemott, et al.[25] | 2007 | one center | LABC | 96 | Baseline, after 1cycle, after 2 cycles, at the midpoint, at the end | after 1 cycle | pCR+pMRD | 34% in ΔSUV | 100 | 66 | | | |
| Berrido-Riedinger, et al.[23] | 2007 | one center | LABC | 50 | Baseline, after 2 cycle | after 2 cycles | 75% or more absence of tumor | 40% in ΔSUV | 77 | 80 | | | |
| Rousseau, et al.[24] | 2006 | one center | LABC | 64 | Baseline, after 1 cycle, after 2 cycles, after 3 cycles, after 6 cycles | after 2 cycles | 50% or more absence of tumor cells | 40% in ΔSUV | 89 | 95 | | 85 | |
| Smith, et al.[19] | 2000 | one center | LABC | 30 | Baseline, after 1cycle, after 2 cycles, after 5 cycles, at the end | after 1 cycle | pCRmicro/macro | 20% in ΔDUR | 90 | 74 | | | |
| Schelling, et al.[18] | 2000 | one center | LABC | 22 | Baseline, after 1 cycle, after 2 cycles | after 1 cycle | pCR and pMRD | 55% in ΔSUV | 100 | 85 | | | |
| Meta-analysis | | | | | | | | | | | | | |
| Authors | Year | Study Type | stage | Population | The timing of PET scans | Evaluation of the timing | Endpoint | Cutoff | Se | Sp | PPV | NPV | Accuracy |
| Wang, et al.[26] | 2011 | meta-analysis | LABC | 920(Total) | Various | Various | Various | Various | 84 | 66 | 50 | 91 | |
| | | | | 347(subset) | Various | After 1-2 cycles | Various | Various | 88 | 70 | 61 | 92 | 76 |
| | | | | 400(subset) | Various | After 3 cycles or later | Various | Various | 81 | 61 | 34 | 93 | 65 |

LABC, Laegelly advanced breast cancer; pCR, pathological complete response; MRD, macroscope residual disease; Se, sensitivity; Sp, specificity; PPV, positive predictive value; NPV, negative predictive value

**Table 1.** Optimal timing of FDG PET during chemotherapy

The high sensitivity and high NPV reported above indicate that FDG-PET may be useful for the identification of nonresponders among patients in the early phases of treatment with neoadjuvant chemotherapy. However, in cases where FDG-PET indicates changes in SUV (responders), decision-making regarding continuation of treatment may still be difficult. This problem has been addressed in research on lymphoma patients. Randomized trials have been conducted to determine whether response-guided treatment using early response to therapy as measured by FDG-PET scans is feasible or useful in decreasing the cumulative dose of potentially cytotoxic agents in nonresponders [27], [28]. These trials aim at treatment modification based on PET response by comparing risk-adapted treatment guided by FDG-PET with standard chemotherapy in these patients [29].

An emerging paradigm for a treatment strategy using FDG-PET has been introduced in addition to traditional assessment of tumor response on the basis of staging and tumor subtyping [30]. A specific treatment was chosen from a number of chemotherapeutic drugs, and the usefulness of FDG-PET was analyzed in comparison to assessment based on staging and subtyping. This new strategy to optimize treatment timing includes staging, subtyping, and response guiding. Staging and subtyping determine favorable treatment options before the initiation of treatment. Functional imaging with FDG-PET offers opportunities to assess tumor response early in the course of treatment. This response-guiding strategy offers the opportunity to revise treatment and improve outcome. FDG-PET not only provides invaluable prognostic information in patients [31] but also supports efforts to switch to more effective treatment options in the early stages of treatment rather than on completion of therapy (Figure 3).

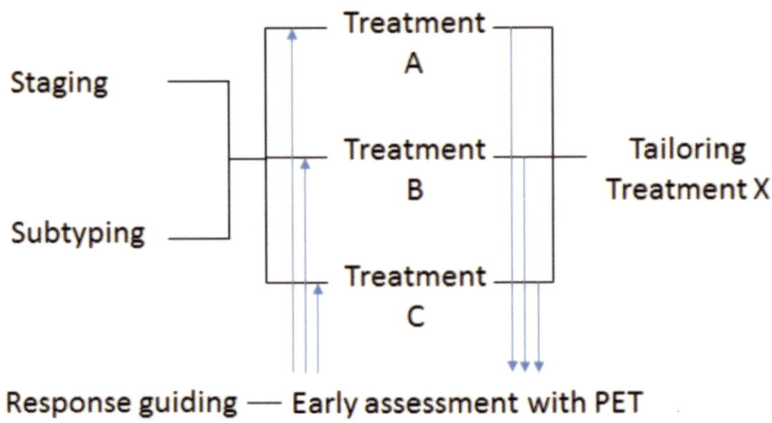


FDG: fluoro-D-glucose; PET: positron emission tomography

**Figure 3.** Treatment strategy options using FDG-PET in conjunction with staging, subtyping, and response-guiding.

## 3. Limitations of FDG-PET

Although tumor FDG uptake is an indicator of the viability of cancer cells [31], [32], it is influenced by many biological factors such as stromal cell activity [33], tumor perfusion [34], immune reaction [35], hypoxia [36], [37], and apoptosis. The acute effect of cytotoxic drugs on tumor FDG uptake occurs as a result of high glucose uptake by inflammatory cells and/or energy demand in the process of acute apoptotic death [38], leading to a transient increase in tumor FDG uptake (so-called "flare response") [39], [40]. Therefore, some authors have claimed that the timing of PET scanning soon after the onset of chemotherapy treatment may be crucial. To avoid the flare response, scanning must be delayed for at least 1–2 weeks after the initiation of chemotherapy [41]. PET may be administered immediately before initiation of the second cycle of chemotherapy.

One cause of confusion regarding the results of FDG-PET is the heterogenous results concerning the pathological criteria of outcome, which distinguishes responders from nonresponders. The overall prognosis of patients remains unconfirmed. In addition, variations in dose and different combinations of drugs add to the confusion. The optimal timing of PET scanning may depend on dose intensity or regimen. If the regimen changes during the course of treatment, the results may be affected because the mechanism of drug sensitivity differs according to tumor characteristics.

The optimal timing of FDG-PET scanning after initiation of chemotherapy for the prediction and elimination of progressive disease (PD) has also not been determined till date. In clinical practice, most physicians are more concerned about tumor progression during neoadjuvant chemotherapy than about achieving pCR. Because chemotherapeutic treatment may increase genomic instability in some tumors, and because chemotherapy resistance may develop in severe cases with hypoxia, neoadjuvant chemotherapy may be contraindicated. However, the role of FDG-PET in the early prediction of PD remains to be established.

The optimal threshold of metabolic change on FDG-PET also remains unclear. A recent draft standard of PERCIST has been advocated as response criteria in solid tumors [7]. It recommends a ≥30% decrease in SUV as a cutoff value for partial metabolic response, which is associated with clinical outcome after chemotherapy. However, specific response criteria for breast cancer must be defined in order to increase the accuracy of prognosis. Further prospective research is needed to determine the optimal cut-off value for predicting tumor response.

Thorough evaluation of cost-effectiveness and prognostic impact of early switching from ineffective neoadjuvant chemotherapy to a more effective regimen is essential. In a simulation study, Schegerin et al. found that early prediction of tumor response using functional imaging devices such as FDG-PET facilitated tailoring of treatment options, which had economic benefits [42]. Further clinical trials must be conducted in order to shed further light on this topic.

Finally, the European Organization for Research and Treatment of Cancer PET study group recommended improvements in the quality of tumor imaging with FDG-PET. Interinstitutional bias is another factor in the usefulness of FDG-PET as a prognostic tool. The available data are insufficient to define the optimal time after injection of FDG and the optimal dose of FDG at which SUV should be measured [41].

## 4. Early changes in metabolism using molecular-targeted drugs and endocrine therapy

Functional imaging devices may be useful in the assessment of the biological activity of molecular-targeted drugs [43]. These agents are predominantly cytostatic in nature, that is, they modulate biological behavior and arrest cell cycling rather than totally killing cancer cells [44]. In cases treated with these agents, the traditional endpoints used to evaluate the effects of cytotoxic drugs, such as RECIST criteria, are insufficient and sometimes inappropriate for the prediction of therapeutic outcome. For example, antagonists of the epidermal growth factor receptor (EGFR), such as trastuzumab and cetuximab, block membranous EGFR in cancer cells, halt cell cycling, and induce apoptosis. These drugs and many others require different evaluation criteria to determine their efficacy. FDG-PET may be useful in establishing these criteria.

Small molecule drugs to block protein kinases, such as gefitinib, have been used for the inhibition of tumor proliferation and neovascularization. A rapid decrease in FDG uptake at 48 hour was seen in lung cancer xenografts treated with gefitinib. Su et al. also reported a very early decrease at 2 hour in gefitinib-sensitive cancer cells and no change in resistant cancer cells [45]. Other reports stated that a reduction in metabolism within 1 week after the commencement of therapy was associated with sensitivity to certain drugs, for example, an epidermal growth factor receptor/human epidermal growth factor receptor 2 (HER2) dual kinase inhibitor (lapatinib) used for the treatment of breast cancer, a c-kit inhibitor (imatinib mesylate) used for the treatment of gastrointestinal stromal tumors (GIST), a mammalian target of rapamycin inhibitor (rapamycin) used for the treatment of GIST, and various other drugs used for the treatment of uterine and neuroendocrine carcinomas and sarcomas [44]. Moreover, in the clinical setting, FDG-PET was reported to be useful for the evaluation of treatment response to sunitinib, a multitarget tyrosine kinase inhibitor, in patients with GIST resistant to treatment with imatinib [46].

Endocrine therapy is one of the most common treatment strategies in patients with estrogen receptor (ER)-positive breast cancer. Successful cytostatic drugs include ER antagonists such as tamoxifen, which induce the deprivation of estrogen production, aromatase inhibitors, ER downregulators, or fulvestrant. In 2011, we reported that changes in SUV at approximately 2 weeks after treatment with letrozole, an aromatase inhibitor, was correlated with a drop in proliferative rate of cancer cells measured by immunohistochemical staining of Ki67 [47]. With a tentative threshold value of a 40% decrease in SUV, Ki67 index values were significantly decreased in metabolic responders. The Immediate Preoperative Anastrozole, Tamoxifen, or Combined with Tamoxifen (IMPACT) randomized trial revealed that 2 weeks of treatment with the aromatase inhibitor anastrozole suppressed the Ki67 index (as compared with a percentage of baseline expression) to a significantly greater extent than did tamoxifen alone or tamoxifen in combination with anastrozole. The affiliated study showed that after 2 weeks of endocrine therapy, Ki67 index values predicted recurrence-free survival in individual patients [48]. A positive correlation between the Ki67 index and tumor SUV has been reported in some studies [32, 49], [50]. Mortazavi-Jehanno et al. investigated the predictive value of metabolic response in patients with metastatic breast cancer after 8 weeks of endocrine therapy, demonstrating that progression-free survival is related to metabolic response [51]. These observations suggest that changes in tumor SUV after endocrine therapy may be associated with favorable prognosis. Therefore, the biological basis of changes in FDG uptake using cytostatic drugs may be associated more with intracellular pathways of metabolism and cell cycling than with cytotoxic agents.

### 4.1. Tumor metabolic flare

Tumor flare reaction denotes a sudden and temporary worsening of tumor-related symptoms after the initiation of treatment [52]. Several studies reported that radiotherapy and some types of chemotherapeutic agents induce diffusely elevated FDG accumulation because of inflammation. Weber suggested a careful inspection of the degree and pattern of FDG uptake to distinguish between radiation-induced inflammation and residual cancer activity [53]. As mentioned earlier, the EORTC PET study group recommends that after baseline FDG-PET scanning and before the initiation of chemotherapy, serial scanning using FDG-PET should be performed 1–2 weeks after the first course [41]. Therefore, the consensus till date has been that a waiting period of 1–2 weeks should be observed after initial drug administration or radiotherapy in order to avoid the inflammatory response and accurately evaluate tumor activity. However, metabolic flare does not necessarily indicate treatment failure or cancer progression. Table 2 lists the imaging studies reporting the association between tumor metabolic flare and tumor response to treatment.

| Animal experiments | Year | Treatment | Cancer type | Origin of cell lines | Tracer | Modality | Animal type | Time of flare reaction occurred | Comments |
|---|---|---|---|---|---|---|---|---|---|
| Furuta, et al.[54] | 1997 | radiotherapy | NNE,GLS,KYG | various | FDG | PET | mice | 2 hours | A flare was observed in radiosensitive tumors |
| Aliga, et al.[56] | 2007 | doxorubicin | MC4L2, MC7L1 | breast | FDG | PET | mice | 7 days | A flare reaction was observed 7 days after treatment of doxorubicin, methotrexate, letrozole, or placebo |
| Aide, et al.[55] | 2009 | cisplatin | NCCIT | testicular | FDG | PET | rats | 2 days | A flare was related to a transient cell cycle arrest and apoptosis but did not reveal refractory disease |
| Bjurberg, et al.[40] | 2009 | cisplatin | HNxSCC24 | head and neck | FDG | PET | mice | 1 day | |
| Bjurberg, et al.[57] | 2010 | cisplatin | HNxSCC24 | head and neck | 2-NBDG | Fluorescene microscope | cell culture | 2 days | A flare occurred early after cisplatin treatment in responding tumors |
| **Clinical studies** | Year | Treatment | Clinical staging | Origin | Tracer | Modality | | Time of flare reaction occurred | Outcome |
| Schneider JA, et al.[58] | 1994 | Paclitaxel | metastatic, bone metastasis | breast | | Scintigraphy | | after 2 cycle (4-6wk) | A flare response of bone metastasis after 2 cycle resulted in improvement on follow-up scan |
| Mortimer JE, et al.[59] | 2001 | Tamoxifen | Advanced/metastatic | breast | FDG, FES | PET | | 7-10 days | Responders had increase in SUV for FDG (28.4±23.3) while non-responders had reduce in SUV (-10.2±16.2) p = 0.0002 |
| Dehdashti, et al.[60] | 2009 | Estradiol | Advanced | breast | FDG, FES | PET | | 1 day | Responders had increase in SUV for FDG (20.9±24.2) while non-responders had reduce in SUV (-4.3±11.0) p < 0.0001 |

**Table 2.** Tumor metabolic flare on very early phase of treatment

In animal experiments, Furuta et al. reported a flare reaction detected by FDG-PET in nude mice with ependymoblastoma, small cell lung cancer, and glioblastoma at 2 h after irradiation with 10 Gy [54]. They claimed that flare intensity was strongest in the ependymoblastoma, the most radiosensitive of these tumors, whereas the two less radiosensitive tumors showed no increase in FDG uptake during the observation period. In human testicular cancer xenografts in nude rats that received cisplatin, Aide et al. reported that FDG-PET scanning detected a peak FDG uptake on day 2, followed by a marked decrease on day 7 despite the lack of change in tumor volume [55]. They observed a transient S and G2/M cell cycle arrest and a marked increase in apoptosis within this phase. A very early increase in FDG uptake may explain the flare reaction that represents increased tumor metabolism in apoptotic cells as well as in cells that exhibit transient cell cycle arrest.

Aliga et al. reported a similar result mice after the administration of doxorubicin to decrease tumor burden in BALB/c mice with breast cancer [56]. They observed a rapid decrease in tumor FDG uptake 24 hour after chemotherapy and a transient accumulation in FDG uptake on day 7. They suggested that a partial agonistic effect of chemotherapy, apoptosis, cell repair mechanisms, or intratumoral inflammation may be responsible for this flare reaction.

Using the fluorescent glucose analog 2-NBDG, Bjurberg et al. reported a very early increase in metabolism in three squamous cell carcinoma cell lines (LU-HNxSCC-7, LU-HNxSCC-24, and LU-CX-2) after exposure to cisplatin [40] [57]. The flare reaction was observed within 3 days after exposure in these cells, whereas FDG uptake in nonmalignant fibroblastic cells was low.

Contrary to recent animal studies revealing a flare phenomenon-associated tumor response, only a few clinical studies have utilized FDG-PET in detecting tumor flare. As early as 1996, Schneiders et al. reported the use of scintigraphy to detect a flare reaction in bone lesions in patients with metastatic disease; the flare reaction occurred despite a favorable overall outcome [58]. This phenomenon may represent enhanced osteoblastic activity, rapid bone repair, and improved blood flow around the responding lesions. Welch et al. conducted an FDG-PET study in which a paradoxical flare phenomenon was detected within 7 to 10 days after the initiation of tamoxifen in patients with breast cancer [59]. An increase in FDG uptake was observed in responding tumors during week 1 after tamoxifen initiation ; however, this was not observed in nonresponding tumors. The transient increase in FDG uptake could reflect hormone receptor-related changes in tumor metabolism, which was predictive of a favorable outcome. Partial agonist–antagonist activity in selective ER modulators such as tamoxifen is known to differ over the treatment course after tissue exposure. The slow onset of action of tamoxifen and the fact that its effects as an estrogen agonist peak 1–2 weeks after the onset of therapy may contribute to the development of the flare reaction. The same group of investigators conducted a clinical study including an estradiol challenge test to predict hormone sensitivity in women with locally advanced or metastatic ER-positive breast cancer. FDG-PET after 30 mg estradiol induced a metabolic flare, showing greater responsiveness to endocrine therapy and better overall survival in flare patients than in non-flare patients [60].

Results of those animal studies lead to the speculation that tumor metabolic flare is related to the following sequence of events: transient cell cycle arrest, apoptosis, induction of the cancer immune system, and hemodynamic reaction. As for estrogen-positive breast cancer and endocrine therapy, estrogen stimulation may be closely associated with an increase in glucose uptake [61]. At lease, this does not necessarily indicate refractory disease.

Taken together, the underlying presumption in these studies is that changes in FDG uptake in response to chemotherapy occur in three phases (Figure 4). In the first phase, cellular damage followed by inflammation and vascular changes occurs within hours or days, resulting in accumulation of FDG and increased uptake in cancer cells and inflammatory cells such as neutrophils (inflammatory phase). In this phase, pro-inflammatory cytokines may be released because of the tumor's response to chemotherapy, and these cytokines accelerate tumor cell proliferation, activate the immune system, and increase blood flow, resulting in accumulation of tumor FDG. Second, apoptosis, cell cycle arrest, and diminishing inflammation, which occur within days or weeks, lead to a decrease in FDG uptake in cancer cells (apoptotic phase). Decreased blood flow due to vascular damage caused by chemotherapy may deteriorate the tumor microenvironment and promote apoptosis. In addition, tumor cells may be replaced by fibrotic cells, shrinking the tumor several weeks after the initiation of chemotherapy. FDG uptake in the tumor then decreases because of volume reduction (volume reduction phase). In this last phase, morphological changes can be identified by CT or magnetic resonance imaging. Therefore, metabolic flare precedes decreased uptake of FDG. This is not necessarily a confounding factor; rather, it provides an insight into pharmacodynamics [62]. Further understanding of cancer metabolic flare in the early phase after chemotherapy can aid in strategic planning of successful therapy.

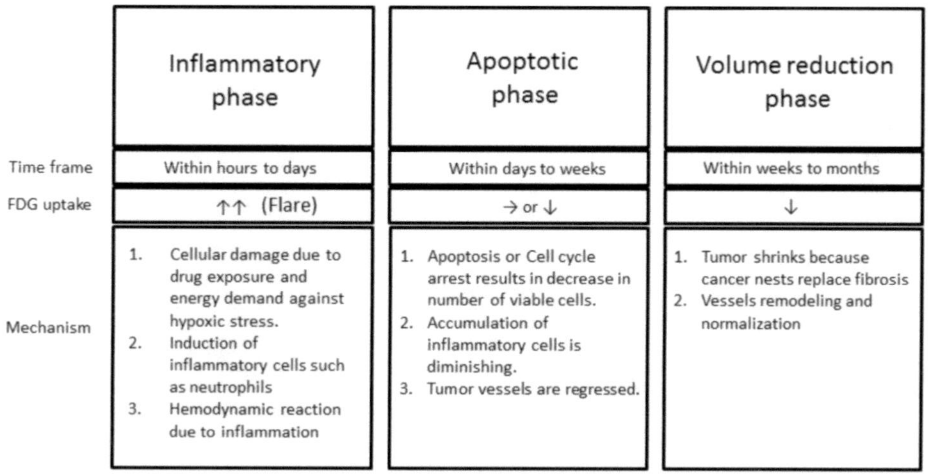


FDG: fluoro-D-glucose

**Figure 4.** Tumor FDG uptake in response to chemotherapy hypothetically occurs in three biological phases. In the first phase, FDG accumulation occurs because of cellular damage, inflammation, and vascular reaction. In the second phase, apoptosis results in decreasing cellularity. In the third phase, the tumor decreases in size.

## 5. Summary

Of late, cancer treatment is frequently optimized on the basis of tumor subtype and stage. Breast cancer is characterized by ER and HER2 status in addition to tumor size and distant metastatic involvement. The advent of commercialized kits containing multiple molecular biomarker assays has shifted the focus in tumor categorization from pathology to molecular analysis. However, rapid development and wide availability of a broad range of new drugs has exceeded the discovery of tumor subtyping methods or the establishment of biomarkers predictive of chemosensitivity. Therefore, a new paradigm that involves response-guided strategies during initial treatment, which can aid in decision-making about the next treatment option, is emerging for cancer treatment. Early response assessment using FDG-PET may eventually be applicable for planning and evaluating future treatment strategies. In future, patients could be allocated to standard or investigational chemotherapy regimens on the basis of metabolic response. Furthermore, in phase 1/2 studies determining the optimal dose of a new drug, nonresponsive patients can be eliminated on the basis of metabolic response. Glucose metabolism analysis using FDG-PET will be one of several critical factors for evaluating tumor response to chemotherapy. Integration of multiple functional imaging systems may also be useful in predicting early tumor response to chemotherapy.

Finally, considering the phenomenon of tumor metabolic flare, clinical trials must be conducted to determine the best timing for the administration of FDG-PET. This information would be useful to predict tumor response in the very early stages of treatment.

## Acknowledgements

We dedicate this review article to the late Dr. Yoshiaki ABE for helpful cooperation with a series of PET studies. We are very grateful to Dr. Hitoshi TSUDA of the National Cancer Institute for his helpful advice and to Dr. Jiro ISHIDA and Dr. Katsumi TAMURA from the Tokorozawa PET Diagnostic Imaging Center for the clinical reading of FDG-PET images.

## Author details

Shigeto Ueda* and Toshiaki Saeki

Department of Breast Oncology, Saitama Medical University, International Medical Center, Saitam, Japan

## References

[1] Juweid ME, Cheson BD: Positron-emission tomography and assessment of cancer therapy. *The New England journal of medicine* 2006, 354(5):496-507.

[2] Cermik TF, Mavi A, Basu S, Alavi A: Impact of FDG PET on the preoperative staging of newly diagnosed breast cancer. *European journal of nuclear medicine and molecular imaging* 2008, 35(3):475-483.

[3] Niikura N, Ueno NT: The Role of F-FDG-Positron Emission Tomography/Computed Tomography in Staging Primary Breast Cancer. *Journal of Cancer* 2010, 1:51-53.

[4] Zhu A, Lee D, Shim H: Metabolic positron emission tomography imaging in cancer detection and therapy response. *Seminars in oncology* 2011, 38(1):55-69.

[5] Weber WA: Assessing tumor response to therapy. *Journal of nuclear medicine : official publication, Society of Nuclear Medicine* 2009, 50 Suppl 1:1S-10S.

[6] Therasse P, Arbuck SG, Eisenhauer EA, Wanders J, Kaplan RS, Rubinstein L, Verweij J, Van Glabbeke M, van Oosterom AT, Christian MC *et al*: New guidelines to evaluate

the response to treatment in solid tumors. European Organization for Research and Treatment of Cancer, National Cancer Institute of the United States, National Cancer Institute of Canada. *Journal of the National Cancer Institute* 2000, 92(3):205-216.

[7] Wahl RL, Jacene H, Kasamon Y, Lodge MA: From RECIST to PERCIST: Evolving Considerations for PET response criteria in solid tumors. *Journal of nuclear medicine : official publication, Society of Nuclear Medicine* 2009, 50 Suppl 1:122S-150S.

[8] MacManus MP, Seymour JF, Hicks RJ: Overview of early response assessment in lymphoma with FDG-PET. *Cancer imaging : the official publication of the International Cancer Imaging Society* 2007, 7:10-18.

[9] Gallamini A, Hutchings M, Rigacci L, Specht L, Merli F, Hansen M, Patti C, Loft A, Di Raimondo F, D'Amore F *et al*: Early interim 2- [18F]fluoro-2-deoxy-D-glucose positron emission tomography is prognostically superior to international prognostic score in advanced-stage Hodgkin's lymphoma: a report from a joint Italian-Danish study. *Journal of clinical oncology : official journal of the American Society of Clinical Oncology* 2007, 25(24):3746-3752.

[10] Schwarz-Dose J, Untch M, Tiling R, Sassen S, Mahner S, Kahlert S, Harbeck N, Lebeau A, Brenner W, Schwaiger M *et al*: Monitoring primary systemic therapy of large and locally advanced breast cancer by using sequential positron emission tomography imaging with [18F]fluorodeoxyglucose. *Journal of clinical oncology : official journal of the American Society of Clinical Oncology* 2009, 27(4):535-541.

[11] Rebollo-Aguirre AC, Ramos-Font C, Villegas Portero R, Cook GJ, Llamas Elvira JM, Romero Tabares A: Is FDG-PET suitable for evaluating neoadjuvant therapy in non-small cell lung cancer? Evidence with systematic review of the literature. *Journal of surgical oncology* 2010, 101(6):486-494.

[12] Lordick F, Ott K, Krause BJ, Weber WA, Becker K, Stein HJ, Lorenzen S, Schuster T, Wieder H, Herrmann K *et al*: PET to assess early metabolic response and to guide treatment of adenocarcinoma of the oesophagogastric junction: the MUNICON phase II trial. *The lancet oncology* 2007, 8(9):797-805.

[13] Kwee RM: Prediction of tumor response to neoadjuvant therapy in patients with esophageal cancer with use of 18F FDG PET: a systematic review. *Radiology* 2010, 254(3):707-717.

[14] Lorenzen S, von Gall C, Stange A, Haag GM, Weitz J, Haberkorn U, Lordick F, Weichert W, Abel U, Debus J *et al*: Sequential FDG-PET and induction chemotherapy in locally advanced adenocarcinoma of the Oesophago-gastric junction (AEG): the Heidelberg Imaging program in Cancer of the oesophago-gastric junction during Neoadjuvant treatment: HICON trial. *BMC cancer* 2011, 11:266.

[15] de Geus-Oei LF, Vriens D, van Laarhoven HW, van der Graaf WT, Oyen WJ: Monitoring and predicting response to therapy with 18F-FDG PET in colorectal cancer: a

systematic review. *Journal of nuclear medicine : official publication, Society of Nuclear Medicine* 2009, 50 Suppl 1:43S-54S.

[16] Wahl RL, Zasadny K, Helvie M, Hutchins GD, Weber B, Cody R: Metabolic monitoring of breast cancer chemohormonotherapy using positron emission tomography: initial evaluation. *Journal of clinical oncology : official journal of the American Society of Clinical Oncology* 1993, 11(11):2101-2111.

[17] Bassa P, Kim EE, Inoue T, Wong FC, Korkmaz M, Yang DJ, Wong WH, Hicks KW, Buzdar AU, Podoloff DA: Evaluation of preoperative chemotherapy using PET with fluorine-18-fluorodeoxyglucose in breast cancer. *Journal of nuclear medicine : official publication, Society of Nuclear Medicine* 1996, 37(6):931-938.

[18] Schelling M, Avril N, Nahrig J, Kuhn W, Romer W, Sattler D, Werner M, Dose J, Janicke F, Graeff H *et al*: Positron emission tomography using [(18)F]Fluorodeoxyglucose for monitoring primary chemotherapy in breast cancer. *Journal of clinical oncology : official journal of the American Society of Clinical Oncology* 2000, 18(8): 1689-1695.

[19] Smith IC, Welch AE, Hutcheon AW, Miller ID, Payne S, Chilcott F, Waikar S, Whitaker T, Ah-See AK, Eremin O *et al*: Positron emission tomography using [(18)F]-fluorodeoxy-D-glucose to predict the pathologic response of breast cancer to primary chemotherapy. *Journal of clinical oncology : official journal of the American Society of Clinical Oncology* 2000, 18(8):1676-1688.

[20] Ueda S, Tsuda H, Saeki T, Osaki A, Shigekawa T, Ishida J, Tamura K, Abe Y, Omata J, Moriya T *et al*: Early reduction in standardized uptake value after one cycle of neoadjuvant chemotherapy measured by sequential FDG PET/CT is an independent predictor of pathological response of primary breast cancer. *The breast journal* 2010, 16(6): 660-662.

[21] Kumar A, Kumar R, Seenu V, Gupta SD, Chawla M, Malhotra A, Mehta SN: The role of 18F-FDG PET/CT in evaluation of early response to neoadjuvant chemotherapy in patients with locally advanced breast cancer. *European radiology* 2009, 19(6):1347-1357.

[22] Martoni AA, Zamagni C, Quercia S, Rosati M, Cacciari N, Bernardi A, Musto A, Fanti S, Santini D, Taffurelli M: Early (18)F-2-fluoro-2-deoxy-d-glucose positron emission tomography may identify a subset of patients with estrogen receptor-positive breast cancer who will not respond optimally to preoperative chemotherapy. *Cancer* 2010, 116(4):805-813.

[23] Berriolo-Riedinger A, Touzery C, Riedinger JM, Toubeau M, Coudert B, Arnould L, Boichot C, Cochet A, Fumoleau P, Brunotte F: [18F]FDG-PET predicts complete pathological response of breast cancer to neoadjuvant chemotherapy. *European journal of nuclear medicine and molecular imaging* 2007, 34(12):1915-1924.

[24] Rousseau C, Devillers A, Sagan C, Ferrer L, Bridji B, Campion L, Ricaud M, Bourbouloux E, Doutriaux I, Clouet M *et al*: Monitoring of early response to neoadjuvant che-

motherapy in stage II and III breast cancer by [18F]fluorodeoxyglucose positron emission tomography. *Journal of clinical oncology : official journal of the American Society of Clinical Oncology* 2006, 24(34):5366-5372.

[25] McDermott GM, Welch A, Staff RT, Gilbert FJ, Schweiger L, Semple SI, Smith TA, Hutcheon AW, Miller ID, Smith IC *et al*: Monitoring primary breast cancer throughout chemotherapy using FDG-PET. *Breast cancer research and treatment* 2007, 102(1): 75-84.

[26] Wang Y, Zhang C, Liu J, Huang G: Is 18F-FDG PET accurate to predict neoadjuvant therapy response in breast cancer? A meta-analysis. *Breast cancer research and treatment* 2012, 131(2):357-369.

[27] Plathow C, Weber WA: Tumor cell metabolism imaging. *Journal of nuclear medicine : official publication, Society of Nuclear Medicine* 2008, 49 Suppl 2:43S-63S.

[28] Dann EJ, Bar-Shalom R, Tamir A, Haim N, Ben-Shachar M, Avivi I, Zuckerman T, Kirschbaum M, Goor O, Libster D *et al*: Risk-adapted BEACOPP regimen can reduce the cumulative dose of chemotherapy for standard and high-risk Hodgkin lymphoma with no impairment of outcome. *Blood* 2007, 109(3):905-909.

[29] Aridgides P, Bogart J, Shapiro A, Gajra A: PET Response-Guided Treatment of Hodgkin's Lymphoma: A Review of the Evidence and Active Clinical Trials. *Advances in hematology* 2011, 2011:309237.

[30] Fleming IN, Gilbert FJ, Miles KA, Cameron D: Opportunities for PET to deliver clinical benefit in cancer: breast cancer as a paradigm. *Cancer imaging : the official publication of the International Cancer Imaging Society* 2010, 10:144-152.

[31] Ueda S, Tsuda H, Asakawa H, Shigekawa T, Fukatsu K, Kondo N, Yamamoto M, Hama Y, Tamura K, Ishida J *et al*: Clinicopathological and prognostic relevance of uptake level using 18F-fluorodeoxyglucose positron emission tomography/computed tomography fusion imaging (18F-FDG PET/CT) in primary breast cancer. *Japanese journal of clinical oncology* 2008, 38(4):250-258.

[32] Ueda S, Kondoh N, Tsuda H, Yamamoto S, Asakawa H, Fukatsu K, Kobayashi T, Yamamoto J, Tamura K, Ishida J *et al*: Expression of centromere protein F (CENP-F) associated with higher FDG uptake on PET/CT, detected by cDNA microarray, predicts high-risk patients with primary breast cancer. *BMC cancer* 2008, 8:384.

[33] Martinez-Outschoorn UE, Pestell RG, Howell A, Tykocinski ML, Nagajyothi F, Machado FS, Tanowitz HB, Sotgia F, Lisanti MP: Energy transfer in "parasitic" cancer metabolism: mitochondria are the powerhouse and Achilles' heel of tumor cells. *Cell Cycle* 2011, 10(24):4208-4216.

[34] Miles KA, Griffiths MR, Keith CJ: Blood flow-metabolic relationships are dependent on tumour size in non-small cell lung cancer: a study using quantitative contrast-en-

hanced computer tomography and positron emission tomography. *European journal of nuclear medicine and molecular imaging* 2006, 33(1):22-28.

[35] Spaepen K, Stroobants S, Dupont P, Bormans G, Balzarini J, Verhoef G, Mortelmans L, Vandenberghe P, De Wolf-Peeters C: [(18)F]FDG PET monitoring of tumour response to chemotherapy: does [(18)F]FDG uptake correlate with the viable tumour cell fraction? *European journal of nuclear medicine and molecular imaging* 2003, 30(5): 682-688.

[36] Goh V, Engledow A, Rodriguez-Justo M, Shastry M, Peck J, Blackman G, Endozo R, Taylor S, Halligan S, Ell P *et al*: The flow-metabolic phenotype of primary colorectal cancer: assessment by integrated 18F-FDG PET/perfusion CT with histopathologic correlation. *Journal of nuclear medicine : official publication, Society of Nuclear Medicine* 2012, 53(5):687-692.

[37] Dooms C, van Baardwijk A, Verbeken E, van Suylen RJ, Stroobants S, De Ruysscher D, Vansteenkiste J: Association between 18F-fluoro-2-deoxy-D-glucose uptake values and tumor vitality: prognostic value of positron emission tomography in early-stage non-small cell lung cancer. *Journal of thoracic oncology : official publication of the International Association for the Study of Lung Cancer* 2009, 4(7):822-828.

[38] Jin S, DiPaola RS, Mathew R, White E: Metabolic catastrophe as a means to cancer cell death. *Journal of cell science* 2007, 120(Pt 3):379-383.

[39] Archer CD, Parton M, Smith IE, Ellis PA, Salter J, Ashley S, Gui G, Sacks N, Ebbs SR, Allum W *et al*: Early changes in apoptosis and proliferation following primary chemotherapy for breast cancer. *British journal of cancer* 2003, 89(6):1035-1041.

[40] Bjurberg M, Henriksson E, Brun E, Ekblad L, Ohlsson T, Brun A, Kjellen E: Early changes in 2-deoxy-2- [18F]fluoro-D-glucose metabolism in squamous-cell carcinoma during chemotherapy in vivo and in vitro. *Cancer biotherapy & radiopharmaceuticals* 2009, 24(3):327-332.

[41] Young H, Baum R, Cremerius U, Herholz K, Hoekstra O, Lammertsma AA, Pruim J, Price P: Measurement of clinical and subclinical tumour response using [18F]-fluorodeoxyglucose and positron emission tomography: review and 1999 EORTC recommendations. European Organization for Research and Treatment of Cancer (EORTC) PET Study Group. *Eur J Cancer* 1999, 35(13):1773-1782.

[42] Schegerin M, Tosteson AN, Kaufman PA, Paulsen KD, Pogue BW: Prognostic imaging in neoadjuvant chemotherapy of locally-advanced breast cancer should be cost-effective. *Breast cancer research and treatment* 2009, 114(3):537-547.

[43] Weber WA, Czernin J, Phelps ME, Herschman HR: Technology Insight: novel imaging of molecular targets is an emerging area crucial to the development of targeted drugs. *Nature clinical practice Oncology* 2008, 5(1):44-54.

[44] Contractor KB, Aboagye EO: Monitoring predominantly cytostatic treatment response with 18F-FDG PET. *Journal of nuclear medicine : official publication, Society of Nuclear Medicine* 2009, 50 Suppl 1:97S-105S.

[45] Su H, Bodenstein C, Dumont RA, Seimbille Y, Dubinett S, Phelps ME, Herschman H, Czernin J, Weber W: Monitoring tumor glucose utilization by positron emission tomography for the prediction of treatment response to epidermal growth factor receptor kinase inhibitors. *Clinical cancer research : an official journal of the American Association for Cancer Research* 2006, 12(19):5659-5667.

[46] Prior JO, Montemurro M, Orcurto MV, Michielin O, Luthi F, Benhattar J, Guillou L, Elsig V, Stupp R, Delaloye AB *et al*: Early prediction of response to sunitinib after imatinib failure by 18F-fluorodeoxyglucose positron emission tomography in patients with gastrointestinal stromal tumor. *Journal of clinical oncology : official journal of the American Society of Clinical Oncology* 2009, 27(3):439-445.

[47] Ueda S, Tsuda H, Saeki T, Omata J, Osaki A, Shigekawa T, Ishida J, Tamura K, Abe Y, Moriya T *et al*: Early metabolic response to neoadjuvant letrozole, measured by FDG PET/CT, is correlated with a decrease in the Ki67 labeling index in patients with hormone receptor-positive primary breast cancer: a pilot study. *Breast Cancer* 2011, 18(4):299-308.

[48] Dowsett M, Smith IE, Ebbs SR, Dixon JM, Skene A, A'Hern R, Salter J, Detre S, Hills M, Walsh G: Prognostic value of Ki67 expression after short-term presurgical endocrine therapy for primary breast cancer. *Journal of the National Cancer Institute* 2007, 99(2):167-170.

[49] Buck A, Schirrmeister H, Kuhn T, Shen C, Kalker T, Kotzerke J, Dankerl A, Glatting G, Reske S, Mattfeldt T: FDG uptake in breast cancer: correlation with biological and clinical prognostic parameters. *European journal of nuclear medicine and molecular imaging* 2002, 29(10):1317-1323.

[50] Shimoda W, Hayashi M, Murakami K, Oyama T, Sunagawa M: The relationship between FDG uptake in PET scans and biological behavior in breast cancer. *Breast Cancer* 2007, 14(3):260-268.

[51] Mortazavi-Jehanno N, Giraudet AL, Champion L, Lerebours F, Le Stanc E, Edeline V, Madar O, Bellet D, Pecking AP, Alberini JL: Assessment of response to endocrine therapy using FDG PET/CT in metastatic breast cancer: a pilot study. *European journal of nuclear medicine and molecular imaging* 2012, 39(3):450-460.

[52] Basu S, Alavi A: Defining co-related parameters between 'metabolic' flare and 'clinical', 'biochemical', and 'osteoblastic' flare and establishing guidelines for assessing response to treatment in cancer. *European journal of nuclear medicine and molecular imaging* 2007, 34(4):441-443.

[53] Weber WA: Use of PET for monitoring cancer therapy and for predicting outcome. *Journal of nuclear medicine : official publication, Society of Nuclear Medicine* 2005, 46(6): 983-995.

[54] Furuta M, Hasegawa M, Hayakawa K, Yamakawa M, Ishikawa H, Nonaka T, Mitsuhashi N, Niibe H: Rapid rise in FDG uptake in an irradiated human tumour xenograft. *European journal of nuclear medicine* 1997, 24(4):435-438.

[55] Aide N, Poulain L, Briand M, Dutoit S, Allouche S, Labiche A, Ngo-Van Do A, Nataf V, Batalla A, Gauduchon P *et al*: Early evaluation of the effects of chemotherapy with longitudinal FDG small-animal PET in human testicular cancer xenografts: early flare response does not reflect refractory disease. *European journal of nuclear medicine and molecular imaging* 2009, 36(3):396-405.

[56] Aliaga A, Rousseau JA, Cadorette J, Croteau E, van Lier JE, Lecomte R, Benard F: A small animal positron emission tomography study of the effect of chemotherapy and hormonal therapy on the uptake of 2-deoxy-2- [F-18]fluoro-D-glucose in murine models of breast cancer. *Molecular imaging and biology : MIB : the official publication of the Academy of Molecular Imaging* 2007, 9(3):144-150.

[57] Bjurberg M, Abedinpour P, Brun E, Baldetorp B, Borgstrom P, Wennerberg J, Kjellen E: Early Metabolic Flare in Squamous Cell Carcinoma after Chemotherapy is a Marker of Treatment Sensitivity In Vitro. *Nuclear medicine and molecular imaging* 2010, 44(3): 165-169.

[58] Schneider JA, Divgi CR, Scott AM, Macapinlac HA, Seidman AD, Goldsmith SJ, Larson SM: Flare on bone scintigraphy following Taxol chemotherapy for metastatic breast cancer. *Journal of nuclear medicine : official publication, Society of Nuclear Medicine* 1994, 35(11):1748-1752.

[59] Mortimer JE, Dehdashti F, Siegel BA, Trinkaus K, Katzenellenbogen JA, Welch MJ: Metabolic flare: indicator of hormone responsiveness in advanced breast cancer. *Journal of clinical oncology : official journal of the American Society of Clinical Oncology* 2001, 19(11):2797-2803.

[60] Dehdashti F, Mortimer JE, Trinkaus K, Naughton MJ, Ellis M, Katzenellenbogen JA, Welch MJ, Siegel BA: PET-based estradiol challenge as a predictive biomarker of response to endocrine therapy in women with estrogen-receptor-positive breast cancer. *Breast cancer research and treatment* 2009, 113(3):509-517.

[61] Fischer WH, Keiwan A, Schmitt E, Stopper H: Increased formation of micronuclei after hormonal stimulation of cell proliferation in human breast cancer cells. *Mutagenesis* 2001, 16(3):209-212.

[62] Trigonis I, Jackson A: Imaging pharmacodynamics in oncology: the potential significance of "flares". *Annals of nuclear medicine* 2010, 24(3):137-147.